RENAL DISEASE IN THE ELDERLY

RENAL DISEASE IN THE ELDERLY

Second Edition, Revised and Expanded

Pierre F. Faubert
Jerome G. Porush

*Brookdale University Hospital and Medical Center
and State University of New York Health Science Center at Brooklyn
Brooklyn, New York*

MARCEL DEKKER, INC. NEW YORK • BASEL • HONG KONG

ISBN: 0-8247-9900-3

This book is printed on acid-free paper.

Headquarters
Marcel Dekker, Inc.
270 Madison Avenue, New York, NY 10016
tel: 212-696-9000; fax: 212-685-4540

Eastern Hemisphere Distribution
Marcel Dekker AG
Hutgasse 4, Postfach 812, CH-4001 Basel, Switzerland
tel: 44-61-261-8482; fax: 44-61-261-8896

World Wide Web
http://www.dekker.com

The publisher offers discounts on this book when ordered in bulk quantities. For more information, write to Special Sales/Professional Marketing at the headquarters address above.

Current printing (last digit):
10 9 8 7 6 5 4 3 2 1

PRINTED IN THE UNITED STATES OF AMERICA

Preface

We decided to write this book because we perceived a need for a comprehensive review of renal disease in the elderly. Although there might not be sufficient data to prove that the elderly are different from other adults, there is a significant amount of specific information concerning the elderly in the nephrological literature, and about subjects over the age of 60 in the general adult literature. We felt that we had a substantial amount of well-documented personal experience to add to the existing literature, and that with this book we could help fill gaps in the present knowledge of this important clinical area.

Renal Disease in the Elderly represents a synthesis of the literature and our experience. We have included most of the subject matter covered in a standard nephrology text. For most subjects, we summarize the existing information on adults in general and then provide information that is specific to the elderly. In all instances, we have been careful to distinguish what we have derived from the literature from what we have learned from our own experience, leaving the reader to draw his or her own conclusions when there is a discrepancy. For the most part, we believe we have achieved our goal of producing a comprehensive review of kidney disease in the elderly.

In this revised, second edition, we have added a significant amount of new data, particularly in Chapters 5, 10, 11, 12, and 13. We have also made changes to improve clarity and readability.

We want to take this opportunity to thank our close colleagues for supporting us in this endeavor. We also would like to gratefully acknowledge the invaluable assistance of Denise Stewart and William Jackson.

Pierre F. Faubert
Jerome G. Porush

Contents

1

Anatomy and Physiology

I. EFFECT OF AGE ON THE ANATOMY OF THE KIDNEY

Like other organs in the body such as the spleen, liver, brain, etc., the kidneys undergo involutional changes with age (1). As seen in Table 1 there is a gradual decline in kidney weight in white males starting after the age of 49 years, with the most marked decrease occurring between the seventh and the eighth decades. Similar observations have been made in females as well as in elderly of other ethnic groups (2–4). The progressive loss of kidney mass appears to affect the renal cortex more than the medulla (5–6a). From birth to age 40 the normal human kidney has an estimated 600,000 to 1,200,000 glomeruli (6). Thereafter, there is a progressive decrease of 30–50% in the number of glomeruli. Ninety-five percent of the normal population below the age of 50 years have less than 10% of sclerotic glomeruli (range 0–7.2%). In subjects older than 50 years, the percentage of sclerotic glomeruli increases, with a range of 0.5–36%, making the distinction between involutional and disease-related sclerosis unclear (7,8). The outer cortical glomeruli are, in general, more extensively involved than the deeper glomeruli. In addition to glomerular sclerosis, there is a gradual increase in interstitial fibrosis. The proximal tubular volume of individual nephrons tends to decrease from a mean of 0.076 mm^3 (range 0.030–0.178 mm^3) at 20–39 years to a mean of 0.050 mm^3 (range 0.020–0.120 mm^3) at 80–101 years (9). Since the loss of glomerular mass is proportional to the loss of tubular mass, glomerulo-

Table 1 Mean Values of Kidney Weights and Some Micromeasuring Data in the Kidney of White Males in Various Age Groups[a]

Age (years)	Under 39	40–49	50–59	60–69	70–79	Above 80
Percent of decrease per decade		10%	6%	3%	8%	10%
Weight of kidneys (g) (144)	432.1 ± 36.4 (12)	388.5 ± 24.5 (23)	365.8 ± 20.2 (20)	355.0 ± 13.7 (35)	327.9 ± 10.9 (32)	294.9 ± 18.4 (22)
Size of glomeruli[b] (μm)(182)	189.5 ± 1.1 (12)	186.4 ± 0.9 (25)	191.9 ± 1.4 (35)	191.2 ± 0.7 (43)	189.2 ± 0.7 (42)	185.1 ± 1.0 (25)
Cell number of glomerular tufts (181)	156.3 ± 4.3 (12)	133.3 ± 2.7 (25)	142.3 ± 2.4 (36)	124.6 ± 1.7 (42)	121.4 ± 1.9 (41)	106.4 ± 2.1 (25)
Number of epithelial cells of convoluted tubules in a given area (125,600 μm^2)(100)	178.1 ± 6.2 (6)	159.3 ± 3.7 (15)	152.4 ± 3.9 (17)	127.2 ± 2.5 (23)	120.5 ± 2.8 (23)	117.9 ± 3.4 (16)
Size of epithelial cell nuclei (μm)(100)[b]	7.08 ± 0.01 (7)	6.85 ± 0.01 (14)	7.07 ± 0.01 (17)	7.02 ± 0.01 (24)	7.18 ± 0.01 (22)	7.27 ± 0.01 (16)

[a]Number of cases examined is indicated in parenthesis.
[b]Square root of value area.
Source: Tauchi H, et al. Age changes in the human kidney of the different races. Gerontologia 1971; 17:87–97.

tubular balance is, in general, well preserved (10). On electron microscopic analysis, there is an increase in reduplication and an increase in focal thickening of both glomerular and tubular basement membranes, probably due to the accumulation of type IV collagen (11).

The increase in the percent of sclerotic glomeruli has been attributed to the protein-rich diet characteristic of modern Western society (12). In the rat this diet induces a state of chronic glomerular hyperfiltration and hyperperfusion, contributing to progressive glomerulosclerosis and age-related decrease in glomerular filtration rate. An increase in the function of residual intact nephrons would be expected to lead to an increase in nephron size; however, no significant correlation is found between glomerular area and glomerulosclerosis (13,14). Another possible explanation for the progressive increase in sclerotic glomeruli with age is glomerular ischemia secondary to the changes in renal blood flow occurring with age. It has been recently demonstrated that both age and vascular disease correlate independently with the percentage of hyalinized glomeruli in the aged (10). Indeed, Hollenberg et al. (15) noted that renal blood flow declined progressively, at a rate of approximately 10% per decade, starting after the 4th decade. The mechanism for the decrease in renal blood flow does not appear to be related to a decrease in cardiac output occurring with age, but is rather anatomical. The interlobar arteries usually become tortuous and spiraling. Furthermore, fibroelastic hyperplasia of arterioles and of arcuate arteries occur progressively with age (16,17). The changes are more pronounced in the cortical vessels, and, as a consequence, the perfusion pressure is relatively well maintained in the juxtamedullary nephrons.

II. EFFECT OF AGE ON THE GLOMERULAR FILTRATION RATE (GFR)

Since total glomerular filtration rate (GFR) is a function of the number of functioning glomeruli, one might expect it to be decreased in the elderly. In cross-sectional and longitudinal studies reported by Davies and Shock (18), a gradual decrease in GFR was noted with age (Table 2). These changes have been confirmed by the longitudinal analysis of Rowe et al. (19) (Table 3) and Lindeman et al. (20) and compiled by Wesson, as shown in Fig. 1 (21).

Based on these data, it has been estimated that after the age of 30 there is a 7.5–8 ml/min decline in the GFR per decade. A nomogram has been constructed by Rowe et al. (22) for age-adjusted standard creatinine clearance and can be computed for males as follows: creatinine clearance (ml/min/1.73 m^2) = 133 × (0.64 × age). For females, multiply the result by 0.93. For instance, a 60-kg male aged 90 years is expected to have a creatinine clearance of 133 × (0.64 × 90) = 75.4 ml/min/1.73 m^2. It should be noted that this formula represents only an estimate, and the error inherent can be substantial since some subjects will

Table 2 Mean Change in GFR and RPF with Age

Age group (years)	Inulin clearance (ml/min/1.73 m²)	Effective renal blood flow (ml/min/1.73 m²)	Filtration fraction (%)
50–59	99.3 ± 14.6	849 ± 123	21 ± 3
60–69	96.0 ± 25.5	775 ± 139	22 ± 3
70–79	89.0 ± 19.9	589 ± 133	26 ± 8
80–89	65.3 ± 20.4	475 ± 141	23 ± 4

Source: Davies DF, Shock NW. Age changes in glomerular filtration rate, effective renal plasma flow and tubular excretory capacity in adult males. J Clin Invest 1950; 29:496–507.

maintain stable renal function while aging (approximately one-third), while a small number will even have an increase in GFR (20,23).

Serum creatinine is the most commonly used marker of kidney function (GFR) in clinical medicine. Kampmann et al. (24) have demonstrated that the decrease in creatinine clearance occurring with age is attended by a parallel reduction in daily creatinine excretion so that there is no change in the serum creatinine level (Table 4). As shown by Forbes et al. (25), adult lean body mass declines by 12 kg in males and by 5 kg in females by age 65–70, so that the decrease in creatinine excretion probably reflects a decrease in muscle mass and creatinine production. Also, since a significant number of elderly suffer from chronic debilitating diseases, including neurogenic diseases, muscle atrophy is quite common. Thus, the serum creatinine may be deceiving in the elderly, and for a more meaningful evaluation of kidney function a creatinine clearance or other measurement of GFR is essential.

Since measurement of creatinine clearance requires a timed urine collection (which are notoriously inaccurate without a bladder catheter), a formula has

Table 3 Age and Creatinine Clearance

Age group (years)	Creatinine clearance (ml/min/1.73 m²)
45–54	128 ± 2
55–64	122 ± 2
65–74	110 ± 3
75–84	97 ± 3

Source: Rowe JW, et al. The effect of age in creatinine clearance in man: a cross-sectional and longitudinal study. J Gerontol 1976; 31:155–163.

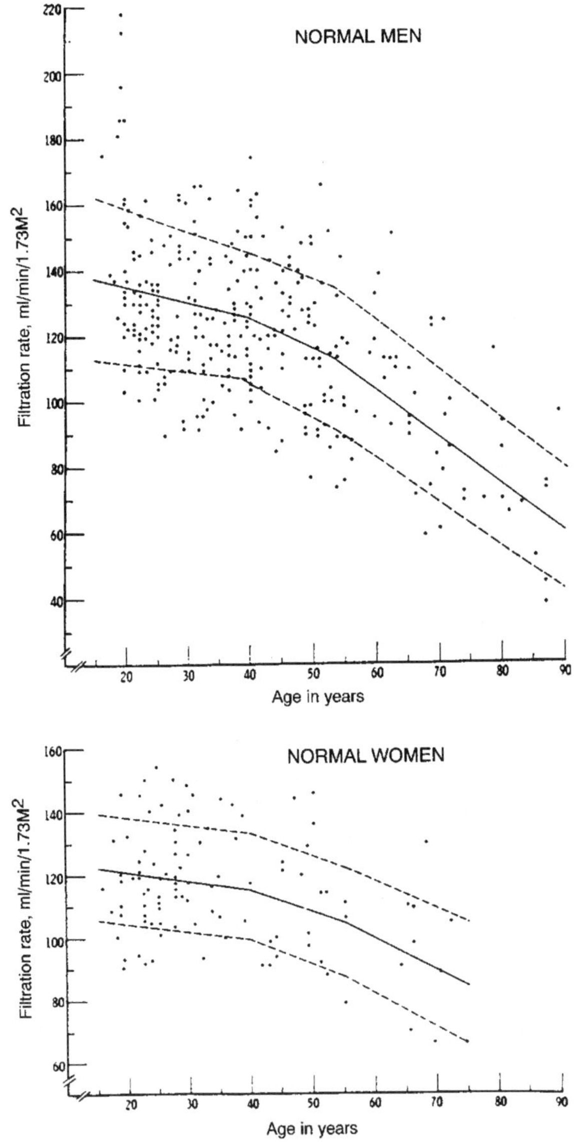

Figure 1 Glomerular filtration rate (inulin clearance) per 1.73 m^2 in normal men and women per decade. Solid and broken lines represent mean value and one standard deviation. (From Wesson LG Jr. Renal hemodynamics in physiological states. In: Physiology of the Human Kidney. New York: Grune & Stratton, 1969: 96–108.

Table 4 Relationship Between Serum and Urine Creatinine and Creatinine Clearance

Age (years)	Serum creatinine (mg/dl)		Urine Creatinine (mg/kg/24 hr)		Creatinine clearance (ml/min/1.73 m²)	
	Male	Female	Male	Female	Male	Female
40–49	1.10	1.00	19.7	17.6	88	81
50–59	1.16	0.99	19.3	14.9	81	74
60–69	1.15	0.97	16.9	12.9	72	63
70–79	1.03	1.02	14.2	11.8	64	54
80–89	1.06	1.05	11.7	10.7	47	46
90–99	1.20	.91	9.4	8.4	34	39

Source: Kampman M, et al. Rapid evolution of creatinine clearance. Acta Med Scand 1974; 196: 517–520.

been developed by Cockcroft and Gault which allows one to calculate the creatinine clearance knowing the subject's age, weight, and serum creatinine (26): estimated creatinine clearance (CrC in ml/min) = [140 − age × weight (kg)] ÷ [72 × serum creatinine (mg/dl)]. For females, multiply the result by 0.8. This formula is applicable as long as the patient has stable kidney function (27). Using this formula, a good correlation has been found between the measured and calculated CrC in the elderly by Gral et al (28), Durakovic (29), Freedman et al. (30), and Hadj-aissa et al. (31), keeping in mind that it overestimates the creatinine clearance in females, the malnourished, and the debilitated (31a). For the latter group, the recent formulas worked out by Sanaka et al. (32) could be used. For males, estimated CrC (ml/min) = [(19 × serum albumin (g/dl) + 32) × weight (kg)] ÷ [100 × serum creatinine (mg/dl)]. For females, CrC (ml/min) = [(13 × serum albumin (g/dl) + 29) × weight (kg)] ÷ [100 × serum creatinine (mg/dl)].

As noted earlier, advancing age is associated with fibroelastic hyperplasia and hyalinization of arterioles and small arteries. It has also been found that blood pressure increases with age. The obvious question is whether the decline in renal function with age is mainly a reflection of the increasing blood pressure. Lindeman et al. (33) found that at a mean arterial pressure (MAP) of less than 107 mmHg, no correlation could be found between creatinine clearance and blood pressure. For pressures above that level, however, there appeared to be a negative correlation between creatinine clearance and MAP. Thus, the progressive decline in GFR with the associated anatomical changes are a function of age per se, but increasing the blood pressure appears to accelerate the decline.

Filtration fraction increases with age due to the fact that the GFR falls less rapidly than renal plasma flow and the higher percentage of functioning deep cortical nephrons in the elderly compared with younger subjects (34).

Infusion of amino acids in the elderly is associated with an increase in GFR, similar to that seen in younger individuals (35). The renal plasma flow response, however, is blunted and less predictable in the elderly, and might be due to the structural changes rather than an alteration in the response to vasodilators such as prostacyclin and nitric oxide. Both these factors have been found to contribute to the renal vasodilatory response to amino acids (36).

Finally, patients over 60 years of age can undergo compensatory hypertrophy to the same extent as younger patients as early as 7 months after unilateral nephrectomy (37,38).

III. EFFECT OF AGE ON TUBULAR FUNCTION

As noted earlier, the anatomical changes affecting the glomeruli are associated with parallel changes in the tubules, so that glomerular–tubular balance is usually well maintained in the elderly (8,31).

A. Sodium Metabolism

1. Low-Sodium Diet

In the study of Weidmann et al. (39), in which 12 patients aged 20–30 years, and 7 patients aged 62–70 years, were placed on a low-sodium diet (<10 mEq/day), overall urinary excretion of Na (measured daily) was similar in the two groups, except on day 9 when the older group showed greater Na excretion. Crane et al. (40) noted that patients older than 50 years of age tend to excrete more Na in the urine when placed on a 10-mEq/day Na diet; however, statistical significance was achieved only in the 70–79 age group. Rather than measuring daily Na excretion in the older age group on a low-Na diet, Epstein and Hollenberg (41) determined the rate at which balance was achieved. They concluded that cumulative Na balance, per se, cannot be used as an index of Na handling by the kidney because of the widely differing starting points due to the variable dietary Na intake beforehand. They found that from age 30 to 60 years dietary Na restriction is associated with a constant half-time for renal Na conservation of 23.4 + 1.1 hr, compared to 30.9 + 2.8 hr for subjects over 60 years of age. Thus, it would appear that age does influence the kidney's capacity to conserve Na (42). The underlying mechanism(s) for this phenomenon is not clear, however. Of interest is that, compared to younger subjects, elderly subjects excreted sodium, potassium, and total solutes at a proportionately higher rate at night (43).

There is experimental evidence that during salt restriction both proximal and distal parts of the nephron participate in the increased reabsorption. The decrease in activity of the autonomic nervous system with age might contribute to the inability of the elderly patient to conserve salt normally, since this system is known to contribute to the increased proximal Na reabsorption noted during salt restriction (44). Despite a reduction in nephron number and cortical blood flow in the elderly, medullary flow is well preserved (39). As a result of this disparate blood flow, medullary washout might take place, reducing the efficacy of the countercurrent system and thereby decreasing the amount of Na removed by the ascending limb of deep nephrons. Plasma renin activity (PRA) and plasma aldosterone (PA) have been measured in different age groups during unrestricted (120 mEq Na/day) and low-sodium (<10 mEq Na/day) diets in the supine and standing position (39,40,45). Both PRA and PA decrease progressively at each decade of life, starting after the fourth decade. The same pattern persists whether subjects are on an unrestricted or a restricted sodium diet, supine or standing. The reduced renin levels may be due in part to the decreased sympathetic activity in the elderly and/or to a decrease in their ability to activate prorennin to renin (46,47). The lower basal aldosterone level can be explained by a decrease in adrenal responsiveness to circulating angiotensin II or the higher baseline circulating plasma atrial natriuretic peptide (ANP) (vide infra) (48). Following salt restriction, PA rises appropriately in the elderly, so that it is unlikely to be responsible for impaired sodium conservation.

2. *Volume Expansion*

As shown by Luft et al. (49), subjects older than 40 years excreted an acute saline load slower than younger subjects, although the plasma Na was similar in both groups. In this particular study creatinine clearance was not measured. Since GFR decreases with age, one explanation for the blunted natriuresis is a decrease in the filtered load. The baseline plasma ANP, a substance which participates in the natriuresis associated with acute and chronic volume expansion, increases with age (50–52), in part due to a decrease in its catabolic rate (53). Since saline loading in the elderly results in a significant rise in ANP (50), the blunted natriuresis cannot be attributed to an inappropriate response, but rather to a possible postreceptor renal resistance to the hormone (50a).

B. Urinary Acidification

The kidneys play a very important role in acid–base homeostasis by reabsorbing the bulk of filtered bicarbonate and generating new bicarbonate through the titration of buffers, the most important being ammonia and titratable acids (phosphate, sulfate). The latter mechanism depends on the active secretion of hydrogen ion (H^+) by tubular cells.

A significant decrease in the plasma bicarbonate concentration and blood pH has been found with aging in subjects on a constant diet. The decrease corelates with the age-related decrease in glomerular filtration rate (54). Despite these changes, both blood pH and bicarbonate levels remain within the normal range and the elderly kidney maintains its ability to maximally acidify the urine in the presence of appropriate stimuli (55). Following a 2-mmol/kg ammonium chloride load, urinary excretion of net acid is significantly lower in elderly compared with younger subjects. The difference could be accounted for solely by a decrease in ammonium excretion, since titratable acid excretion is unchanged. This impairment of ammonium excretion represents a reduction in the maximum capacity of the tubular cells to synthesize ammonia (56).

C. Urinary Concentration

Rowe et al. (57) noted after 12 hr of water deprivation the elderly (mean age 68 years) achieve a mean urine osmolality of 882 compared with 1051 in a group of middle-aged subjects (mean age 49 years) and 1109 mOsm/kg H_2O in a younger group of subjects (mean age 33). The differences among the three groups were statistically different. The authors concluded that aging is associated with a decrease in the ability to maximally concentrate the urine. Identical conclusions have been reached by Dontas et al. (10). To achieve maximal urine concentration the following features should prevail.

1. A normally functioning hypothalamic-hypophyseal axis. If anything, it has been shown that there is a significant age-related increase in osmoreceptor sensitivity. For the same osmolar stimulus, elderly subjects tend to release twice as much antidiuretic hormone (ADH) as younger subjects (58).
2. Adequate fluid delivery to the distal segment of the nephron. The GFR decreases with age; however, no significant relationship has been found between creatinine clearance and urine osmolality, suggesting that fluid delivery to the distal nephron is not a limiting factor (57).
3. A collecting tubule that is responsive to ADH. Although maximum urine osmolality following infusion of large doses of vasopressin is decreased in the elderly undergoing a water diuresis, urine osmolality responds normally to stepwise incremental doses of vasopressin insufficient to maximally concentrate the urine, ruling out any significant impairment in the ability of the collecting duct to respond to vasopressin (59,60).
4. A normally functioning ascending limb of Henle. There are suggestions of a defect in sodium reabsorption in the ascending limb of Henle's loop in elderly subjects. This defect, coupled with a state of relative medullary washout (61), leads to a significant reduction in medullary tonicity, and consequently, the maximum urinary concen-

tration. In summary, it appears that the impaired ability of the elderly kidney to maximally concentrate the urine results from a reduced medullary tonicity.

D. Urinary Dilution

During water loading, the minimum urine osmolality achieved by the elderly has been found to be higher than that of younger subjects by some (10), but not by others (62). In the latter study, the hourly free water clearance was lower in the elderly; however, the recovery of serum osmolality to baseline was slower. The observed delayed water excretion could be explained by the lower GFR and subsequent increase solute load per nephron and to some extent may be related to the reduction in the renal synthesis of prostaglandins seen with aging (63), which may be associated with enhanced ADH responsiveness.

E. Tubular Reabsorption of Glucose

The effects of age on the maximal rate of renal tubular reabsorption of glucose have been examined by Miller and co-workers (64), who demonstrated a linear decrease with age. Since GFR decreases as well, glycosuria does not occur at normal plasma levels.

REFERENCES

1. Westking, D, Pushparaj N, O'Toole K. Morbidity and mortality in the aged. Hosp Prac 1982;17:97–109.
2. Tauchi H, Tsuboi K, Okutomi J. Age changes in the human kidney of the different races. Gerontologia 1971;17:87–97.
3. DeLeon W, Garcia A, DeJesus PI. Normal weight of visceral organs in adult Filipinos. Philip J Sci 1933;52:111–127.
4. McLachlan MSF, Wasserman P. Changes in sizes and distensibility of the aging kidney. Br J Radiol 1981;54:488–491.
5. Griffiths GJ, et al. Loss of renal tissue in the elderly. Br J Radiol 1976;49:111–117.
6. Moore RA. The total number of glomeruli in the normal human kidney. Anat Rec 1931;48:153–168.
6a. Ishikawa I, et al. Renal cortex visualization and analysis of dynamic CT curves of the kidney. J Comput Assist Tomogr 1981;5:695–701.
7. Kappel B, Olsen S. Cortical interstitial tissue and sclerosed glomeruli in the normal human kidney, related to age and sex: a quantitative study. Virchows Arch A Path Anat Histol 1980;387:271–277.
8. Kaplan C, et al. Age-related incidence of sclerotic glomeruli in human kidneys. Am J Pathol 1975;80:227–234.
9. Darmady EM, Offer J, Woodhouse MA. The parameters of the aging kidney. J Pathol 1973;109:195–207.
10. Dontas AS, Marketos SG, Papanayiotou P. Mechanisms of renal tubular defects in old age. Postgrad Med J 1972;48:295–303.

11. Langeveld JPM, et al. Chemical characterization of glomerular and tubular basement membrane of men of different ages. Kidney Int 1981;20:104–114.
12. Brenner B, Meyer TW, Hostetter TH. Dietary protein intake and the progressive nature of kidney disease: The role of hemodynamically mediated glomerular injury in the pathogenesis of progressive glomerular sclerosis in aging, renal ablation and intrinsic renal disease. N Engl J Med 1982;307:652–659.
13. Kasiske BL. Relationship between vascular disease and age associated changes in the human kidney. Kidney Int 1987;31:1153–1159.
14. Baylis C. Age-dependent glomerular damage in the rat: dissociation between glomerular injury and both glomerular hypertension and hypertrophy. Male gender as a primary risk factor. J Clin Invest 1994;94:1823–1829.
15. Hollenberg NK, et al. Senescence and the renal vasculature in normal man. Circ Res 1974;34:309–316.
16. McLachlan MSF, et al. Vascular and glomerular changes in the aging kidney. J Pathol 1977;121:65–78.
17. Yamaguchi T, Omae T, Katsuki S. Quantitative determination of renal vascular changes related to age and hypertension. Jpn Heart J 1969;10:248–258.
18. Davies DF, Shock NW. Age changes in glomerular filtration rate: effective renal plasma flow and tubular excretory capacity in adult males. J Clin Invest 1950;29: 496–507.
19. Rowe JW, et al. The effect of age on creatinine clearance in man: a cross-sectional and longitudinal study. J Gerontol 1976;31:155–163.
20. Lindeman RD, Tobin J, Shock NW. Longitudinal studies on the rate of decline in renal function with age. J Am Geriatr Soc 1985;33:278–285.
21. Wesson LG Jr. Renal hemodynamics in physiological states. In: Physiology of the Human Kidney. New York: Grune & Stratton, 1969:96–108.
22. Rowe JW, et al. Age-adjusted standards for creatinine clearance. Ann Intern Med 1976;84:567–569.
23. Feinfeld DA, et al. Sequential changes in renal function tests in the old: results from the Bronx longitudinal aging study. J Am Geriatr Soc 1995;43:412–414.
24. Kampman J, et al. Rapid evaluation of creatinine clearance. Acta Med Scand 1974;196:517–520.
25. Forbes GB, Reina JC. Adult lean body mass declines with age: Some longitudinal observations. Metabolism 1970;19:653–663.
26. Cockcroft DW, Gault MH. Prediction of creatinine clearance from serum creatinine. Nephron 1976;16:31–41.
27. Drusano GL, et al. Commonly used methods of estimating creatinine clearance are inadequate for elderly debilitated nursing home patients. J Am Geriatr Soc 1988; 36:437–441.
28. Gral T, Young M. Measured versus estimated creatinine clearance in the elderly as an index of renal function. J Am Geriatr Soc 1980;28:492–496.
29. Durakovic Z. Creatinine clearance in the elderly: a comparison of direct measurement and calculation from serum creatinine. Nephron 1986;44:66–69.
30. Friedman JR, Norman DC, Yoshikawa TT. Correlation of estimated renal function parameters versus 24-hour creatinine clearance in ambulatory elderly. J Am Geriatr Soc 1989;37:1485–1489.

31. Hadj-Aissa A, et al. Renal function in the elderly. Nephron 1990;54:364–365.
31a. Malarose LC, et al. Measured versus estimated creatinine clearance in a high-functioning elderly sample. MacArthur foundation study of successful aging. J Am Geriatr Soc 1993;41:715–721.
32. Sanaka M, et al. Serum albumin for estimating creatinine clearance in the elderly with muscle atrophy. Nephron 1996;73:137–144.
33. Lindeman RD, Tobin JD, Shock NW. Association between blood pressure and the rate of decline in renal function with age. Kidney Int 1984;26:861–868.
34. Sarris E, Wilkinson R. Aging and the kidney. J Nephrol 1991;2:67–74.
35. Fliser D, et al. Renal functional reserve in healthy elderly subjects. J Am Soc Nephrol 1993;3:1371–1377.
36. Baylis C, Schmidt R. The aging glomerulus. Sem Nephrol 1996;16:265–276.
37. Boner G, Shery J, Riesebach RE. Hypertrophy of the normal human kidney following contralateral nephrectomy. Nephron 1972;9:364–370.
38. Eklund L, Gothlin J. Compensatory renal enlargement in older patients. J Roentgenol 1976;127:713–715.
39. Weidman P, et al. Effect of aging on plasma renin and aldosterone in normal man. Kidney Int 1975;8:325–333.
40. Crane MG, Harris JJ. Effect of aging on renin activity and aldosterone excretion. J Lab Clin Med 1976;87:947–959.
41. Epstein M, Hollenberg NK. Age as a determinant of renal sodium conservation in normal men. J Lab Clin Med 1976;87:411–417.
42. Macias Nuñea JF, et al. Renal handling of sodium in old people. A functional study. Age and Aging 1980;7:178–181.
43. Kirkland JL, et al. Patterns of urine flow and electrolyte excretion in healthy elderly people. Br Med J 1983;287:1665–1667.
44. Gottschalk CW. Renal nerves and sodium excretion. Ann Rev Physiol 1979;41: 229–240.
45. Flood C, et al. The metabolism and secretion of aldosterone in elderly subjects. J Clin Invest 1967;46:960–966.
46. Tsunoda K, et al. Effect of age on the renin-angiotensin-aldosterone system in normal subjects: Simultaneous measurement of active and inactive renin, renin substrate and aldosterone in plasma. J Clin Endocrinol Metab 1986;62:384–389.
47. Higaki J, et al. Effects of aging on human plasma renin: simultaneous multiple assays of enzyme activity and immunoactivity of plasma renin. Acta Endocrinol 1989; 120:81–86.
48. Duggan J, et al. Aging and human hormonal and pressor responsiveness to angiotensin II infusion with simultaneous measurements of exogenous and endogenous AII. Am J Hypertens 1993;6:641–647.
49. Luft FC, et al. Effects of volume expansion and contraction in normotensive whites, blacks and subjects of different ages. Circulation 1979;59:643–650.
50. Ohashi M, et al. High plasma concentration of human natriuretic polypeptide in aged man. J Clin Endorinol Metab 1987;64:81–85.
50a. Leosco D, et al. Effects of age on the role of a trial natriuretic factor in renal adaptation to physiologic variations of dietary salt intake. J Am Soc Nephrol 1996;7: 1045–1051.

51. Clark BA, Elahi D, Epstein FH. Age and dose related differences in response to atrial natriuretic peptide in man. Kidney Int 1989;35:282A.
52. Haller BGD, et al. Effects of posture and aging on circulating atrial natriuretic peptide levels in man. J Hypertens 1987;5:551–556.
53. Tan AC, et al. Kinetics of atrial natriuretic peptide in young and elderly subjects. Eur J Clin Pharmacol 1992;42:449–452.
54. Frassetto LA, Morris RC Jr. Sebastian A. Effect of age on blood acid-base composition in adult humans: role of age-related renal functional decline. Am J Physiol 1996;271:F1114–1122.
55. Agarwal BN, Cabebe FG. Renal acidification in elderly subjects. Nephron 1980; 26:291–295.
56. Yamada H, Sacktor B, Kinsella J. Age-associated changes in ammoniagenesis in isolated rat renal tubule segments. Am J Physiol 1992;262:F600–F605.
57. Rowe JW, Shock NW, DeFronzo RA. The influence of age on the renal response to water deprivation in man. Nephron 1976;17:270–278.
58. Helderman JH, et al. The response of arginine vasopressin to intravenous ethanol and hypertonic saline in man: the impact of aging. J Gerontol 1978;33:39–47.
59. Bengele HH, et al. Urinary concentrating defect in the aged rat. Am J Physiol 1981; F147–F150.
60. Miller JH, Shock NW. Age differences in the renal tubular response to antidiuretic hormone. J Gerontol 1953;8:446–450.
61. Takazakura E, et al. Intrarenal vascular changes with age and disease. Kidney Int 1972;2:224–230.
62. Clark BA, et al. Increased susceptibility to thiazide-induced hyponatremia in the elderly. J Am Soc Nephrol 1994;5:1106–1111.
63. Clark BA, et al. Decline in urinary excretion of dopamine and PGE_2 with age. Clin Res 1991;39:226A.
64. Miller JH, McDonald RK, Shock NW. Age changes in the maximal rate of renal tubular reabsorption of glucose. J Gerontol 1952;7:196–200.

2

Disorders of Water and Salt Metabolism

Normally, plasma osmolality is maintained within a narrow range despite wide daily variations in water intake. More than 90% of the osmotic pressure of plasma (and other extracellular fluids) is accounted for by sodium (Na) and its anions, with urea and glucose providing the remainder. The constancy of plasma osmolality is maintained by rapid adjustments in water excretion or intake to oppose any changes in the plasma concentration of Na and its anions. Changes in osmolality are perceived quite rapidly by neurons located in the anterior hypothalamus, where there is integration and transmission of the neural signals to cells of the supraoptic and paraventricular nuclei responsible for antidiuretic hormone (ADH) synthesis, and to the so-called thirst centers. The secretion of ADH serves to retain water by increasing its reabsorption by the kidneys. Its absence will have the opposite effect. The system is sensitive enough to perceive changes in plasma osmolality as small as 1%, although the mechanism(s) responsible for such a response is not yet entirely clear (1).

Besides changes in osmolality, nonosmotic stimuli can also independently affect ADH release, including: (a) hemodynamic events (hypotension and/or hypovolemia), mediated primarily by pressure-sensitive receptors located in the left atrium and large arteries of the chest and neck (2); (b) drugs such as barbiturates, opiates, chlorpropamide, tolbutamide, vinca alkaloids, carbamazepine, and clofibrate; (c) others, such as catecholamines and acetylcholine (3); (d) pain and nausea (4). The different factors involved in water excretion are summarized in Fig. 1. How does this apply to the elderly? Both serum osmolality and plasma Na are well maintained in the elderly; however, there are alterations in the physiological patterns outlined in Fig. 1 which make the elderly subject more susceptible to disorders of water balance.

1. A decrease in thirst with hypodypsia related to a defect in the opioid-associated drinking drive has been found in the elderly subjected to 24 hr of water deprivation (5,6).
2. In general, ADH synthesis increases with age, apparently due to a decrease in receptor sensitivity. Although the linear relationship between ADH and serum osmolality is maintained in most elderly healthy subjects, in some the osmotic regulation of the plasma ADH level is lost (7,8). Since water loading in such individuals will not necessarily suppress ADH, one would expect them to be more prone to hyponatremia.
3. The ADH response to changes in volume-pressure (nonosmotic stimuli), as estimated by orthostasis, is also blunted in the elderly. This defect appears to be between the vasomotor center and the supraoptic and paraventricular nuclei of the hypothalamus, since norepinephrine release is intact (9).

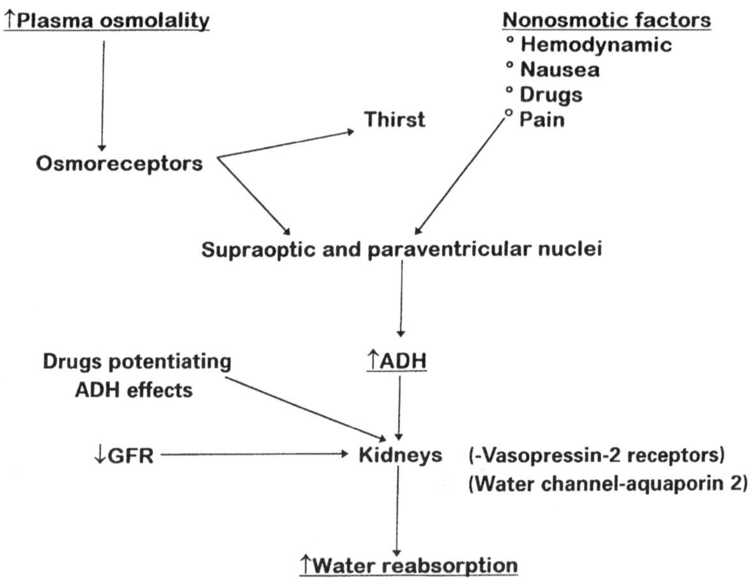

Figure 1 Factors involved in water excretion.

I. HYPONATREMIA

A. Incidence and Prevalence

In a study of all patients hospitalized over a 3-month period in their institution, Baran and Hutchinson (10) found 78 patients with a serum Na less than or equal to 128 mEq/L. Sixty percent were over the age of 60, with 31% aged 61–70 years, 24% 71–80 years, and 5% over 80 years. Of 683 patients admitted to an acute geriatric unit over a 10-month period, 77 (11.3%) had a plasma Na concentration below 130 mEq/L (11). Kleinfeld et al. (12), in a random sampling of plasma Na of 160 patients in a chronic care facility, reported that 36 patients (22.5%) had chronic hyponatremia. In another study, 53% of nursing home residents developed hyponatremia over a 12-month period (13). It appears from these data that hyponatremia is a rather common event in the elderly. Indeed, in a prospective study of patients with hyponatremia admitted to the Hospital of the University of Colorado Health Sciences Center, the mean age varied between 57 and 63 years in the different groups studied (14). Of 22 patients with symptomatic hyponatremia reported by Cogan et al. (15), most were elderly.

B. Pathogenesis

Before a diagnosis of hyponatremia is made, pseudohyponatremia due to hyperlipidemia or hyperproteinemia must be eliminated (16). In the case of hyperlipidemia and hyperproteinemia, serum osmolality will be normal in the face of hyponatremia. Hyponatremia could also occur with hyperglycemia and with the presence in the serum of exogenous osmoles such as mannitol; ethanol, or ethylene glycol. In the case of hyperglycemia, for each 100 mg/dl increment in serum glucose, there is a decrement of 1.6 mEq/L in serum Na (17). In the presence of exogenous osmoles, the difference between the measured and calculated serum osmolality will be more than 10 mOsm/kg/H_2O (18). Once these conditions are ruled out, the hyponatremic patient can be classified as normovolemic, edematous, or hypovolemic, depending on the clinical assessment of the extracellular fluid volume (Table 1) (14). Whereas the diagnosis of edematous hyponatremia can be easily made at the bedside, differentiating between normovolemic and hypovolemic hyponatremia may be difficult on clinical grounds, especially in the bed-ridden elderly, where useful signs of hypovolemia such as poor skin turgor or orthostasis may be absent. A low sodium (<20 mEq/L) in a spot urine specimen strongly suggests a hypovolemic state, whereas the urine sodium is usually > 40 mEq/L in the normovolemic hyponatremic patient (19).

1. Normovolemic Hyponatremia

The syndrome of inappropriate secretion of ADH (SIADH) and diuretic administration constitute the most common causes in the elderly, accounting for 59% of the cases (20).

Table 1 Classification of Hyponatremia

A.	Normovolemic
	Syndrome of inappropriate secretion of ADH (SIADH)
	Diuretic induced
	Postoperative
	Others—hypothyroidism, adrenal insufficiency, acute respiratory failure
B.	Edematous
	Congestive heart failure
	Liver disease
	Nephrotic syndrome
	Chronic obstructive pulmonary disease
C.	Hypovolemic
D.	Hypoalbuminemic hyponatremia—a syndrome of variable etiology in the elderly

a. SIADH. Several conditions have been associated with this syndrome (Table 2). In the series of Sunderam et al. (11), stroke, chest infection, and carcinoma were most common. Of the 13 patients over the age of 60 reported by Kleinfeld et al. (12), 3 had a cerebrovascular accident, 3 were taking pharmacological agents known to impair water excretion, 2 had malignancy, and the remaining 5 had a variety of disorders. These latter 5 patients may have had an idiopathic form, as described by Goldstein et al. (21), who reported one patient with SIADH without any associated disease and found 9 other previously reported cases. Edward et al. (22) subsequently described an 86-year-old patient with the syndrome. This form might be present in 26–39% of elderly with SIADH, as recently reported by Miller et al. and by Hirshberg and Ben-Yehuda (20,20a). The mechanism for ADH release in these patients is not clear, but in some patients stress or orthostatic hypotension might serve as stimuli (20a,23). Such patients, however, should be followed carefully, since clinically detectable malignancy has been identified several months after the diagnosis of "idiopathic" SIADH has been made (24,25).

Several pharmacological agents have been associated with SIADH, including fluoxetine, sertraline, vinblastine, phenothiazines, monoamine oxidase (MAO) inhibitors, clofibrate, chlorpropamide, and carbamazepine. Among this list, the latter two are commonly used in the elderly for the management of

Table 2 Cause of Inappropriate Secretion of ADH

Central nervous system: vascular abnormalities, infections
Intrathoracic disorders: malignancy, infections
Idiopathic
Drug-induced: chlorpropamide, carbamazepine, vinca alkaloids, phenothiazines, clofibrate, fluoxetine, sertraline

adult-onset diabetes mellitus and tic douloureux (trigeminal neuralgia), respectively. Of the 5 patients with chlorpropamide hyponatremia studied by Weissman et al. (26), 4 were over the age of 60. The majority of patients who developed SIADH due to fluoxetine were also elderly (26a). Elevated plasma ADH levels in SIADH has been confirmed by Zerbe et al. (27) in 79 patients. They have shown plasma ADH levels that are inappropriate in relation to the hypotonicity of body fluids (Fig. 2). The changes in serum Na concentration are accounted for primarily by changes in solute and water balance, as shown by Cooke et al. (28). Atrial natriuretic factor is elevated acutely and chronically during SIADH and may be responsible, in part, for the natriuresis seen early in this syndrome (29). In some patients with SIADH, salt wasting due to an inability of the distal part of the nephron to maximally reabsorb sodium has been reported (30). These patients differ markedly from those with the more common "pure" form of SIADH in that water restriction, associated with continued loss of sodium in the urine, can result in severe volume contraction. It is important to diagnose these patients, since they generally require administration of large doses of mineralo-corticoids (31).

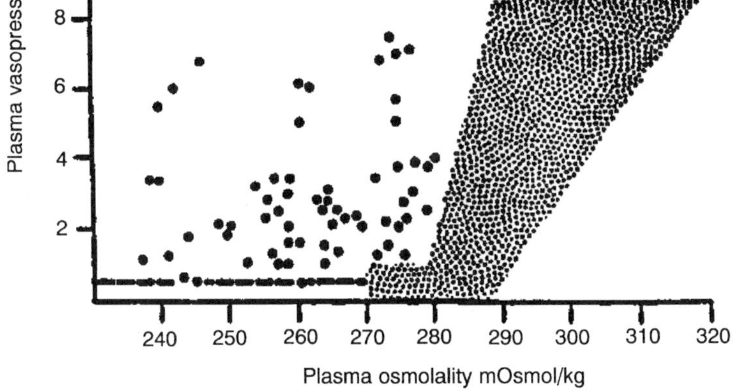

Figure 2 Relationship between plasma vasopressin and osmolality in 79 patients with clinical features of SIADH (shaded area represents the range of normal values). (From Zerbe R, Stropes L, Robertson G. Vasoressin function in the syndrome of inappropriate antidiuresis. Ann Rev Med 1980; 31:315–327.

Besides hyponatremia, hypouremia is commonly encountered in patients with SIADH, which is secondary to both an increase in urinary losses of urea and body fluid dilution (32,33). Beck (34) reported a mean serum urate concentration of 2.9 ± 4 mg/dl in patients with SIADH, compared with 7.7 ± 0.8 mg/dl in other forms of hyponatremia. Hypouricemia has been demonstrated by others and attributed to increased tubular secretion of uric acid (35) and a decrease in the post-secretory reabsorption rate (36).

a. Diuretic-Induced Hyponatremia. The true incidence of diuretic-induced hyponatremia in the elderly is not known. Of 48 episodes of hyponatremia studied retrospectively by Abramow and Cogan (37), 14 instances (29%) were explained solely on the basis of diuretic use. Seven of 59 patients with severe hyponatremia (mean Na of 112 mEq/L) reported by Booker (23) were taking a diuretic. The thiazide group of diuretics and, rarely, indapamide (38) or the potassium-sparing diuretics such as triamterene or amiloride may be responsible for the syndrome, which is seen most often in elderly females. Seventy-seven percent of reported patients were over 60, with 85% females, as reported by Grenfell (39). In the series of Abramow and Cogan (37), the mean age was 76.5 years and 11 of the 12 patients (92%) were females. The reason(s) why diuretic-induced hyponatremia is more prevalent in elderly females is not clear. Approximately 60% of the patients come to medical attention because of symptomatic hyponatremia, ranging from nausea and vomiting to confusion, seizures, or coma. The mechanisms responsible for the hyponatremia are probably multiple and include potassium depletion (40,41) and urinary Na losses associated with increase in water intake (42). It should be noted, however, that hypokalemia is not present in all reported patients. The inappropriate release of ADH has also been suggested as a cause of diuretic-induced hyponatremia (43,44). Finally, there is experimental evidence that a sulfonamide diuretic can potentiate the effect of ADH on the collecting tubule (45). In the presence of a submaximal concentration of ADH (2.5 mU/ml), indapamide (a sulfonamide diuretic) significantly increases the hydraulic permeability of the isolated cortical collecting tubule. Figure 3 describes schematically how the above factors play a role in diuretic-induced hyponatremia.

Another reason why diuretic-induced hyponatremia is seen most commonly with thiazides could be related to their different effect on prostaglandins compared to furosemide (46). Furosemide increases urinary prostaglandin excretion, which antagonizes the hydroosmotic effect of ADH, whereas the thiazides have no effect on prostaglandin release (47).

b. Postoperative Hyponatremia. In younger individuals, postoperative antinatriuresis is usually a transient phenomenon secondary to ADH release due to pain, analgesic use, etc. In the elderly, by contrast, this problem may be severe and prolonged. Deutsch et al. (48) reported a group of patients (average age was 75 years) in whom symptoms of hyponatremia, including moderate to marked

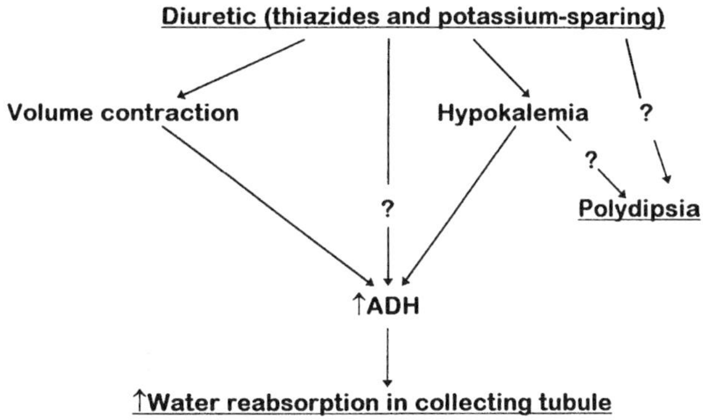

Figure 3 Mechanisms of diuretic-induced hyponatremia.

changes in the level of consciousness, occurred within the first 5 postoperative days. Likely contributing factors include narcotic use during the pre-, peri-, and postoperative periods and excessive hypotonic fluid administration in the presence of non-osmotic-stimulated secretion of ADH (49). Based on these findings, fluid replacement in the postoperative elderly patient should be planned carefully, and limited to replacing losses on an hourly basis, if possible. In these patients, serum electrolytes should be measured periodically or wherever a change in the level of consciousness is noted.

Hyponatremia has also been reported following transurethral prostatic resection. The true incidence of this problem is not known; however, in a prospective study carried out by Rhymer et al. (50), 7 of 100 patients developed significant hyponatremia (range 103–133 mEqL). They found a significant correlation between the weight of the prostate resected and the postoperative decrease in serum Na, as well as between the weight of the gland resected and the volume of irrigation fluid (glycine) used. Since the hyponatremia most likely represents reabsorption of electrolyte-free solution by the open prostatic veins (51), the larger the gland and the longer the surgery the more irrigating solution will be reabsorbed. Another contributing factor to the amount of irrigating solution reabsorbed is the irrigating pressure. It is recommended that the latter be kept below 60 mmHg during the procedure (52). Symptoms usually appear near the end or immediately following surgery and include increasing apprehension, disorientation, blood pressure elevation, bradycardia, irritability, twitching, nausea, vomiting, and convulsions. In general, the prognosis is good, but it depends on the rate at which serum Na is lowered. Six of the 7 patients reported by Rhymer et al. (50) recovered within 48 hr. Sunderrajan et al. (52) noted a mortality rate as high as 50% for the group with a rapid fall in serum Na. Our patients who developed hyponatremia postprostatic resection were usually on a low-Na diet and continued diuretic therapy for hypertension, so that preoperative volume contraction with persistent ADH release might have contributed to their postoperative water retention.

c. Other. Endocrine disorders such as hypothyroidism and adrenal insufficiency can be associated with hyponatremia. It is not known how often this complication is seen in the elderly with these disorders. In both situations, persistent release of ADH, although playing a significant role, does not entirely explain the water retention (53). It is important to note that transient asymptomatic hyperthyroxinemia can occur during hyponatremia (54) and that hypothyroidism has been reported to affect as many as 10% of elderly patients (55).

Acute respiratory failure has also been found to be associated with hyponatremia. Szatalowicz et al. (56) reported 13 patients with acute respiratory failure with an average age of 59 years whose serum ADH levels were significantly elevated. The nonosmotic stimulus for the ADH release in these patients is not clear. The hyponatremia observed was mild (plasma Na 133 ± 1 mEq/L) and reversible upon correction of the acute problem. It would seem prudent to administer hypotonic fluid cautiously to patients with acute respiratory failure in order to avoid severe hyponatremia.

2. *Edematous Hyponatremia*

a. Congestive Heart Failure. Hyponatremia is not an uncommon finding in patients with congestive heart failure (57,58). Dzau et al. (59) compared biochemical and hemodynamic parameters in hyponatremic and normonatremic patients with congestive heart failure. Ejection fraction was similar in both groups; however, plasma angiotensin II, renin activity, aldosterone, and prostaglandins (PGE_2 and 6 keto-PGF_1 alpha) were higher in the hyponatremic group. In patients with congestive heart failure, kidney function is decreased in those with hyponatremia compared to normonatremic patients (60). Rondeau et al. (61) found that plasma ADH levels were higher in 31 elderly patients with heart failure compared to age-matched controls, although plasma Na and osmolality were lower in the heart failure group. The nonosmotic stimulation of ADH release in heart failure does not appear to be dependent on the renin-angiotensin system, since plasma renin activity does not correlate with plasma ADH (62). The hyponatremia of congestive heart failure is multifactorial and depends on: (a) increased water intake secondary to the dipsogenic effect of increased angiotensin II (63); (b) intrarenal factors; and (c) nonosmotic release of ADH. As a rule, the more severe the heart failure, the higher is the plasma ADH. Since the level of ADH decreases with improvement in cardiac function, the latter might represent the main determinant for the nonosmotic release of the hormone (64). In milder forms of the disease, control of the heart failure will correct the hyponatremia; however, in more severe states, the combined use of furosemide (daily dose tailored to the patient's diuretic response) and an angiotensin-converting enzyme inhibitor (started at an initial low dose and titrated to achieve a maximal hemodynamic response) have been found to be very helpful and should be used in these patients (65,66).

b. Liver Disease. The hyponatremia of chronic liver disease is also multifactorial. Renal hemodynamics have been found by Lancestremere et al. (67) to play a role. Plasma ADH levels are usually elevated in hyponatremic patients with cirrhosis (68), but diuresis can occur without concomitant suppression of ADH in some patients, suggesting that the hormone may represent a "permissive" rather than a pivotal factor in the impaired water excretion (69). A decrease in effective arterial blood volume has been theorized as being the nonosmotic stimulus for the ADH release, since the latter can be suppressed by head-out water immersion, a maneuver associated with central blood volume expansion (70,71). The importance of ineffective blood volume and catecholamines, which have been suggested to play a role in the hyponatremia in cirrhosis (72,73), are still a matter of controversy, however. Recently, urinary PGE_2 was found to be lower in cirrhotic patients with hyponatremia compared to those with normonatremia (74). As noted, PGE_2 modulates the effect of ADH in the cortical collecting tubule, so that a lower PGE_2 level would result in the reabsorption of a larger percentage of the water presented to this site. The reason for the decreased urinary excretion of PGE_2 in these patients is not known.

The management of hyponatremia in the cirrhotic patient consists mainly of water and moderate salt restriction and gentle diuresis. Demeclocycline has been tried, but the incidence of side effects is rather high in this patient population. Oral urea (see below) is worth trying in recalcitrant cases.

c. Nephrotic Syndrome. Hyponatremia has not been a common occurrence in the elderly with nephrotic syndrome (less than 1%). Three (8.3%) of Kleinfeld's patients with hyponatremia had nephrotic syndrome (12). Usberti et al. (75) found an inverse correlation between blood volume or plasma volume and the ability to excrete a water load. Expansion of blood volume with 20% albumin reduced the plasma level of ADH and promoted a water diuresis. Bichet et al. (76) also found a lower GFR, lower fractional excretion of Na, higher plasma renin activity, higher plasma aldosterone and catecholamines, and impaired water excretion in patients with nephrotic syndrome, suggesting that a decrease in blood volume might be the nonosmotic stimulus for ADH release.

d. Chronic Lung Disease (COPD). Farber et al. (77) have reported a high incidence of hyponatremia in edematous patients with COPD and respiratory failure (mean age was 57 ± 7 years). When compared to controls, these patients had a lower effective renal plasma flow and GFR together with elevated PRA and PA. Plasma ADH could not be suppressed despite the lower plasma osmolality. It appears that the hyponatremia is a consequence of both intrarenal hemodynamics and persistent ADH release. Again, the cause for nonosmotic release of ADH is not clear. Therefore, one should be cautious about the amount of hypotonic solution infused in such patients. Even in normonatremia patients, the percentage of a water load excreted may be significantly lower than in normal subjects.

3. *Hypovolemic Hyponatremia*

The hyponatremia in this group is the result of release of ADH due to a persistent volume stimulus in a patient with free access to water. The source of volume losses is usually the gastrointestinal tract (severe diarrhea) or the kidneys (osmotic diuresis of hyperglycemia and glycosuria, continued use of a diuretic and low-salt diet in the elderly hypertensive hospitalized for other problems, and overdiuresis for congestive heart failure). The diagnosis is not difficult in most patients, when physical signs of volume contraction such as weight loss, orthostatic drop in blood pressure, and poor skin turgor are usually present. However, the signs of hypovolemia may be difficult to detect in the elderly, as noted earlier. A combined low fractional excretion of Na (<0.5%) and urea (<55%) have been shown to better predict volume contraction and response to saline infusion in these patients (78). When renal failure is present, the BUN is usually disproportionately higher than the serum creatinine. Therapy should be directed at correcting the cause of the fluid losses and expansion of the extracellular volume with a saline solution.

4. *Hypoalbuminemic Hyponatremia*

Dandona et al. (79) have described 6 patients with severe hyponatremia and pronounced hypoalbuminemia. The age was given for only three of the 6 patients, all of whom were older than 60 years. The explanation for the inability of these patients to excrete water is not clear; however, since the hypoosmolality could be corrected by plasma albumin infusion, hypovolemia might have been the stimulus for persistent ADH release. We have seen 12 patients (all elderly females) with hypoalbuminemia (range 1.5–2.0 gm/dl) and hyponatremia (110–120 mEq/L). All were patients hospitalized for either cerebrovascular disease or advanced dementia (possibly the stimulus for ADH release), receiving large volumes of nasogastric feedings low in Na. Three of these patients were edematous with a normal PRA and PA. These patients responded well to water restriction. After correction of the hyponatremia, NaCl (2 g daily) was added to their tube feeding without any further problems. In another 3 patients, edema was absent and PRA and PA were both elevated, suggesting volume contraction. The addition of 4 g of NaCl to their feeding resulted in prompt correction of the hyponatremia.

C. Clinical Manifestations

Studies by Arieff et al. (80) have demonstrated that symptoms, which are due to cerebral edema, are related to both the magnitude and the rate of development of hyponatremia. Of the 36 patients reported by Kleinfeld et al. (12), 9 were asymptomatic, and in the remaining 27 the various symptoms present were to a great extent secondary to the underlying disease. The clinical features attributable to hyponatremia are summarized in Table 3, from Sunderam et al. (11).

D. Treatment

1. Asymptomatic Patients

The therapy for hyponatremia depends on the clinical situation. The traditional method in the asymptomatic patient consists of fluid restriction. When a drug is the cause, it should be discontinued. Unfortunately, normonatremia is difficult to maintain with fluid restriction alone, so other therapies may be necessary in patients with chronic hyponatremia as in SIADH. Several approaches have been recommended.

a. Lithium. Lithium carbonate can produce a nephrogenic diabetes insipidus by downregulating aquaporin-2 water channel expression (81); however, its effectiveness is limited to only a minority of patients and it is potentially toxic, limiting its usefulness in the elderly, in whom the half-life of the drug is prolonged (81a,82).

b. Demeclocycline. This tetracycline antibiotic inhibits the action of ADH in the cortical collecting tubule. Doses of 600–1200 mg per day are generally used. The drug is well tolerated, but its use in patients with preexisting kidney or liver disease is limited (81,83–85). Side effects include nausea, photosensitivity, and extracellular fluid volume contraction (86).

c. Urea. Oral urea (0.5 g/kg) in two divided doses has been reported by Decaux et al. (87–90) to be of benefit in the long-term management of patients with SIADH or the hyponatremia associated with liver disease. The drug has

Table 3 Clinical Features Attributable to Hyponatremia in 77 Patients

Clinical feature	No. of patients
Weakness	28
Confusion	21
Postural hypotension	17
Falls	13
Transient hemiparesis	1
Seizures	2

Source: Sunderam SG, Mankikar GD. Hyponatremia in the elderly. Age & Aging 1983; 12:77–80.

both an antinatriuretic and diuretic effect. According to the passive countercurrent model, the antinatriuretic action is secondary to increased NaCl reabsorption in the thin ascending limb of Henle (87). Its diuretic effect is due to the osmotic force of unabsorbed urea. To maximize response, water restriction should be continued. Urea should not be used in patients with active peptic ulcer, advanced liver, or renal insufficiency (BUN > 80 mg/dl).

d. Phenytoin. At a dose of 100 mg thrice daily orally, this drug has been used successfully for up to 8 months in one patient (91). It acts by inhibiting the release of ADH from the hypophysis (92). Since its therapeutic efficacy is unpredictable, a trial in a large number of patients is necessary before recommending its routine use.

e. Furosemide. The combination of furosemide (40 mg daily) and supplementary dietary salt (3 g daily) have been used long term by Decaux et al. (90,93) with good results, particularly in those patients with a urine osmolality equal to or greater than 600 mOsm/kgH_2O.

f. ADH Analogs. The advent of new analogs of ADH with specific antagonist activity against the antidiuretic properties of this hormone will allow for a more specific therapy of SIADH and other chronic hyponatremic states (94).

2. Symptomatic Patients

The presence of symptoms related to hyponatremia depends on the rapidity with which hypotonicity occurs, as well as the absolute level of the serum Na. When a patient has symptoms such as delirium, seizures, new onset of focal neurological signs, or coma, rapid correction is indicated. To estimate the Na deficit in these patients, the following formula has been recommended: Desired Na concentration − observed Na concentration × (0.6 × body weight). However, from Table 4, it is evident that in the elderly total body water represents 45–50% of body weight, so using 60% will tend to overestimate the Na deficit, as discussed recently by Shankel (95). This question is of more than academic interest, since overcorrection has been associated with central pontine myelinolysis, also called osmotic demyelination syndrome (96,97). Clinical manifestations of this syndrome vary from minimal to severe neurological deficits with flaccid quadriplegia and facial weakness. The incidence of this syndrome in the overtreated hyponatremic patient is a matter of controversy, however (98). Once the decision to treat the hyponatremia is made, some authors have advised rapid correction at rates approaching 2 mEq/L/hr (99,100); however, patients corrected slower usually do as well (90,101). Ashouri (102) reported 8 symptomatic patients with diuretic-induced hyponatremia corrected at a rate of 0.78 ± 0.26 mEq/L/hr and requiring 28.8 ± 6 hr. All the patients recovered with complete resolution of their neurological symptoms. Recent evidence suggests that an increase in plasma sodium of 20 mEq/L or less in the first 24 hr of therapy is associated with re-

Table 4 Body Water Compartments (as Percent of Body Weight)

Age	Sex	Body weight (kg)	Total body water (%)	Extra-cellular water (%)	Intra-cellular water (%)
0–11 days			76.4	41.6	34.8
11–180 days			72.8	34.9	39.9
6 months–2 years			62.2	27.5	34.7
2–7 years			65.5	25.6	36.9
7–14 years			64.2	17.5	46.7
23-54 years	Male	72.5	54.3 ±1.4[a]	23.4 ±0.6	30.9 ±0.9
23–51 years	Female	59.3	48.6 ±1.5	22.7 ±0.5	25.9 ±1.0
71–84 years	Male	68.1	50.8 ±1.6	25.4 ±1.4	25.4 ±0.6
61–74 years	Female	63.9	43.4 ±1.3	21.4 ±0.5	22.4 ±1.0

[a]Standard error of the mean.

Source: Weitzman R, Kleeman CR. Water metabolism and the neurohypophyseal hormones. In: Maxwell MH, Kleeman CR, eds., Clinical Disorders of Fluid and Electrolyte Metabolism. 3d ed. New York: McGraw-Hill, 1980: 531–645.

covery without sequalae in most patients (103). Our approach consists of reaching a serum Na of 120–125 mEq/L, corrected at a rate of 0.5 to 0.8 mEq/L/hr, using hypertonic NaCl alone (514 mM/L) for the volume-depleted patient. Intermittent doses of intravenous furosemide (1 mg/kg body weight), as recommended by Hantman et al. (104), is added for patients with SIADH or patients with edema. In the latter group, diuresis should be initiated with furosemide before any salt is infused. If hypokalemia is present, it should be corrected as well, particularly after furosemide administration.

E. Mortality in Hyponatremic Patients

The mortality rate associated with hyponatremia in the ambulatory geriatric patient is similar to that of the normonatremic patient (20). In the hospitalized patient the fatality rate for patients with hyponatremia is 11.2%, compared to 0.19% for the remainder of the patient population examined during the same period of time (14); however, as is the case for other published series as well as our own experience, hyponatremia is often a marker for severe underlying disease, which generally carries a rather poor prognosis.

II. HYPERNATREMIA

Hypernatremia is less common in the elderly than hyponatremia. For instance, among 14,133 patients over the age of 60 seen over a 3-year period in a Veterans Administration hospital, 212 or 1.5% had a serum Na greater than 148 mEq/L (105). Hypernatremia is seen more frequently in the elderly compared to younger patients, particularly if the hypernatremia developed prior to hospital admission (106). A decrease in thirst perception as well as an inability to maximally concentrate the urine predispose the elderly to hypernatremia (107).

A. Etiology

Hypernatremia is the result of either the addition of a hypertonic Na solution to the extracellular fluid or hypotonic fluid losses. Extracellular hypertonic fluid gain is seen mainly following the infusion of Na bicarbonate during cardiopulmonary resuscitation. Accidental ingestion of salt is rather rare in the elderly. Hypotonic fluid losses through the gastrointestinal tract secondary due to diarrhea is the most common cause of hypernatremia in the elderly (105). In our experience, the most common cause of the diarrhea in a hospital setting has been hyperosmolar tube feeding and lactulose administration in patients with portal-systemic encephalopathy (108,109) or constipation. Renal loss of water due to a concentrating defect, particularly when associated with diuretic use, renal insufficiency, glycosuria (mainly in patients with the hyperglycemic hyperosmolar syndrome), mannitol or glycerol infusion, or high-protein tube feeding, is the next most common cause of hypernatremia (105,106,110).

B. Clinical Manifestations

The clinical manifestations associated with hypernatremia are usually those of the underlying disease. In one large series, the conditions most often seen were dementia (32%), pneumonia (27%), sepsis (25%), heart failure (20%), and stroke (8%) (105). Occasionally an acute confusional state due to the hyperosmolar state will bring the patient to medical attention (111). The sensation of thirst, which is probably present in many of these patients, may not be verbalized, since those patients affected frequently have a depressed sensorium. With hypotonic losses from the gastrointestinal tract, evidence of volume contraction will be found on physical examination. It should be noted, however, that changes usually associated with dehydration, such as poor skin tone and sunken eye sockets, may be seen in aging per se. Urinary Na concentration will usually be less than 20 mEq/L, unless the patient has chronic renal failure, develops acute tubular necrosis due to accompanying shock, or the hypernatremia is marked (112). In the patient who has received Na bicarbonate, the history should be helpful and the urinary Na concentration will usually be greater than 60 mEq/L. The urinary osmolality will generally be greater than twice the plasma osmolality unless there is some degree of resistance to ADH due to superimposed acute or chronic renal insufficiency. In our experience this combination (hypotonic losses through the GI tract and renal insufficiency) has been the rule rather than the exception in the elderly with severe extracellular fluid volume losses. Hypernatremia secondary to water losses through osmotic diuresis should be suspected in patients on high-protein tube feeding, receiving an osmotic diuretic such as mannitol (aortic aneurysm, surgery, or cerebrovascular accident), or having severe hyperglycemia and glycosuria. In these situations the urine Na tends to be above 30 mEq/L and the urine osmolality close to isotonicity.

C. Treatment

Water losses should be estimated before institution of therapy. Several formulas have been described, but we have found the following most helpful: $BW_2 = Na_1 \times BW_1/Na_2$, where BW_2 represents the current body water, Na_1 the normal serum Na (145 mEq/L), BW_1 the original volume of body water (50% of the body weight for the elderly), and Na_2 the current serum Na. The water loss is the difference between BW_1 and BW_2. For instance, in a 70-kg man with a serum Na of 165 mEq/L, $BW_2 = 145 \times 35/165 = 5075/165 = 31$ L. The water deficit is then $35 - 31 = 4$ L.

1. Type of Solution

Dextrose in water should be used for the patient with hypernatremia secondary to Na excesses, with careful monitoring of the urinary output. If the patient is oliguric, intravenous furosemide can be tried. In post-cardiac arrest patients with acute oliguric renal failure in whom large volumes of sodium bicarbonate were infused, dialysis should be initiated. For the patient with hypotonic fluid losses and hypotension, rapid expansion of the extracellular fluid can be achieved with 0.9% NaCl infusion. Once normotension is achieved, one can switch to any of the hypotonic solutions available (we usually base our decision on determination of the urine Na).

2. Rate of Infusion

It is recommended that calculated losses be repaired in 48–72 hr. In Snyder's series (105), the mortality rate in patients who had their deficit replaced in 48–72 hr was 31%, compared to 66% in those corrected within 24 hr. The marked difference was attributed to the probable development of cerebral edema. The overall mortality rate in hypernatremic patients is around 40–50% (105, 106,113). The severity of the hypernatremia does not appear to contribute directly to the mortality rate (Table 5). When other problems such as chronic renal failure, ischemic heart disease, surgery, or pneumonia were present concurrently, the mortality rate increased, which suggests that hypernatremia in the elderly often represents a marker for more serious illness, as does hyponatremia.

Table 5 Association of Clinical Characteristics with Mortality in 162 Elderly Patients with Hypernatremia

Measure of severity hypernatremia	Survivors	Nonsurvivors
Serum sodium levels (mEq/L)		
Peak	154	153
Mean (for entire episode)	151	151
Total body water deficit at time of peak sodium level (%)	10.7	9.5
Duration of episode (days)	2.1	1.9
Age (years)[a]	78 ± 9	77 ± 9
Sex (%)		
Women	41	42
Men	59	58
Race (%)		
White	69	72
Black	26	22
Other	5	6

[a]Value given as mean ± SD.
Source: Snyder NA, Feigel DW, Arieff AI. Hypernatremia in elderly patients. A heterogenous, morbid and iatrogenic entity. Ann Intern Med 1987; 107:309–319.

III. DIABETES INSIPIDUS

A. Incidence

New-onset diabetes insipidus (DI) is rare in the elderly. Of 85 adult patients reported in the literature, only 3 were 60 years and older (114–121).

B. Etiology

DI is secondary to either a deficiency in ADH synthesis by the pituitary (neurogenic DI) or an inability of the cells of the renal collecting tubule to respond to circulating ADH (nephrogenic DI). The causes of these two varieties of DI are outlined in Table 6.

C. Clinical Manifestations

DI should be suspected in any elderly patient presenting with polyuria and hypotonic urine. The most important diagnosis to rule out is psychogenic polydypsia (compulsive water drinking), a condition more common in this age group than DI. Patients with psychogenic polydypsia are usually women who have a history of psychiatric disease (122). In some patients (mostly males), the syn-

Table 6 Causes of Diabetes Insipidus

Neurogenic diabetes insipidus
Hypophysectomy
Intracranial surgery
Head trauma
Intracranial tumors
Primary—suprasellar or intrasellar
Metastatic—breast or lung carcinoma; myeloproliferative disorders
Granulomatous disease
Tuberculosis
Sarcoidosis
Vascular abnormalities—aneurysms
Infections (viral)
"Empty sella" syndrome
Nephrogenic diabetes insipidus
Congenital
Chronic renal insufficiency
Electrolyte disorders
Hypokalemia
Hypercalcemia
Drugs
Lithium
Demeclocycline
Other?

drome develops on a background of chronic alcoholism, and in others chronic hiccups is the reason for excessive drinking (123). In contrast with DI patients, who are, in general, normo- or even hypernatremic, patients with compulsive water drinking are hyponatremic, at times severe and symptomatic. Laboratory evidence for rhabdomyolysis has been reported (123), the mechanism of which is not clear. The diagnosis of psychogenic polydypsia can be confirmed by water restriction, which leads to an increase in plasma ADH and urine osmolality (to greater than plasma osmolality) as free water clearance becomes negative. In some patients, ADH is released and urine osmolality increases while the plasma osmolality remains relatively low, suggestive of a resetting of the osmostat. Besides a defect in the excretion of ADH, patients with psychogenic polydypsia exhibit unexplained deficits in urinary dilution and osmoregulation of water intake (124).

In psychotic patients, increase in water intake tends to occur during exacerbations of the psychiatric problem and improves with therapeutic intervention. During water deprivation, patients with neurogenic DI will achieve a urinary osmolality above that of plasma after ADH administration. A dose of 5 IU of aqueous ADH is used subcutaneously. The plasma ADH concentration and osmolality after administration of hypertonic (5%) saline infused at a rate of 0.05–0.06 ml/kg body weight will also help differentiate neurogenic from nephrogenic DI (120), keeping in mind that in elderly subjects there may be no correlation between plasma ADH and osmolality because of the higher basal ADH levels, as noted earlier.

D. Treatment

The therapy of choice for neurogenic DI consists of intranasal administration of dDAVP. A starting dose of 2.5 mg once daily has been suggested, with gradual increases until polyuria is adequately controlled (119). Certain patients will require a divided dose. The drug is generally well tolerated, and only an occasional patient will develop resistance to its effect. In patients who cannot tolerate dDAVP and those with congenital nephrogenic DI or chronic renal insufficiency, the urine volume can be significantly decreased by the use of indomethacin, a thiazide diuretic, and salt restriction. Care must be taken to avoid excessive volume contraction with postural hypotension or a further decrease in kidney function. Since nephrogenic DI in the elderly is most likely secondary (Table 6), management is that of the underlying problem. Therapy of lithium-induced DI is discussed in Chapter 11.

E. Prognosis and Mortality

Both prognosis and mortality rate in patients with DI depend primarily on the underlying disease; however, in the elderly, who may not be able to replace water losses because of decreased mentation and the inability to comprehend or respond to thirst or the inability to take liquids because of infirmity and lack of attention, severe volume contraction and even shock may occur, leading to significant morbidity and even mortality.

REFERENCES

1. Robertson GL, et al. Development and clinical application of a new method for the radioimmunoassay of arginine vasopressin in human plasma. J Clin Invest 1973;52: 2340–2352.
2. Robertson GL. Osmotic and hemodynamic control of vasopressin. Functional and anatomical relationships. In: Takacs L, ed., Advances in Physiological Sciences. Vol II. Kidneys and Body Fluids. Budapest: Akademiai Kiado and Pergamon Press, 1981.
3. Sklar AH, Schrier RW. Central nervous system mediators of vasopressin release. Physiol Rev 1983;63:1243–1280.
4. Rowe JW, et al. Influence of the emetic reflex on vasopressin release in man. Kidney Int 1979;16:729–735.

5. Silver AJ, Morley JE. Role of the opioid in hypodipsia with aging. J Am Geriatr Soc 1992;40:556–560.
6. Phillips PA, et al. Reduced thirst after water deprivation in healthy elderly men. N Engl J Med 1984;311:753–759.
7. Duggan J, et al. The association of age with plasma arginine vasopressin and plasma osmolality. Age & Aging 1993;22:332–336.
8. Johnson AG, et al. Arginine vasopressin and osmolality in the elderly. J Am Geriatr Soc 1994;42:399–404.
9. Rowe JW, et al. Age related failure of volume-pressure mediated vasopressin release. J Clin Endocrinol Metab 1982;54:661–664.
10. Baran D, Hutchinson TA. The outcome of hyponatremia in a general hospital population. Clin Nephrol 1984;22:72–76.
11. Sunderam SG, Mankikar GD. Hyponatremia in the elderly. Age & Aging 1983; 12:77–80.
12. Kleinfeld M, Casimir M, Borra S. Hyponatremia as observed in a chronic disease facility. J Am Geriatr Soc 1979;27:156–161.
13. Miller M, Morley JE, Rubenstein LZ. Hyponatremia in a nursing home population. J Am Geriatr Soc 1995;43:1410–1413.
14. Anderson RJ, et al. Hyponatremia a prospective analysis of its epidemiology and the pathogenic role of vasopressin. Ann Intern Med 1985;02:164–168.
15. Cogan E, Abramow M. Transient hyperthyroxinemia in symptomatic hyponatremic patients. Arch Intern Med 1986;146:545–547.
16. Weisberg LS. Pseudohyponatremia: a reappraisal. Am J Med 1989;86:313–318.
17. Katz M. Hyperglycemia-induced hyponatremia. Calculation of expected serum sodium depression. N Engl J Med 1973;289:843–844.
18. Glasser L, et al. Serum osmolality and its applicability to drug overdose. Am J Clin Pathol 1973;60:695–699.
19. Chung, HM, et al. Clinical assessment of extracellular fluid volume in hyponatremia. Am J Med 1987;83:905–908.
20. Miller M, et al. Apparent idiopathic hyponatremia in an ambulatory geriatric population. J Am Geriatr Soc 1996;44:404–408.
20a. Hirshberg B, Ben-Yehuda A. The syndrome of inappropriate antidiuretic hormone secretion in the elderly. Am J Med 1997;103:270–273.
21. Goldstein CS, Braunstein S, Goldbfarb S. Idiopathic syndrome of inappropriate antidiuretic hormone secretion possibly related to advanced age. Ann Intern Med 1983;99:185–188.
22. Edward K, Barken F, Lovold JA. Age and inappropriate antidiuretic hormone secretion. Ann Intern Med 1984;100:766.
23. Booker JA. Severe symptomatic hyponatremia in elderly outpatients. The role of thiazide therapy and stress. J Am Geriatr Soc 1984;32:108–113.
24. Martinez-Maldonado M. Inappropriate antidiuretic hormone secretion of unknown origin. Kidney Int 1980;17:554–567.
25. Verbalis JG: Tumoral hyponatremia. Arch Intern Med 1986;146:1686–1687.
26. Weissman PN, Shenkman L, Gregerman RI. Chlorpropamide hyponatremia. N Engl J Med 1971;284:65–71.

26a. TenHolt WL, et al. Severe hyponatremia during therapy with fluoxetine. Arch Intern Med 1996;156:681–682.
27. Zerbe R, Stropes L, Robertson G. Vasopressin function in the syndrome of inappropriate antidiuresis. Ann Rev Med 1980;31:315–327.
28. Cooke RC, Turin MD, Walker GW. The syndrome of inappropriate antidiuretic hormone secretion (SIADH): pathophysiologic mechanisms in solute and volume regulation. Medicine 1979;58:240–251.
29. Cogan E, et al. Natriuresis and atrial natriuretic factor. Secretion during inappropriate anti-diuresis. Am J Med 1988;84:409–417.
30. Al-Mufti, Arieff Al. Hyponatremia due to central salt-wasting syndrome. Combined cerebral and distal tubular lesion. Am J Med 1984;77:740–746.
31. Ishikawa SE, et al. Hyponatremia responsive to fludrocortisone acetate in elderly patients after head injury. Ann Intern Med 1987;146:187–191.
32. Barter FC, Schwartz WB. The syndrome of inappropriate secretion of antidiuretic hormone. Am J Med 1967;42:790–806.
33. Decaux G, Genette F, Mockel J. Hypouremia in the syndrome of inappropriate secretion of antidiuretic hormone. Ann Intern Med 1980;93:716–717.
34. Beck LH. Hypouricemia in the syndrome of inappropriate secretion of antidiuretic hormone. N Engl J Med 1979;301:528–530.
35. Shichiri M, et al. Renal handling of urate in the syndrome of inappropriate secretion of antidiuretic hormone. Arch Intern Med 1985;145:2045–2047.
36. Decaux G, et al. Mechanisms of hypouricemia in the syndrome of inappropriate secretion of antidiuretic hormone. Nephron 1985;39:164–168.
37. Abramow M, Cogan E. Clinical aspects and pathophysiology of diuretic- induced hyponatremia. Adv Nephrol 1984;13:1–28.
38. Chan TY. Indapamide-induced severe hyponatremia and hypokalemia. Ann Pharmacother 1995;29:1124–1128.
39. Grenfell RF. Hyponatremia with the administration of diuretics. In: Puschett JB, Greenberg A, eds., Diuretics II. Chemistry Pharmacology, and Clinical Applications. New York: Elsevier, 1986.
40. Ashraf N, Locksley R, Arieff AI. Thiazide-induced hyponatremia associated with death or neurologic damage in outpatients. Am J Med 1981;70:1163–1168.
41. Fichman MP, et al. Diuretic-induced hyponatremia. Ann Intern Med 1971;75:853–863.
42. Friedman E, et al. Thiazide induced hyponatremia. Reproducibility by single dose rechallenge and an analysis of pathogenesis. Ann Intern Med 1989;110:24–30.
43. Hamburger S, et al. Thiazide-induced syndrome of inappropriate secretion of antidiuretic hormone. Time course of resolution. JAMA 1981;246:1235–1236.
44. Sonnenblick M, Algur N, Rosin A. Thiazide induced hyponatremia and vasopressin release. Ann Intern Med 1989;110:751.
45. Abramow M, Dratwa M. Interaction of vasopressin and diuretics in the isolated collecting tubule. Eur J Clin Invest 1974;4:353.
46. Clark BA, et al. Increased susceptibility to thiazide-induced hyponatremia in the elderly. J Am Soc Nephrol 1994;5:1106–1111.
47. Keischi A, et al. Effect of furosemide on urinary excretion of prostaglandin E in normal volunteers and patients with essential hypertension. Prostaglandins 1977; 14:513–521.

48. Deutsch S, Goldberg M, Dripps RD. Postoperative hyponatremia with the inappropriate release of antidiuretic hormone. Anesthesiology 1966;27:250–256.
49. Chung H-M, et al. Postoperative hyponatremia. A prospective study. Arch Intern Med 1986;146:333–336.
50. Rhymer JC, et al. Hyponatremia following transurethral resection of the prostate. Br J Urol 1985;57:450–452.
51. Griffin M. Toxic symptoms accompanied by hemolysis during transurethral prostatectomy. J Urol 1984;59:431–436.
52. Sunderrajan S, et al. Post-transurethral prostatic resection hyponatremic syndrome. Case report and review of the literature. Am J Kidney Dis 1984;4:80–84.
53. Weiss JM, Robertson GL. Water metabolism in endocrine disorders. Sem Nephrol 1984;4:303–315.
54. Cogan E, Abramow M. Transient hyperthyroxinemia in symptomatic hyponatremic patients. Arch Intern Med 1986;146:545–547.
55. Sawin CT, et al. The aging thyroid: increased prevalence of elevated serum thyrotropin levels in the elderly. JAMA 1979;242:247.
56. Szatalowitz VL, Goldberg JP, Anderson RJ. Plasma antidiuretic hormone in acute respiratory failure. Am J Med 1982;72:583–587.
57. Weston RE, et al. The pathogenesis and treatment of hyponatremia in congestive heart failure. Am J Med 1958;25:558–572.
58. Bell NH, Schedl HP, Bartter FC. An explanation for abnormal water retention and hypoosmolality in congestive heart failure. Am J Med 1964;36:351–360.
59. Dzau VJ, et al. Prostaglandins in severe congestive heart failure. Relation to activation of the renin-angiotensin system and hyponatremia. N Engl J Med 1984;310: 347–352.
60. Szatalowitz VL, et al. Radioimmunoassay of plasma arginine vasopressin in hyponatremic patients with congestive heart failure. N Engl J Med 1981;305:263–266.
61. Rondeau E, et al. High plasma antidiuretic hormone in patients with cardiac failure: influence of age. Min Electrol Metab 1982;8:267–274.
62. Korfas C, et al. Non-osmotic stimulation of vasopressin (ADH) is independent of the renin-angiotensin (RAS) in severe congestive heart failure (CHF) in man. Am Soc Nephrol 18th Ann Meeting 1985;44A.
63. Johnson AK, et al. Plasma angiotensin II concentration and experimentally induced thirst. Am J Physiol 1981;240:R229–R234.
64. Bichet DG, et al. Modulation of plasma and platelet vasopressin by cardiac function in patients with heart failure. Kidney Int 1986;29:1188–1196.
65. Dzau VJ, Hollenberg NK. Renal response to captopril in severe heart failure: role of furosemide in natriuresis and reversal of hyponatremia. Ann Intern Med 1984; 100:772–782.
66. Packer M, Medina N, Yushak M. Correction of dilutional hyponatremia in severe chronic heart failure by converting enzyme inhibition. Ann Intern Med 1984;100: 782–789.
67. Lancestremere RG, et al. Renal failure in Laennec's cirrhosis: III. Diuretic response to administered water. J Lab Clin Med 1962;60:967–975.
68. Bichet D, et al. Role of vasopressin in abnormal water excretion in cirrhotic humans. Ann Intern Med 1982;96:413–416.

69. Epstein M, et al. Relationship between plasma arginine vasopressin and renal water handling in decompensated cirrhosis. Min Electr Metab 1984;10:155–165.
70. Bichet DG, Groves BM, Schrier RW. Mechanisms of improvement of water and sodium excretion by immersion in decompensated cirrhotic patients. Kidney Int 1983;24:788–794.
71. Shapiro MD, et al. Interrelationship between cardiac output and vascular resistance as determinants of effective arterial blood volume in cirrhotic patients. Kidney Int 1985;26:206–211.
72. Bichet DG, Van Patten VJ, Schrier RW. Potential role of increased sympathetic activity in impaired sodium and water excretion in cirrhosis. N Engl J Med 1982;307:1552–1557.
73. Epstein M, Larios O, Johnson O. Effects of water immersion on plasma catecholamines in decompensated cirrhosis. Implications for deranged sodium and water homeostasis. Min Electr Metab 1985;11:25–34.
74. Perez-Ayuso RM, et al. Evidence that renal prostaglandins are involved in renal water metabolism in cirrhosis. Kidney Int 1984;26:72–80.
75. Usberti M, et al. Role of plasma vasopressin in the impairment of water excretion in nephrotic syndrome. Kidney Int 1984;25:522–429.
76. Bichet DG, Schrier RW. Water metabolism in edematous disorders. Sem Nephrol 1984;4:325–333.
77. Farber MO, et al. Abnormalities of sodium and water handling in chronic obstructive lung disease. Arch Intern Med 1982;142:1326–1330.
78. Musch W, et al. Combined fractional excretion of sodium and urea better predicts response to saline in hyponatremia than do usual biochemical parameters. Am J Med 1995;99:348–354.
79. Dandona P, Fanseca V Baron DN. Hypoalbuminemic hyponatremia: a new syndrome? Br Med J 1985;291:1253–1255.
80. Arieff A, Llack F, Massry S. Neurologic manifestations and morbidity of hyponatremia: correlation with brain water and electrolytes. Medicine 1976;55:121–129.
81. Marples D, et al. Lithium-induced downregulation of aquaporin—2: water channel expression in rat kidney medulla. J Clin Invest 1995;95:1838–1845.
81a. Forrest JN, et al. Superiority of demeclocycline over lithium in the treatment of chronic syndrome of inappropriate antidiuretic hormone. N Engl J Med 1978;298:173–177.
82. Chapron DJ, Cameron IR, White LD. Observations on lithium disposition in the elderly. J Am Geriatr Soc 1982;30:651–655.
83. DeTroyer A. Demeclocycline treatment for the syndrome of inappropriate antidiuretic hormone secretion. JAMA 1977;237:2723–2726.
84. Miller PD, Linas SL, Schrier RW. Plasma demeclocycline levels and nephrotoxicity. Correlation in hyponatremic cirrhotic patients. JAMA 1980;243:2513–2515.
85. Geheb M, Cox M. Renal effects of demeclocycline. JAMA 1980;243:2519–2520.
86. Danovitch G, LeRoith D, Glick S. Renal function during treatment of inappropriate secretion of antidiuretic hormone with demeclocycline. Isr J Med Sci 1978;14: 852–857.
87. Decaux G, Unger J, Mockel J. Urea therapy for inappropriate antidiuretic hormone secretion from tuberculous meningitis. JAMA 1980;244:589–590.

88. Decaux G, et al. Treatment of the syndrome of inappropriate secretion of antidiuretic hormone by urea. Am J Med 1980;69:99–106.
89. Decaux G, et al. Five-year treatment of the chronic syndrome of inappropriate secretion of ADH with oral urea. Nephron 1993;63:468–470.
90. Soupart A, Decaux G. Therapeutic recommendations for management of severe hypnonatremia; current concepts on pathogenesis and prevention of neurologic complications. Clin Nephrol 1996;46:149–169.
91. Taney A, et al. Long-term treatment of the syndrome of inappropriate antidiuretic hormone secretion with phenytoin. Ann Intern Med 1979;90:50–52.
92. Fichman MP, Bethune JE, Kleeman CR. Inhibition of antidiuretic hormone by diphenylhydantoin (abstr). Clin Res 1967;15:141.
93. Decaux G, et al. Treatment of the syndrome of inappropriate secretion of antidiuretic hormone with furosemide. N Engl J Med 1981;304:329–330.
94. Shimizu K. Aquaretic effects of the non-peptide V_2 antagonist OPC-31260 in hydropenic patients. Kidney Int 1995;48:220–226.
95. Shankel SW. A new formula for correction of hyponatremia. Am Soc Nephrol 19th Ann Meeting 1986;59A.
96. Sterns RH, Riggs JE, Schochet SS Jr. Osmotic demyelination syndrome following correction of hyponatremia. N Engl J Med 1986;314:1535–1542.
97. Ayus JC. Diuretic-induced hyponatremia. Arch Intern Med 1986;146:1295–1296.
98. Norenberg MD. Treatment of hyponatremia: the case for a more conservative approach. Dubois GD, Arieff AI. Treatment of hyponatremia: The case for rapid correction. In: Narins RG, ed. Controversies in Nephrology and Hypertension. New York: Churchill Livingstone, 1984.
99. Ayus JC, Olivero JJ, Frommer JP. Rapid correction of severe hyponatremia with intravenous hypertonic saline solution. Am J Med 1982;72:43–48.
100. Ayus JC, Krothapalli RK, Arieff AI. Changing concepts in treatment of severe symptomatic hyponatremia: rapid correction and possible relation to central pontine myelinolysis. Am J Med 1985;78:897–902.
101. Stern RH. Severe symptomatic hyponatremia: Treatment and outcome. A study of 64 cases. Ann Intern Med 1987;107:656–664.
102. Ashouri OS. Severe diuretic-induced hyponatremia in the elderly. A series of eight patients. Arch Intern Med 1986;146:1355–1357.
103. Ayus JC, Krothapolli RK, Arieff AI. Treatment of symptomatic hyponatremia and its relation to brain damage: a prospective study. N Engl J Med 1987;317:1190–1195.
104. Hantman D, et al. Rapid correction of hyponatremia in the syndrome of inappropriate secretion of antidiuretic hormone. An alternative treatment to hypertonic saline. Ann Intern Med 1973;78:870–875.
105. Snyder NA, Feigal DW, Arieff AI. Hypernatremia in elderly patients. A heterogenous, morbid and iatrogenic entity. Ann Intern Med 1987;107:309–319.
106. Palevsky PM, Bhagrath RV, Greenberg A. Hypernatremia in hospitalized patients. Ann Intern Med 1996;124:197–208.
107. Mack GW, et al. Body fluid balance in dehydrated healthy older men: thirst and renal osmoregulation. J Appl Physiol 1994;76:1615–1623.
108. Nelson DC, McGrew WRG Jr, Hoyumpa AM Jr. Hypernatremia and lactulose therapy. JAMA 1983;249:1295–1298.

109. Warren SE, Mitas JA II, Swerdlin AHR. Hypernatremia in hepatic failure. JAMA 1980;243:1257–1261.
110. Gault MH, et al. Hypernatremia, azotemia and dehydration due to high-protein tube feeding. Ann Intern Med 1968;68:778–791.
111. Jana DK, Romano-Jana L. Hypernatremic psychosis in the elderly. Case reports. J Am Geriatr Soc 1973;21:473–477.
112. Ross EJ, Christie SBM. Hypernatremia. Medicine 1969;48:441–467.
113. Himmelstein DV, Jones AA, Woolhandler S. Hypernatremic dehydration in nursing home patients: an indicator of neglect. J Am Geriatr Soc 1983;31:466–471.
114. Vavra I, et al. Effect of a synthetic analogue of vasopressin in animal and in patients with diabetes insipidus. Lancet 1968;1:948–952.
115. Andersson KE, Arner B. Effects of DDAVP, a synthetic analogue of vasopressin in patients with cranial diabetes insipidus. Acta Med Scand 1972;192:21–27.
116. Edwards CRW, et al. Vasopressin analogue DDAVP in diabetes insipidus: clinical and laboratory studies. Br Med J 1973;375–378.
117. Ward MK, Fraser TR. DDAVP in treatment of vasopressin-sensitive diabetes insipidus. Br Med J 1974;3:86–89.
118. Robinson AG. DDAVP in the treatment of central diabetes insipidus. N Engl J Med 1976;294:507–511.
119. Cobb WE, Spare S, Reichlin S. Neurogenic diabetes insipidus: management with dDavp (1-desamino-8-D-Arginine vasopressin). Ann Intern Med 1978;88: 131–188.
120. Zerbe RL, Robertson GL. A comparison of plasma vasopressin measurements with a standard indirect test in the differential diagnosis of polyuria. N Engl J Med 1981;305:1539–1546.
121. Milles JL, Spruce B, Baylis PH. A comparison of diagnostic methods to differentiate diabetes insipidus from primary polydypsia, a review of 21 patients. Acta Endocrinol 1983;104:410–416.
122. Hariprasad MK, Eisinger RP, Nadler IM. Hyponatremia in psychogenic polydypsia. Arch Intern Med 1980;140:1639–1642.
123. Cronin RE. Psychogenic polydypsia with hyponatremia: report of eleven cases. Am J Kidney Dis 1987;9:410–416.
124. Goldman MB, Luchins DJ, Robertson GL. Mechanisms of altered water metabolism in psychotic patients with polydipsia and hyponatremia. N Engl J Med 1988;318:397–403.

3

Disorders of Potassium Metabolism

I. NORMAL PHYSIOLOGY

Serum potassium (K) in the normal individual is maintained within the narrow range of 3.5–5.5 mEq/L, despite wide fluctuation in intake. Both extrarenal and renal mechanisms are involved in K homeostasis. During the first few hours after a K load, it is estimated that 50% will be disposed of by extrarenal mechanisms and the remainder by the kidney.

II. EXTRARENAL MECHANISMS OF POTASSIUM HOMEOSTASIS

A. Gastrointestinal Tract

In response to K loading, the colonic surface mucosal cells undergo structural changes leading to increased excretion. The basolateral membrane Na/K-ATPase may increase as much as 40%, with the serum aldosterone and plasma K concentration the two main regulators (1,2).

B. Insulin

Insulin exerts its effect by shifting K from the extra- to the intracellular space, mainly in hepatocytes (accounting for 70% of the insulin effect), with other peripheral tissues such as muscle and fat accounting for the remainder. Insulin acts directly on plasma membranes, resulting in an increase in Na/K-ATPase-dependent pumps (3).

C. Adrenergic Nervous System

The effector organ appears to be muscle cells, with the membrane beta-2-adrenergic receptor primarily involved (4). The entry of K into these cells requires activation of membrane-bound adenylate cyclase and stimulation of Na/K-ATPase-dependent pumps, leading to K entry into the cell. The alpha-adrenergic system has been found to have the opposite effect (5). The decline in beta-adrenergic response seen with aging might explain, in part, a higher plasma K seen in the elderly athletic subject following exercise (6).

D. Mineralocorticoids

In addition to its effect on the colon, aldosterone participates in extrarenal K homeostasis (7) through mechanisms yet to be completely elucidated (8).

E. Glucagon

Glucagon has been found to induce a transient mobilization of K from the splanchnic region (9). The contribution of glucagon and glucocorticoids to the day-to-day maintenance of extrarenal K homeostasis is not entirely clear, however.

III. RENAL MECHANISM OF POTASSIUM HOMEOSTASIS

Since virtually all of the filtered K is reabsorbed in the proximal portion of the nephron, the urinary K excretion reflects the secretion of K in the distal nephron. In experimental animals the principal cells of the cortical collecting tubules have been shown to undergo surface density changes in the basolateral membrane under varying K loads (10). Potassium present in the surrounding plasma and interstitial fluid is actively transported by these cells via an ATP-driven Na–K exchange pump across the basolateral membrane, while K diffuses passively across the luminal membrane. Also, during adaption to K loading, the cells of the papillary collecting duct undergo an increase in luminal membrane surface area with no change in the basolateral surface (11). Several factors are involved in the regulation of K secretion by the distal nephron.

A. Plasma Factors

1. Serum Potassium

The higher the plasma K level, the greater is the K secretion.

2. *Aldosterone*

By increasing sodium reabsorption in the cortical collecting tubule, aldosterone induces a depolarization of the luminal membrane, thereby amplifying the electrochemical driving force for K movement from cell to lumen.

3. *Acid–Base Status*

Changes in blood pH influence changes in plasma K which vary among the cardinal acid–base disorders. The intra- to extracellular shift of K is maximal during metabolic acidosis and minimal during respiratory acidosis. Acute organic acid acidosis is not associated with any measurable changes in plasma K concentration. During metabolic and respiratory alkalosis, K moves intracellularly (12,12a).

4. *Antidiuretic Hormone*

Antidiuretic hormone has been found to increase K secretion by the distal nephron in the rat (13).

B. Luminal Factors

1. *Flow Rate*

Increasing tubular flow rate has been shown to stimulate K secretion in the rat (14).

2. *Changes in Transepithelial Voltage*

The presence of a large concentration of either endogenous (bicarbonate) or exogenous nonreabsorbable anions (e.g., carbenicillin) will increase K secretion by making the luminal fluid more negative (15).

3. *Luminal Chloride Concentration*

Potassium secretion is stimulated in the presence of a low luminal chloride concentration (16).

4. *Potassium Recycling*

It has been shown in the rat that the pars recta and/or the descending limb of Henle can secrete K (17). The magnitude of K secreted varies with the K status of the animal (18,19), and results from the coordinated activity of both apical Na channels and the apical and basolateral K channels (20).

IV. CHANGES IN POTASSIUM METABOLISM WITH AGE

Total body potassium decreases as muscle mass decreases with age. Table 1 summarizes the average total body K according to age, as described by Novak (21). Serum K in the healthy elderly is maintained within the same narrow range of 3.5–5.5 mEq/L found in younger individuals, despite the progressive decrease in glomerular filtration rate seen with advancing age. Therefore, both extrarenal and

Table 1 Average Total Body Potassium in Different Age Groups

	Body potassium (mEq)	
Age	Male (± SD)	Female (± SD)
45–55	3775 (425)	2575 (291)
55–65	3607 (433)	2403 (287)
65–85	3168 (234)	2351 (200)

Source: Novak LP. Aging, total body potassium fat-free mass and cell mass in males and females between ages 18 and 85 years. J Gerontol 1972; 27:438–443.

renal mechanisms involved in the K homeostasis must remain intact to adapt to the progressive nephron loss.

V. HYPOKALEMIA

A. Incidence and Prevalence

In a survey of 3684 hospitalized patients, Morgan et al. (22) found 70 (1.9%) with hypokalemia. The incidence was 1.4% among newly admitted cases. The mean age was 61 years, with 57% over the age of 65 at a time when 41% of the inpatient population was over 65 years. Between 1.1% and 16% of reported acutely hospitalized geriatric patients are hypokalemic (23–25). The incidence of hypokalemia in the outpatient elderly is not known; however, given the frequency of hypertension, heart failure, and the use of diuretics in this age group, it must be relatively common. Twenty-two percent of the hypokalemia patients reported by Nasar and Lyle (25) were on diuretics.

B. Etiology

There is very little specific information available on the distribution of etiological factors causing hypokalemia in elderly inpatients. In 100 elderly patients seen at our hospital, the etiology of hypokalemia (serum K < 3.0 mEq/L) was renal losses in 53%, gastrointestinal tract losses in 15%, mixed in 13%—more common in patients with severe hypokalemia (serum K < 1.5 mEq/L). Ten percent had K redistribution from the extracellular to the intracellular fluid; others (9%) included injury, acute transient hypokalemia, and hypokalemia with no obvious cause (Table 2).

Table 2 Etiology of Hypokalemia in 100 Consecutive Elderly Seen at The Brookdale University Hospital and Medical Center

1. Potassium losses through the kidneys
   a. Diuretics: thiazides, furosemide, diamox
   b. Other drugs: carbenicillin, bicarbonate, aminoglycosides, amphotericin B, cisplatin
   c. Magnesium deficiency: diarrhea, aminoglycosides
   d. Mineralcorticoid excess
2. Potassium losses through the gastrointestinal tract
   a. Diarrhea
3. Potassium losses through both kidneys and gastrointestinal tract
4. Potassium redistribution from the extracellular to the intracellular fluid
   a. Respiratory alkalosis
   b. Hyperalimentation

C. Pathogenesis

Diuretics (thiazides and loop diuretics) induce hypokalemia by increasing tubular flow and sodium delivery to the distal convoluted tubule and also by producing chloride depletion. There is also some experimental evidence suggesting that furosemide might stimulate renal tubular K secretion directly (26). Acetazolamide increases K losses by its effect on proximal tubular bicarbonate and the increased delivery of this relatively nonresorbable anion to the distal tubule. Some of our patients were receiving acetozolamide and large doses of intravenous bicarbonate to alkalinize the urine for uric acid stones. In these patients, the presence of bicarbonate in the distal nephron as well as an increase in urinary volume serve as stimuli for increased K secretion. In diuretic-induced hypokalemia the urinary K is usually greater than 30–40 mEq/L while the patient is still on the drug. If the history of diuretic use is not elicited, the clinical picture might suggest Bartter's syndrome. This entity, however, is initially diagnosed earlier in life (27,28). In cases where the diuretic has been recently discontinued, urinary K may be low (< 10 mEq/L).

The hypokalemia associated with sodium carbenicillin is due to the carbenicillin, which is a nonreabsorbable anion inducing a favorable electrical gradient for K secretion in the distal nephron. Hypokalemia associated with aminoglycosides and cisplatin is discussed in Chapter 5. The causes of hypokalemia associated with hypomagnesemia are not entirely clear, but probably include both proximal and distal (aldosterone) tubular mechanisms (see Chapter 5). The presence of hypokalemic metabolic alkalosis with a high urinary chloride and K in a normotensive elderly should lead to the suspicion of mineralocorticoid excess, frequently due to licorice ingestion (29). Our patients were usually females who generally did not volunteer that they ate large amounts of licorice unless specifically asked. Severe diarrhea is the most common cause of gastrointestinal K losses. Significant hyperchloremic metabolic acidosis with evidence of volume contraction are generally present. The urinary K in those patients tends to be low, less than 20 mEq/L. Patients with intestinal obstruction requiring prolonged nasogastric suction develop hypokalemia associated with both gastrointestinal and urinary K losses. These patients have a metabolic alkalosis and low urinary chloride (< 10 mEq/L), with most of the K lost in the urine during the initiation phase of the alkalosis, when there is significant bicarbonaturia.

The hypokalemia related to transcellular shifts occurred in patients with respiratory alkalosis or those receiving hypertonic glucose and insulin during hyperalimentation.

The postulated mechanism for the so-called acute transient hypokalemia is an intracellular shift of K, most likely secondary to an increase in catecholamine secretion which might be expected in acutely ill patients (4,22). In some, however, prior thiazide therapy may have been playing a role, since it has been shown that this diuretic can increase catecholamine-induced hypokalemia (30). Indeed, a similar mechanism could also be invoked in the hypokalemia which develops in patients with acute myocardial infarction (31–33).

D. Clinical Manifestations

Moderate to severe K deficiency may have important effects on cardiac, skeletal, and smooth muscle, intermediary metabolism (carbohydrate and protein), and the kidney's ability to maximally concentrate the urine (34,35). Severe manifestations of hypokalemia are, fortunately, uncommon in the elderly in our experience. Furthermore, most of our patients were acutely ill, so the overwhelming clinical manifestations were mainly those of the underlying disease. The elderly ambulatory patient with hypokalemia is usually asymptomatic, although a small minority have ill-defined complaints of musculoskeletal origin, reversible upon K replacement.

E. Therapy and Prognosis

Since most of the total body K is stored in muscle, direct muscle K measurement represents the most accurate way of assessing deficits. This is, however, impractical in clinical practice. Sterns et al. (36), by analyzing pure K depletion in humans, concluded that a decrease in plasma K of 0.3 mEq/L is, in general, associated with an average total body deficit of 100 mEq. This data is compatible with studies where muscle K was measured in patients on diuretic therapy (37–39).

Patients with acute transient hypokalemia can be watched for several days if there are no specific symptoms, as most will become normokalemic within a week. In the absence of spontaneous correction, oral or parenteral supplementation may be required.

Those patients with acute myocardial infarction and hypokalemia present a more difficult problem, since the incidence of ventricular fibrillation in this group appears to be significantly higher than in those with normal serum K (31,33,40,41). It is not clear whether the hypokalemia serves as a marker or is etiologically responsible for the ventricular arrhythmia, since the latter is not necessarily prevented by K supplementation. Intravenous administration of a nonselective beta-blocker has been recommended and used with some success in these patients (42).

Parenteral administration of KCl is frequently necessary in hospitalized patients with increased losses through the kidneys and/or the gastrointestinal tract. In those patients with associated renal insufficiency (acute or chronic), careful monitoring of the serum K is mandatory to avoid hyperkalemia. In most patients, normokalemia, once corrected, is maintained except for those with associated hypomagnesemia, in whom long-term oral therapy may be required. In elderly ambulatory patients on diuretics the hypokalemia is usually well tolerated, although controversy exists as to whether the incidence of ventricular arrhythmia is increased (43,44). Some authors recommend supplementation for every patient on a diuretic, in view of the fact that the cellular concentration of K may be significantly decreased even with a normal serum K (45). Furthermore, it has been shown in a short-term study that the addition of KCl to the diuretic regimen of an hypertensive patient may induce a significant fall in blood pressure (46). Based these data, we recommend treating or preventing hypokalemia only in those elderly patients taking a diuretic who have heart disease, a history of previous arrhythmias, or taking digitalis. Hypokalemia can be prevented or treated in these patients with either the use of one of the several KCL preparations available or with K-sparing agents such as aldactone, triamterene, or amiloride. When these agents are used, the K level should be monitored, particularly if a drug known to interfere with K metabolism, such as converting enzyme inhibitors, beta-blockers, or nonsteroidal antiinflammatory drugs (NSAID) are used concurrently or if the patient has diabetes mellitus or renal insufficiency.

The amount of KCl required to achieve normokalemia in diuretic-treated patients is quite variable. In one study of a small group of patients, 60 mEq/day of KCl effectively corrected hypokalemia in 80% of the patients (47). In another study, a dose as high as 96 mEq/day was required (48). Our practice is to start with 20 mEq twice a day and gradually increase the dose until normokalemia is achieved. Gastrointestinal upset has been the most common side effect encountered. A slow-release tablet containing 8 mEq of KCl is available for use, which has the advantage of a lower incidence of ulcerative lesions of the gastrointestinal tract. The price and the large number of tablets required to correct the hypokalemia with this preparation is a major drawback for the elderly, however.

Spironolactone acts by binding competitively to the aldosterone receptor site and thereby preventing its action. The most common side effect associated with its use is hyperkalemia, which occurs in 10% of patients (49). At greatest risk for this complication are patients with renal insufficiency and/or those concurrently taking either KCL supplements or other drugs known to produce an increase in serum K. The required dose is 25–150 mg/day. Therapy should be initiated with the smallest dose, since a significant elevation of the plasma K may be seen even with the daily ingestion of 25 mg. The drug is relatively expensive (50).

Triamterene and amiloride both act by blocking the entry of Na into the renal tubular cell by reversibly inhibiting amiloride-sensitive Na channels. This leads to a decrease in the amount of Na extruded across the basolateral cell membrane, with a concomitant decrease in K uptake by the cell (51). In addition, both drugs decrease the electrochemical driving force for cell to lumen efflux of K by making the cell interior more electrically negative (52). The recommended dose for triamterene is 100–300 mg/day in divided doses. Elevation of serum creatinine, acute renal failure (when combined with indomethacin), and nephrolithiasis are reported side effects (53,54). The amiloride dose is 5–20 mg/day, as a single dose. Hyperkalemia is the most common side effect, particularly in diabetic patients. Either drug will add a substantial burden to the already limited budget of many elderly patients. It is estimated that the elderly patient fills an average of 12 prescriptions per year (55), so one alternative to treating diuretic-induced hypokalemia is the use of one of the available K-sparing agents combined with the diuretic. Spironolactone-hydrochlorothiazide and triamterene-hydrochlorothiazide have been tried in the elderly and found to be relatively well tolerated (56). An amiloride-hydrochlorothiazide combination is also available and might be preferable in patients for whom maintenance of glomerular filtration rate is prostaglandin dependent (heart failure, liver cirrhosis, etc.). Urinary PGE_2 excretion was found to increase in patients receiving amiloride-hydrochlorothiazide, whereas in the group receiving triamterene-hydrochlorothiazide, urinary PGE_2 may decrease (57). The required dose should be established by individual titration of each component before switching to the combination. Again, it cannot be emphasized enough that KCl supplementation should not be used together with a K-sparing agent in the elderly because of the possibility of fatal hyperkalemia. In patients where there is difficulty correcting the hypokalemia, primarily hospitalized patients on diuretics or with diarrhea, the serum magnesium should be measured, since normokalemia can be achieved only after hypomagnesemia (if present) is corrected (58).

VI. HYPERKALEMIA

A. Incidence and Prevalence

The true incidence of hyperkalemia in the geriatric population is not known; however, the frequency of this complication does increase with age. Significant hyperkalemia was found in 406 (1.4%) of 29,063 hospitalized patients in a Scottish hospital (59). The average age of these patients was 58 ± 1.6 years, significantly older than 1218 randomly selected controls. Of 4921 patients receiving potassium chloride, hyperkalemia developed in 179 (3.6%). The age distribution of these hyperkalemic patients is summarized in Table 3 and shows a disproportionate number 60 years or older. Similarly, the patients with hyperkalemia reported by Shemer et al. (60) were also significantly older than the control group (66.8 ± 13.7 vessus 56.0 ± 19.1 years). The reason the elderly patient is more prone to hyperkalemia is not clear, but probably is related to the existence in a given subject of several risk factors such as renal insufficiency, multiple drug interactions, and a blunted aldosterone response to K-loading (60,61).

B. Etiology and Pathogenesis

The etiology of hyperkalemia in the elderly is similar to that in younger patients. Pseudohyperkalemia related to hemolysis, leukocytosis, or thrombocytosis should be ruled out first in every patient with an elevated serum K. The etiology of hyperkalemia in 100 consecutive elderly patients seen by us is summarized in Table 4.

1. Drug-Induced Hyperkalemia

Drug-induced hyperkalemia was the most common cause of hyperkalemia in our series, with KCl replacement the cause in 40%. Normal subjects can handle diets containing as much as 300 mEq of K per day without the development of hyperkalemia (62). A shift in sodium reabsorption from a proximal to a distal nephron site as well as an elevated aldosterone level are key factors in the adaptation to the high-K diet (62). In the elderly, however, decreased aldosterone levels and associated blunted aldosterone response to various stimuli most likely contribute to making them more prone to KCl-induced hyperkalemia. In addition, the BUN tends to be higher in the elderly on KCl replacement with hyperkalemia than in those who are normokalemic, suggesting that renal insufficiency may also play a role (59).

Table 3 Frequency of Hyperkalemia According to Age

Age (years)	Hyperkalemia (%)
< 50	0.8
50–59	4.2
60–69	4.3
70–79	4.6
80+	6.0

Source: Lawson DH. Adverse reactions to potassium chloride. Quart J Med 1974; 171:433–440.

Table 4 Etiology of Hyperkalemia in 100 Consecutive Elderly Seen at The Brookdale University Hospital and Medical Center

Drug-induced
KCl replacement
K-sparing diuretic
Nonsteroidal antiinflammatory agents
Converting enzyme inhibitors
Trimethoprim-sulfamethoxazole
Beta-blockers
Heparin
Renal tubular hyperkalemia
Renal failure
Acute
Chronic
Disturbed intra-extracellular gradient
Hyperglycemia
Acid–base disturbance

Potassium-sparing diuretics produce hyperkalemia by interfering with K secretion in the distal part of the nephron, as discussed earlier.

Since NSAIDs are commonly used in the elderly, hyperkalemia related to these agents is relatively common. For some reason this complication is seen mainly with the use of indomethacin, although occasionally piroxicam and ibuprofen have been implicated (63–66). The exact frequency of this problem is not known; however, in one reported prospective study of 50 patients on indomethacin, the serum K concentration exceeded 5.0 mEq/L in 23 patients (46%) (67). Older age and mild preexisting renal insufficiency were significant risk factors for the development of hyperkalemia. Of 22 patients reported in the literature, 15 (68%) were over the age of 60, further suggesting a higher prevalence of this complication in the elderly (63–75). Mild elevation in BUN and serum creatinine were present in the majority of the patients prior to starting NSAIDs. Hyperkalemia may develop any time after starting the drug (average 3–4 days), and dose did not appear to play a role. In addition to hyperkalemia, worsening in kidney function with oliguric renal failure and hyperchloremic metabolic acidosis are also quite common following NSAIDs (63,66,71,73,74). The fact that the hyperkalemia and renal failure are easily reversible upon discontinuing the offending agent favors a functional mechanism rather than a structural alteration. Indeed, it has been shown that indomethacin, by decreasing renal PGE_2 production, induces a hyporenin-hypoaldosterone state which may explain the hyperkalemia (69,70). McCarthy et al. (75) have suggested a possible direct role of these agents in inhibiting the excretion as well as cellular uptake of K. The inhibition of renal prostaglandin synthesis could also explain the renal failure, since under conditions of circulatory stress prostaglandins appear to play a major role in the maintenance of glomerular filtration rate. Thus, it appears to be a good practice to monitor serum K and kidney function in any elderly patient on NSAIDs. If one of these agents is necessary, it appears that sulindac is the safest (76). It should be noted, however, that the risk of acute renal failure, particularly in patients with concomitant cardiovascular and renal problems, is increased with this drug (77).

Hyperkalemia associated with the use of converting enzyme inhibitors is becoming the most common cause of drug-induced hyperkalemia, given their widespread use in the therapy for congestive heart failure and diabetic nephropathy. Preexisting impairment in kidney function is a major risk factor (78). Therefore, care should be taken in using these drugs in the elderly with renal insufficiency. Concomitant use of a beta-blocker will substantially increase the likelihood of hyperkalemia in the presence of renal impairment.

Standard doses of sulfamethoxazole, an antibiotic commonly used for the treatment of urinary tract infection in the elderly, has been associated with hyperkalemia in 21% of patients, particularly if there is concurrent renal insufficiency (79). This antibiotic acts by blocking apical membrane amiloride-sensitive sodium channels in the distal nephron (80,80a). As a result, the transepithelial voltage is reduced and K secretion inhibited. The hyperkalemia usually corrects following discontinuation of the drug. Patients should be kept well hydrated during the course of therapy (80a).

Isolated beta-blocker-induced hyperkalemia is rare. We have seen it in only one elderly patient with severe renal insufficiency (creatinine 4.2 mg/dl). Normokalemia followed withdrawal of the drug, and hyperkalemia reappeared after the drug was inadvertently reinstituted. A similar problem was reported by Swenson (81) in an elderly man treated for glaucoma with timolol maleate. In general, elderly patients with severe renal insufficiency are at risk for developing hyperkalemia secondary to beta-blockers (82). The rise in serum K is most likely due to the inhibition of its translocation from the extracellular to the intracellular fluid compartment.

Parenteral or subcutaneous administration of heparin causes hypoaldosteronism by inhibiting the conversion of cortisone to 18-hydroxycorticosterone (83,84). The development of hyperkalemia, however, is rather rare with this agent. Patients with chronic renal insufficiency or uncontrolled diabetes mellitus are particularly at risk and deserve to have their serum K monitored regularly while receiving heparin (85,86). Hyperkalemia can be noted as early as 5 days and up to months after initiation of therapy. Hyperchloremic metabolic acidosis is a frequent associated abnormality, probably a consequence of the elevated K (see below).

2. *Renal Tubular Hyperkalemia*

A defect in the tubular secretion of K (87) is the second most common cause of hyperkalemia in the elderly (Table 4). Seventy-four percent of patients reported in the literature were over age 60 (88–96). Patients are usually asymptomatic with mild to moderate hyperkalemia (5.6–6.0 mEq/L). Renal insufficiency (creatinine 2.0–5.0 mg/dl) is universally present. Diabetic nephropathy or tubulo-interstitial nephropathy of various etiologies is usually responsible for the renal insufficiency. Obstructive uropathy should be ruled out in these patients, particularly if the etiology of the renal failure is obscure (97). Hyperchloremic metabolic acidosis is found in 50% of the patients. The acidosis is explained, in part, by a decrease in ammonia production and delivery to the loop of Henle, with subsequent lowering of the concentration gradient between the loop and the inner medullary collecting duct (98,99). The rate of H^+ secretion in the medullary collecting duct is also decreased due to a decrease in distal sodium delivery, as well as a decrease in pump activity, a direct effect of aldosterone deficiency (98,100). The underlying defect responsible for the syndrome may be an abnormality in the production of renin, aldosterone, or both. Some patients, however, will have a normal renin-angiotensin-aldosterone axis, with an isolated defect in tubular K secretion. In others, both these factors might be at play, as summarized in Table 5.

This syndrome may be due to a variety of structural or physiological problems, including: (a) sclerosis of the juxtaglomerular apparatus due to the underlying kidney disease (101); (b) defective conversion of inactive renin to active renin (102,103); (c) abnormality in the synthesis of prostaglandin E_2 and kallikrein (104); (d) deficiency in prostacyclin (105); (e) suppression of renin production (and aldosterone) by volume expansion, resulting from the renal insufficiency

Table 5 PRA, PA, and Urinary pH in the Three Forms of Renal Tubular Hyperkalemia[a]

	PRA (ng/ml/hr)			PA (ng/dl)			
Defect	Baseline	Standing	Post-Furosemide	Baseline	Post-ACTH	Post-AII	Urine pH
Renin production	Low	—	—	Low/normal	↑	↑	Can reach 5.5 or less
Aldosterone synthesis	Low/normal	↑	↑	Low	—	—	As above
Tubular K secretion	Normal	↑	↑	Normal	↑	↑	> 6.0

[a]PRA = plasma renin activity; PA = plasma aldosterone; ACTH = adrenocorticotropic hormone; AII = angiotensin II; — = unchanged; ↑ = increase.

found in practically all these patients, and associated with an increase in atrial natriuretic peptide (106); and (f) the "chloride shunt" (107). In the latter form of renal tubular hyperkalemia, the distal tubule has a higher than usual Cl reabsorption. As a consequence, volume expansion ensues, with subsequent suppression of the renin-aldosterone axis. In fact, following furosemide administration, plasma renin increases out of the range found in normals. In this group, the glomerular filtration rate is normal and hypertension is frequently present (70%). This problem must be rather rare in the elderly, as none of the 28 patients reported in the literature and reviewed by Gordon (108) was over 60 years and only 3 were in their fifth decade of life.

A tubular defect in K secretion occurs less commonly than hyporenin-hypoaldosteronism (109). In patients with a tubular defect, urinary pH remains above 6.0 in the presence of acidosis, compared with patients with hyporenin-hypoaldosteronism in whom the urine pH may be 5.5 or less (110). Whereas patients with hyporenin-hypoaldosteronism will increase their fractional excretion of K after administration of a mineralocorticoid or sodium sulfate, those with a defect in tubular secretion will be unresponsive. Because of the similarity to the effect of amiloride, this form of hyperkalemic acidosis has been labeled a voltage-dependent type of renal tubular acidosis (111).

None of our patients had Addison's disease; however, this problem should be kept in mind when evaluating a hyperkalemic patient, particularly if marked volume contraction exists.

3. Renal Failure

Hyperkalemia may be seen in acute oliguric renal failure of diverse etiology. In some of these patients, hemolysis and increased tissue breakdown (rhabdomyolysis) are probably contributing factors by increasing the K load. Some patients have advanced chronic insufficiency (creatinine > 5.0 mg/dl), which, together with the ingestion of a salt substitute (the K content of these substitutes varies between 10 and 13 mEq/g), causes hyperkalemia.

4. Disturbed Intra–Extracellular Gradient

a. Hyperglycemia. If a 50-g dose of glucose is given to an insulin-dependent diabetic, plasma K increases by an average of 1.3 mEq/L, peaking at 30–60 min following the load (112,113). If the patient also has superimposed hypoaldosteronism and/or renal insufficiency, one might expect the serum K to rise even more. Plasma aldosterone concentration has been found to be decreased in these patients. The hyperkalemia might be quite severe at times, so care should be exercised in administering glucose to a comatose diabetic patient (114–117).

b. Acid–Base Disturbances. Hyperkalemia can complicate acute metabolic acidosis in the elderly. When H^+ is added to the extracellular fluid, it undergoes buffering by intracellular proteins, leaving K free to be redistributed from the intra- to the extracellular fluid. The extent of K movement depends on the quantity of acid buffered rather than the arterial pH. In general, the rise in serum K associated with acidosis due to an increase in organic acids (such as lactate) tends to be less than with acidosis related to mineral acids (such as chloride) (118). Since organic anions tend to accumulate in the cell with subsequent cell swelling, some K will remain intracellular (119). Hyperkalemia can also occur with respiratory acidosis.

C. Clinical Manifestations

The clinical manifestations of hyperkalemia relate primarily to interference with the electrophysiological events underlying muscle contraction. Even though all muscle groups may be involved, cardiac tissue is exceptionally vulnerable to hyperkalemia. The magnitude of the hyperkalemia as well as the rate at which it develops determine cardiotoxicity. Since it is very difficult to predict the progression to fatal cardiotoxicity, the presence of any electrocardiographic abnormality is an indication for immediate therapy. The earliest ECG change is symmetrical peaking of the T wave, followed by widening of the QRS complex and prolongation of the PR interval. Heart block, atrial standstill, and a sine wave configuration (due to the merging of QRS complex with the T wave) is a late event, often followed by ventricular fibrillation or asystole.

D. Treatment

1. General

Several measures are available for the management of cardiotoxicity in the hyperkalemic patient. These fall into three broad categories and, in order to maximize the chances of full recovery, may be undertaken simultaneously.

a. Calcium. The infusion of calcium restores a more normal differential between the threshold and resting transmembrane potential. The usual approach is the infusion of 10–30 ml of 10% calcium gluconate under constant EKG monitoring. This form of therapy does not change the serum K, but it can rapidly reverse EKG changes. Caution should be exercised, however, in using this therapy in patients on digoxin.

b. Sodium Bicarbonate. One or two ampules (44 mEq/50 ml) infused over a 10-min period may be used initially. Additional amounts should be administered, depending on the presence and severity of acidosis.

c. Glucose and Insulin. The usual approach is to administer 50 ml of 50% glucose followed by a continuous infusion of 10% glucose until the K level normalizes. Insulin can be added to the glucose infusion at the rate of 10–20 units of regular insulin for each 100 g of glucose. This form of therapy is the most efficient way of rapidly lowering serum K in the patient with end-stage kidney disease, pending the initiation of hemodialysis (120). The latter two forms of therapy act by redistributing K from the extracellular to the intracellular compartment. By so doing, the transmembrane potential is increased toward normal. Nebulized albuterol at a dose of 10–20 mg has also been used successfully in these patients (121). This approach, however, might not be very helpful in the elderly, given the reduced sensitivity of their beta-receptors to the beta-agonists (6,122). In addition to the above, which act relatively rapidly, measures to remove the excess K from the body can be initiated. These include: (a) sodium polystyrene sulfonate (a K-exchange resin), 15–30 g administered in liquid suspension given orally, or 50–100 g in 200 ml of water used as a retention enema; (b) hemo- or peritoneal dialysis with a zero-K bath may be necessary in patients with significant renal insufficiency.

2. *Specific*

Once the serum K is brought to a normal level, more specific measures should be undertaken for the long-term management of the patient. In patients with drug-induced hyperkalemia, the offending agent should be discontinued. For those with renal failure, dialytic therapy may be necessary. On occasion, patients on maintenance hemodialysis will require interdialytic administration of alkali (for those who tend to maintain a serum bicarbonate below 15 mEq/L) or sodium polysterene sulfonate (15–30 g twice a day) might be necessary. Oral sodium bicarbonate can be used; however, compliance, in our experience, is generally poor, because of gastric complaints.

Once the diagnosis of hyporenin-hypoaldosteronism is made, correction of systemic acidosis and hyperkalemia can be sustained by administration of fludrocortisone in daily doses of 0.1–0.3 mg (95). Side effects, such as extracellular fluid retention and hypertension, might limit the use of this drug, however. Other alternatives which can be used for the patient with "voltage-dependent" tubular acidosis and hyperkalemia include: (a) administration of alkali (1.5–2.0 mEq of sodium bicarbonate per kilogram per day) combined with dietary K restriction (2 g K diet); (b) potassium-binding resins (see above for dose); and (c) furosemide administration, with the dose dependent on the level of kidney function (123). Since the aciduric response to furosemide is somewhat attenuated by aldosterone deficiency, in those patients with both "voltage-dependent" and hypoaldosteronism hyperkalemia, furosemide in combination with fludrocortisone may be useful, as long as no contraindication for the use of the mineralocorticoid exists (124,125).

E. Prognosis

Acutely, the prognosis depends on how rapidly the cardiotoxicity of hyperkalemia is reversed. Otherwise the mortality is based mainly on the underlying disease. None of our 100 patients died as a direct result of hyperkalemia.

REFERENCES

1. Hirsch DJ, Hayslett JP. Adaptation to potassium. NIPS 1986;1:54–57.
2. Sweiry JC, Binder HJ. Characterization of aldosterone-induced potassium secretion in rat distal colon. J Clin Invest 1989;83:844–851.
3. Gavryck WA, Moore RD, Thompson RC. Effect of insulin upon membrane-bound (Na^++K+)-ATPase extracted from frog skeletal muscle. J Physiol 1975;252: 43–58.
4. Brown MJ, Brown DC, Murphy MB. Hypokalemia from ß2-receptor stimulation by circulating epinephrine. N Engl J Med 1983;309:1414–1419.
5. Williams ME, et al. Impairment of extrarenal potassium disposal by adrenergic stimulation. N Engl J Med 1984;311:145–149.
6. Ford GA, et al. Effect of aging on changes in plasma potassium during exercise. J Gerontol 1993;48:M140–M145.
7. Bia MJ, DeFronzo RA. Extrarenal potassium homeostasis. Am J Physiol 1981;240: F257–F268.
8. Cox M, Sterns RH, Singer I. The defense against hyperkalemia: the roles of insulin and aldosterone. N Engl J Med 1978;299:525–532.
9. Massara F, et al. Pathophysiological doses of glucagon cause a transient increase of the hepatic vein potassium concentration in man. Miner Electr Metab 1986;12: 142–146.
10. Stanton BA, et al. Structural and functional study of the rat distal nephron: effects of potassium adaptation and depletion. Kidney Int 1981;19:36–48.
11. Rastegar A, et al. Changes in membrane surfaces of collecting duct cells in potassium adaptation. Kidney Int 1980;18:293–301.
12. Sterns RH, Spital A. Disorders of internal potassium balance. Sem Nephrol 1987;7: 206–222.

12a. Adrogué HJ. Madias NE. Changes in plasma potassium concentration during acute acid-base disturbances. Am J Med 1981;71:456–467.

13. Field MJ, Stanton BA, Giebisch GH. Influence of ADH on renal potassium handling: a micropuncture and microperfusion study. Kidney Int 1984;25:502–511.
14. Good DW, Wright FS. Luminal influences of K secretion: sodium concentration and fluid flow rate. Am J Physiol 1979;236:F192–F205.
15. Sullivan LP. Effect of Na and impermeant anions on renal K transport during stopped flow. Am J Phsyiol 1961;201:774–780.
16. Velazquez H, Wright FS, Good DW. Luminal influences on potassium secretion: chloride replacement with sulfate. Am J Physiol 1982;242:F46–F55.
17. Jamison RL, et al. Potassium secretion by the descending limb of pars recta of the juxtamedullary nephron in vivo. Kidney Int 1976;9:323–332.
18. Battilana CA, et al. Effect of chronic potassium loading on potassium secretion by the pars recta or descending limb of the juxtamedullary nephron in the rat. J Clin Invest 1978;62:1093–1103.
19. Arrascue JF, Dobyan DC, Jamison RL. Potassium recycling in the renal medulla: effects of acute potassium chloride administration to rats fed a potassium-free diet. Kidney Int 1981;20:348–352.
20. Giebisch G. Renal potassium channels: an overview. Kidney Int 1995;48:1004–1009.

21. Novak LP. Aging, total body potassium, fat free mass and cell mass in males and females between ages 18 and 85 years. J Geront 1972;27:438–443.
22. Morgan DB, Young RM. Acute transient hypokalemia: new interpretation of a common event. Lancet 1982;2:751–752.
23. McCarthy ST. Body fluid, electrolytes and diuretics. Curr Med Res Opin 1982;7: 87–95.
24. Sorensen IJ, Matzen LE. Serum electrolytes and drug therapy of patients admitted to a geriatric department. Ugeskr Laeger 1993;155:3921–3924.
25. Nasar MA, Lyle EM. Hypokalemia in the elderly: is it always diuretic induced? Br J Clin Pract 1994;48:19–21.
26. Tannen RL, Gerrits L. Response of the renal K conserving mechanism to a kaliuretic stimuli: evidence for a direct kaliuretic effect of furosemide. Clin Res 1983; 31:752A.
27. Tannen RL. Potassium metabolism. In: Gonick HC, ed. Current Nephrology. Vol. 6. New York: Wiley, and Sons. 1983.
28. Jamison RL, et al. Surreptitious diuretic ingestion and pseudo-Bartter's syndrome. Am J Med 1982;73:142–147.
29. Conn JW, Rovner DR, Cohen EL. Licorice-induced pseudoaldosteronism. JAMA 1968;205:492–496.
30. Struthers AD, Whitesmith R, Reid JL. Prior thiazide diuretic treatment increases adrenaline-induced hypokalaemia. Lancet 1983;1:1358–1361.
31. Solomon RJ. Ventricular arrythmias in patients with myocardial infarctions and ischemia. Relationship to serum potassium and magnesium. Drugs 1984;28(suppl 1):66–76.
32. Nordrehang JE, Johannessen KA, Von der Lippe G. Serum potassium concentrations as a risk factor of ventricular arrythmias early in acute myocardial infarction. Circulation 1985;71:645–649.
33. Reuben SR, Thomas RD. The relationship between serum potassium and cardiac arrythmias following cardiac infarction in patients aged over 65 years. Curr Med Res Bull 1982;7(suppl 1):79–82.
34. Knochel JP. Hypokalemia. Adv Intern Med 1984;30:317–335.
35. Halevy J, Gunsherowitz M, Rosenfeld JB. Life-threatening hypokalemia in hospitalized patients. Miner Elec Metab 1988;14:163–167.
36. Sterns RM, et al. Internal potassium balance and the control of the plasma potassium concentration. Medicine 1981;60:339–354.
37. Villamil MF, et al. Effect of long term treatment with hydrochlorothiazide on water and electrolytes of muscle in hypertensive subjects. Am Heart J 1963;65:294–302.
38. Bergstrom J, Hultman E. The effect of thiazides, chlorthalidone and furosemide on muscle electrolytes and muscle glycogen in normal subjects. Acta Med Scand 1966;180:363–376.
39. Morgan DB, Davidson C: Hypokalemia and diuetics: an analysis of publications. Br Med J 1980;280:905–908.
40. Nordrehang JE, Von der Lippe G. Hypokalemia and ventricular fibrillation in acute myocardial infarction. Br Heart J 1983;50:525–529.
41. Higham PD, et al. Plasma potassium, serum magnesium and ventricular fibrillation: a prospective study. Quart J Med 1993;86:609–617.

42. Norris RM, et al. Prevention of ventricular fibrillation during acute myocardial infarction by intravenous propranolol. Lancet 1984;2:883–886.
43. Kassirer JP, Harrington JT. Fending off the potassium pushers. N Engl J Med 1985;312:785–787.
44. Kaplan NM. Our appropriate concern about hypokalemia. Am J Med 1984;77:1–4.
45. Abraham AS, et al. Intracellular cations and diuretic therapy following acute myocardial infarction. Arch Intern Med 1986;146:1301–1303.
46. Kaplan NM, et al. Potassium supplementation in hypertensive patients with diuretic-induced hypokalemia. N Engl J Med 1985;312:746–749.
47. Schwartz AB, Swartz CD. Dosage of potassium chloride elixir to correct thiazide-induced hypokalemia. JAMA 1974;230:702–704.
48. Papademetrion V, et al. Effectiveness of potassium chloride or triamterene in thiazide hypokalemia. Arch Intern Med 1985;145:1986–1990.
49. Greenblat DJ, Koch-Weser J. Adverse reactions to spironolactone. A report from the Boston Collaborative Drug Surveillance Program. JAMA 1973;225:40–43.
50. Ramsay LE, et al. Amiloride spirono-lactone and potassium chloride in thiazide-treated hypertensive patients. Clin Pharmacol Ther 1980;27:533–543.
51. Benos DJ. The biology of amiloride-sensitive sodium channels. Hosp Prac 1989;24:149–164.
52. Cannon-Babb ML, Schwartz AB: Drug induced hyperkalemia. Hosp Prac 1986;21: 99–127.
53. Sica DA, Gehr TWB. Triamterene and the kidney. Nephron 1989;51:454–461.
54. Weinberg MS, et al. Anuric renal failure precipitated by indocin and triamterene. Nephron 1985;40:216–218.
55. Williams P, Rush DR. Geriatric polypharmacy. Hosp Prac 1986;6:104–120.
56. Finnegan TP, Spence JD, Cape RD. Potassium sparing diuretics interaction with digoxin in elderly men. J Am Geriatr Soc 1984;32:129–131.
57. Zawada ET Jr. Antihypertensive therapy with triamterene-hydrochloro-thiazide vs. amiloride-hydrochlorothiazide. Arch Intern Med 1986;146:1312–1314.
58. Whang R, et al. Magnesium depletion as a cause of refractory potassium depletion. Arch Intern Med 1985;145:1686–1688.
59. Paice B, et al. Hyperkalemia in patients in hospital. Br Med J 1983;286:1189–1192.
60. Shemer J, et al. Incidence of hyperkalemia in hospitalized patients. Isr J Med Sci 1983;19:659–661.
61. Mulkerrin E, Epstein FH, Clark BA. Aldosterone responses to hyperkalemia in healthy elderly humans. J Am Soc Nephrol 1995;6:1459–1462.
62. Hené RJ, et al. Adaption to chronic potassium loading in normal man. Miner Electr Metab 1986;12:165–172.
63. Frais MA, Burgers ED, Mitchell LB. Piroxicam-induced renal failure and hyperkalemia. Ann Intern Med 1980;99:129.
64. Grossman LA, Moss S. Piroxicam and hyperkalemic acidosis. Ann Intern Med 1983;99:282.
65. Miller KP, Lazar EJ, Fotino S. Severe hyperkalemia during piroxicam therapy. Arch Intern Med 1984;144:2414–2415.
66. Corwin HL, Bonventre JV. Renal insufficiency associated with nonsteroidal anti-inflammatory agents. Am J Kidney Dis 1984;4:147–152.

67. Aimran A, et al: Incidence of hyperkalemia induced by indomethacin in a hospital population. Br Med J 1985;291:107–108.
68. Findling JW, et al. Indomethacin-induced hyperkalemia in three patients with gouty arthritis. JAMA 1980;244:1127–1128.
69. Tan SY, et al. Indomethacin-induced prostaglandin inhibition with hyperkalemia. Ann Intern Md 1979;90:783–785.
70. Beroniade V, Corneille L, Haraoui B. Indomethacin induced inhibition of prostaglandin with hyperkalemia. Ann Intern Med 1979;91:499–500.
71. Kimberly RP, et al. Reduction of renal function by newer nonsteroidal anti-inflammatory drugs. Am J Med 1978;64:804–807.
72. Meier DE, et al. Indomethacin-associated hyperkalemia in the elderly. J Am Geriatr Soc 1983;31:371–373.
73. Geller M, Folkert VW, Schlondorff D. Reversible acute renal insufficiency and hyperkalemia following indomethacin therapy. JAMA 1981;246:154–155.
74. Goldszer RC, et al. Hyperkalemia associated with indomethacin. Arch Intern Med 1981;141:802.
75. MacCarthy EP, Frost GW, Stokes GS. Indomethacin-induced hyperkalemia. Med J Austral 1979;1:550.
76. Swainson CP, Griffiths P. Acute and chronic effects of sulindac on renal function in chronic renal disease. Clin Pharmacol Ther 1985;37:298–300.
77. Nescher G, Zimran A, Hershkoc C. Reduced incidence of hyperkalemia and azotemia in patients receiving sulindac compared with indomethacin. Nephron 1988;48:291–295.
78. Textor SC, et al. Hyperkalemia in azotemic patients during angiotensin-converting enzyme inhibition and aldosterone reduction with captopril. Am J Med 1982;73: 719–725.
79. Alappan R, Perazella MA, Buller GK. Hyperkalemia in hospitalized patients treated with trimethoprim-sulfamethoxazole. Ann Intern Med 1996;124:316–320.
80. Velazquez H, et al. Renal mechanism of trimethoprim-induced hyperkalemia. Ann Intern Med 1993;119:296–301.
80a. Reiser I, et al. Reversal of trimethoprim-induced antikaluresis. Kidney Int 1996;50: 2063–2069.
81. Swenson ER. Severe hyperkalemia as a complication of timolol, a topically applied β-adrenergic antagonist. Arch Intern Med 1986;146:1220–1221.
82. Yang WC, et al. Beta adrenergic-mediated extrarenal potassium disposal in patients with end-stage renal disease: Effect of propranolol. Miner Electr Metab 1986;12:186–193.
83. Coun JW, et al. Inhibition of heparinoid of aldosterone biosynthesis in man. J. Clin Endocrinol Metab 1966;26:527–532.
84. Sherman RA, Ruddy MC. Suppression of aldosterone production by low-dose heparin. Am J Nephrol 1986;6:165–168.
85. Leehy D, Gantt C, Lim V. Heparin-induced hypoaldosternism. JAMA 1981;246: 2189–2190.
86. Edes TE, Sunderrajan EV. Heparin-induced hyperkalemia. Arch Intern Med 1985; 145:1070–1072.
87. Perez GO, Pelleys R, Oster JR. Renal-tubular hyperkalemia. Am J Nephrol 1982;2: 109–114.

88. Gerstein AR, et al. Aldosterone deficiency in chronic renal failure. Nephron 1968; 5:90–105.
89. McGiff JC, et al. Interrelationships of renin and aldosterone in a patient with hypoaldosteronism. Am J Med 1970;48:247–253.
90. Perez G, Siegel L, Schreiner GE. Selective hypoaldosteronism with hyperkalemia. Ann Intern Med 1972;76:757–763.
91. Gossain VV, et al. Impaired renin responsiveness with secondary hyperaldosteronism. Arch Intern Med 1973;132:885–890.
92. Weidmann P, et al. Syndrome of hyporeninemic hypoaldosteronism in renal disease. J Clin Endocrinol Metab 1973;36:965–977.
93. Oh MS, et al. A mechanism for hyporeninemic hypoaldosteronism in chronic renal disease. Metabolism 1974;23:1157–1166.
94. DeLeiva A, et al. Big renin and biosynthetic defect of aldosterone in diabetes mellitus. N Engl J Med 1976;295:639–643.
95. Sebastian A, et al. Amelioration of metabolic acidosis with fluodrocortisone therapy in hyporeninemic hypoaldosteronism. N Engl J Med 1977;297:576–583.
96. Schambelan M, Sebastian A, Biglieri EG. Prevalence, pathogenesis and functional significance of aldosterone deficiency in hyperkalemic patients with chronic renal insufficiency. Kidney Int 1980;17:89–101.
97. Battle DC, Arruda JAL, Kurtzman NA. Hyperkalemic distal renal tubular acidosis associated with obstructive uropathy. N Engl J Med 1981;304:373–380.
98. Dubose TD, Coflisch CR. Effect of selective aldosterone deficiency on acidification in nephron segments of the rat inner medulla. J Clin Invest 1988;82: 1624–1632.
99. Szylman P, et al. Role of hyperkalemia in the metabolic acidosis of isolated hyperaldosteronism. N Engl J Med 1976;294:361–465.
101. Sebastian A, et al. Effect of mineralocorticoid replacement therapy in renal acid-base homeostasis in adrenalectomized patients. Kidney Int 1980;18:767–769.
102. Phelps KRR, et al. Pathophysiology of the syndrome of hyporeninemic hypoaldosteronism. Metabolism 1980;29:186–199.
103. Tan SY, Antonipillae I, Mulrow PJ. Inactive renin and prostaglandin E2 production in hyporeninemic hypoaldosteronism. J Clin Endocrinol Metab 1980;51:849–853.
104. Tuck ML, Mayes DM. Mineralocorticoid biosynthesis in patients with hyporeninemic hypoaldosteronism. J Clin Endocrinol Metab 1980;50:341–347.
105. Kaufman JS, et al. Isolated hypoaldosteronism and abnormalities in renin, kallikrein and prostaglandin. Nephron 1986;43:203–210.
106. Nadler JL, et al. Evidence of prostacyclin deficiency in the syndrome of hyporeninemic hypoaldosteronism. N Engl J Med 1986;314:1015–1020.
107. Williams GH. Hyporeninemic hypoaldosteronism. N Engl J Med 1986;314: 1041–1042.
108. Schambelan M, Sebastian A, Rector F. Mineralocorticoid resistant renal hyperkalemia without salt wasting (type II pseudohypoaldosteronism): role of increased renal chloride reabsorption. Kidney Int 1981;19:716–727.
109. Gordon RD. Syndrome of hypertension and hyperkalemia with normal glomerular filtration rate. Hypertension 1986;8:93–102.

110. Arruda JAL, et al. Hyperkalemia and renal insufficiency: role of selective aldosterone deficiency and tubular unresponsiveness to aldosterone. Am J Nephrol 1981;1:160–167.
111. Battle DC. Hyperkalemic hyperchloremic metabolic acidosis associated with selective aldosterone deficiency and distal renal tubular acidosis. Sem Nephrol 1981; 1:260–274.
112. Arruda JAL, et al. Voltage-dependent distal acidification defect induced by amiloride. J Lab Clin Med 1980;95:407–416.
113. Viberti GC. Glucose-induced hyperkalemia: a hazard for diabetics? Lancet 1978;1: 690–691.
114. Nicolio GL, et al. Glucose-induced hyperkalemia in diabetic subjects. Arch Intern Med 1981;141:49–53.
115. Goldfarb S, et al. Paradoxical glucose-induced hyperkalemia. Am J Med 1975;59: 744–750.
116. Goldfarb S, et al. Acute hyperkalemia induced by hyperglycemia: hormonal mechanisms. Ann Intern Med 1976;84:426–432.
117. Ammon RA, May SW, Nightingale SD. Glucose-induced hyperkalemia with normal aldosterone levels. Ann Intern Med 1978;89:349–351.
118. Montolin J, Revert L. Lethal hyperkalemia associated with severe hyperglycemia in diabetic patients with renal failure. Am J Kidney Dis 1985;1:47–48.
119. Adrogué HJ, Madias NE. Changes in plasma potassium concentration during acute acid-base disturbances. Am J Med 1981;71:456–467.
120. Oster JR, et al. Plasma potassium response to acute metabolic acidosis induced by mineral and non-mineral acids. Miner Electr Metab 1980;4:28–36.
121. Blumberg A, et al. Effect of various therapeutic approaches on plasma potassium and major regulating factors in terminal renal failure. Am J Med 1988;85:507–512.
122. Allon M, Dunlay R, Copkney C. Nebulized albuterol for acute hyperkalemia in patients on hemodialysis. Ann Intern Med 1989;110:426–429.
123. Vestral RE, Wood AJJ, Shand DG. Reduced beta-adrenoreceptor sensitivity in the elderly. Clin Pharmacol Ther 1979;26:181–186.
124. Rastogi SP, et al. Effect of furosemide on urinary acidification in distal renal tubular acidosis. J Lab Clin Med 1984;104:271–282.
125. Sebastian A, Schambelan M, Sutton JM. Amelioration of hyperchloremic acidosis with furosemide therapy in patients with chronic renal insufficiency and type 4 renal tubular acidosis. Am J Nephrol 1984;4:287–300.

4

Acid–Base Disorders

I. INTRODUCTION

The maintenance of acid–base balance in humans depends on the balance between hydrogen ion (H) production and excretion. Hydrogen ion production, primarily a consequence of cellular metabolism, consists of two components: carbonic acid (H_2CO_3) and fixed acids. The former is excreted by the lungs as CO_2 and the latter by the kidney. Under normal circumstances, net daily fixed acid production is 50–100 mM (1 mM/kg). In addition to cellular metabolism, dietary foodstuffs (protein, fat, carbohydrate), absorption by the gut of available base equivalents, and buffering by bone also contribute to net acid production (1).

The kidneys participate in the excretion of fixed acids through their regulation of bicarbonate (a major extracellular buffer) absorption and excretion, NH_3 production, and titrable acid excretion.

II. RENAL BICARBONATE REGULATION

Bicarbonate (HCO_3) is freely filtered through the glomerular capillary wall at a rate related to the plasma HCO_3 concentration and the glomerular filtration rate (GFR). In the proximal tubule, HCO_3 reabsorption is linked to the luminal secretion of H as shown by the following reaction:

$$H + HCO_3 \rightleftharpoons H_2CO_3 \rightleftharpoons H_2O + CO_2$$

The dissociation of H_2CO_3 to $H_2O + CO_2$ is almost immediate, due to the presence of carbonic anhydrase (CA) in the proximal tubule brush border. The CO_2 produced diffuses back into the cell to participate in the formation of HCO_3, which then diffuses into the peritubular interstitial space, and H, which will be secreted into the lumen, completing the cycle:

$$CO_2 + H_2O \underset{}{\overset{CA}{\rightleftharpoons}} H_2CO_3 \overset{CA}{\rightleftharpoons} HCO_3 + H$$

Eighty to eighty-five percent of the filtered HCO_3 is reabsorbed this way in the early segments of the proximal tubule. An increase in luminal HCO_3 concentration, luminal flow rate, or arterial pCO_2 stimulates proximal HCO_3 reabsorption. Renal nerve stimulation and angiotensin II also increase HCO_3 reabsorption. On the other hand, an increase in peritubular HCO_3 concentration inhibits HCO_3 reabsorption (2).

Both the medullary and cortical segments of the thick ascending limb of Henle participate in HCO_3 reabsorption through an active process requiring CA. The process can be stimulated by metabolic acidosis or an increase in dietary sodium and is inhibited by metabolic alkalosis, low-sodium diet, vasopressin, and medullary hypertonicity (3). A large part of the HCO_3 escaping proximal tubular reabsorption is reabsorbed in this segment.

Both the inner and the outer medullary collecting ducts also participate in HCO_3 reabsorption (4,5), which can be modulated by mineralocorticoids and various peptide hormones via cyclic AMP (6).

III. AMMONIA PRODUCTION

The regeneration of HCO_3 and the adaptation to changes in acid–base balance occur mainly through variations in the synthesis of ammonia (NH_3) from amino acids (chiefly glutamine) by the cells of the early proximal tubular segment. NH_3 excretion increases during metabolic acidosis and decreases during metabolic alkalosis. Besides changes in peritubular H concentration, luminal flow rate and K concentration are important regulators of NH_3 synthesis. The synthesis of NH_3 from glutamine also results in the formation of HCO_3. The latter is preferentially transported across the basolateral membrane of the proximal tubule into the systemic blood, whereas the NH_3 formed is secreted into the tubular fluid, much of which is reabsorbed in the thick ascending limb, leading to its accumulation in the medulla by countercurrent multiplication. From the medullary interstitium, NH_3 is passively secreted across the collecting duct epithelium, where it combines with H secreted actively, resulting in the formation of ammonium (NH_4), which is excreted in the final urine (7).

IV. TITRABLE ACID EXCRETION

The titrable acids (TA) consist of all the filtered buffers present in the urine (with the exception of NH_3) combined with H. These buffers are usually organic acids such as phosphate, creatinine, or beta-hydroxybutyrate. Phosphate accounts for the bulk of titrable acid and is generated mainly in the proximal tubule through the conversion of Na_2HPO_4 to NaH_2PO_4. Under ordinary circumstances, 33–50% of the total H load is excreted as titrable acid (8). Factors known to affect the rate of formation and excretion of titrable acids include the degree of acidosis and the concentration and pK of the filtered buffer. In summary, net acid excretion (NAE) is the sum of the NH_3 and TA excreted minus any HCO_3 loss: $NAE = NH_4 + TA - HCO_3$.

V. EFFECTS OF AGE ON ACID–BASE METABOLISM

Blood pH and plasma HCO_3 remain within normal ranges in the aged (9). Therefore, the aging kidney is able to maintain acid–base homeostasis under basal conditions; however, when subjected to an acute acid load, the elderly do not increase NAE to the same degree as younger subjects (see Chapter 1). This phenomenon is secondary to a lower NH_4 excretion, which cannot be accounted for solely by the progressive decrease in GFR seen with age. Additional factor(s), not yet elucidated, must be responsible for this impairment.

VI. ACID–BASE DISORDERS

Judging from our own experience with a large number of elderly, acid–base disorders are rather common. The true incidence, however, is not known. In 7433 abnormal blood gases obtained from patients of various ages reported by Hodgkins et al. (10), metabolic alkalosis was present in 36%, respiratory alkalosis in 21%, mixed abnormalities in 19%, respiratory acidosis in 16%, and metabolic acidosis in 8%. We retrospectively analyzed 300 consecutive abnormal arterial blood gas determinations obtained from elderly hospitalized patients. Metabolic acidosis was present in 30%, mixed abnormalities in 23%, respiratory acidosis in 18%, metabolic alkalosis in 17%, and respiratory alkalosis in 12%, suggesting differences in acid–base metabolism in the elderly and/or different medical problems associated with these metabolic disturbances. Most of the data presented in this section are drawn from this experience, since there is relatively little available in the literature that specifically addresses acid–base disturbances in the elderly.

A. Metabolic Acidosis

1. Etiology

The etiology of metabolic acidosis is dependent on the type of acidosis present, which is classified in the elderly similarly as in younger patients: (a) increased anion gap acidosis, due (in decreasing order of frequency) to severe chronic renal insufficiency, lactic acidosis, ketoacidosis, drugs, or poisons; or (b) non-anion gap acidosis, due to mild or moderate chronic renal insufficiency (with or without tubular hyperkalemia), HCO_3 losses through the gastrointestinal tract, drugs, renal tubular acidosis, or diabetes mellitus.

2. Clinical Manifestations and Pathogenesis

In general, the clinical manifestations in patients with metabolic acidosis are those of the associated disease state. The conscious patient might complain of shortness of breath. Upon physical examination, Kussmaul breathing may be present, as well as asterixis, particularly if the acidosis is severe. The pathogenesis of the acidosis (both anion gap and non-anion gap varieties) associated with renal insufficiency (which is responsible for over 30% of elderly patients with metabolic acidosis) is discussed in Chapters 3 and 11.

Lactic acidosis is generally found in states of poor tissue perfusion (e.g., septic or cardiogenic shock) and results from an imbalance between production (by the poorly perfused organs) and utilization (by an ischemic liver and other tissues) (11). It may be present in a pure form or associated with other anion or non-anion gap acidosis. An increase in the blood lactate level with acidosis has also been reported in elderly patients with certain types of malignancy, such as lymphomas and carcinoma of the breast, lung, and bowel (12). The exact mechanism(s) responsible for the increase in lactate production in these patients has not been completely elucidated (13). Lactic acidosis can also be associated with a number of other conditions, such as seizures, short bowel syndrome, and hereditary defects (14), but their occurrence in the elderly is rather rare. In the appropriate setting, the diagnosis of lactic acidosis is confirmed by a plasma lactate level >5 mmol/L.

Metformin, a drug which lowers blood glucose by inhibiting hepatic glucose production and improving peripheral insulin sensitivity, has been associated with lactic acidosis in the elderly (14a). Hypotension and/or evidence of tissue hypoxia is present in the majority of these patients. True type B (aerobic) lactic acidosis is rare (14b). Neither the mortality rate, which is approximately 50% (14c), nor the severity of the acidosis correlate with metformin blood levels (14b). Since renal insufficiency (serum creatinine >1.7 mg/dl), cardiac failure, peripheral vascular disease, or the use of parenteral iodinated contrast agents appear to be risk factors in 54% of the reported cases, it is recommended that the drug not be used in these situations or temporarily discontinued (14a, 14d).

Ketoacidosis occurs in diabetes mellitus, starvation, and alcoholism; the inorganic acids generated endogenously are beta-hydroxybutyric (from incompletely burned body fat) and acetoacetic.

Of the various drugs and chemicals (salicylate, methanol, ethylene glycol, paraldehyde, acetominophen) capable of causing an anion gap acidosis (15–18) when ingested either accidentally or in a suicide attempt, salycylate poisoning is the only one of significant clinical importance in the elderly. In the absence of a definite history of salycylate ingestion, the clinical picture can be easily confused with other clinical states seen in the elderly, such as a primary central nervous system event, alcoholic intoxication, or sepsis (19). The presence of a mixed acid–base picture (respiratory alkalosis and metabolic acidosis) should raise suspicion of this diagnosis, which is confirmed by measuring the plasma salicylate level. A level of 40–60 mg/dl is associated with mild toxicity, 60–100 mg/dl with moderate intoxication, and greater than 100 mg/dl with severe intoxication. The acidosis is secondary to the accumulation of ketones and lactate in the extracellular fluid, resulting from disturbed carbohydrate metabolism which is a consequence of uncoupling of mitochondrial oxidative phosphorylation by salicylates. In addition, the salycilate itself contributes to the increase in the anion gap (20,21).

Gastrointestinal losses of HCO_3 secondary to diarrhea constitute the second most common cause of non-anion gap acidosis in the elderly (mild to moderate renal insufficiency being the most common). At the time of diagnosis, renal failure (acute or chronic), severe volume contraction, hypophosphatemia, and hypophosphaturia were usually present in our patients. Since renal failure decreases NH_3 availability, a low distal Na delivery associated with volume contraction interferes with H secretion, and hypophosphaturia limits urinary TA, the kidneys probably contribute to the acidosis in many of these patients.

Hyperchloremic acidosis of varying severity occurs in 55% of elderly patients treated with carbonic anhydrase inhibitors (e.g., acetazolamide) for glaucoma (22,23). This high incidence in the elderly may be due, in part, to a higher blood concentration of the drug at the commonly prescribed doses than seen in younger patients (23). Since these drugs act by inhibiting tubular HCO_3 secretion, the urine pH during the early phase of therapy is greater than 7. During more chronic administration, however, a lower pH (5–6) may be found. Other drugs, such as amiloride, spirolonactone, and the converting enzyme inhibitors, can also produce a non-anion gap acidosis, although in our experience this has been rare.

Defective urinary acidification occurring in either the proximal or the distal portion of the nephron is classified under the term renal tubular acidosis (RTA). In proximal RTA (type II), massive urinary HCO_3 losses lead to a steady-state metabolic acidosis in association with a normal NAE. A first morning urine pH in these patients is characteristically less than 6.0 and can be as low as 5.3

following an acid load. In addition to HCO_3, other solutes usually absorbed in the proximal tubule, such as glucose, phosphate, uric acid, and amino acids, may also be lost. In patients with distal RTA (type I), the first morning urine pH is usually greater than 6.0 and remains greater than 5.3 following a acid load. Hypercalciuria and hypocitruria associated with nephrolithiasis are common in these patients. In both forms of RTA, hypokalemia is common. Hyperkalemic distal RTA, also referred to as type IV RTA, is commonly seen in the elderly as discussed in Chapter 3, but pure type I RTA is rare in this age group. In one recent review of 40 adults with type I RTA, only 2 (5%) were over the age of 60 (24). Type I RTA in the elderly is almost always secondary to other diseases such as amyloidosis, multiple myeloma, rheumatoid arthritis, or Sjögren's syndrome. Type II RTA is even less common than type 1 in the elderly.

Hyperchloremic metabolic acidosis may be seen in the uncontrolled diabetic at the time of presentation to the hospital or following treatment for ketoacidosis (25). These patients are usually not severely volume depleted; therefore the renal losses of keto-anions will exceed the capacity of the kidneys to regenerate alkali, resulting in a net loss of HCO_3 precursors (26).

It is possible to use a variety of guidelines and formulas to diagnose a pure metabolic acidosis. During steady-state metabolic acidosis the ventilatory response is usually quite predictable and can be calculated from the formula $pCO_2 = 1.54 \times \text{serum } HCO_3 + 8.36$, or derived from the relationship that for each 1-mEq/L decrease in serum HCO_3 there is a 1.1-mmHg decrease in pCO_2. If the measured pCO_2 is 2 mmHg or more over the calculated pCO_2, there is probably an accompanying respiratory acidosis; whereas if it is 2 mmHg or more less, a primary respiratory alkalosis is likely present.

3. *Treatment*

$NaHCO_3$ administration remains the mainstay of treatment for metabolic acidosis. The distribution space of HCO_3 is estimated to be 50% of total body weight for a serum HCO_3 above 5 mEq/L and 80–100% for values below this range. In patients with severe acute acidosis, we usually attempt to increase the serum HCO_3 concentration to 10–12 mEq/L. The amount required for a given patient should be infused as an isotonic or hypotonic solution rather than "bolus pushes," which are hypertonic. Since this regimen requires the administration of a significant amount of fluid, if volume overload is a danger, furosemide may be given in conjunction with the $NaHCO_3$. Dialysis may be necessary in patients with associated severe renal and/or heart failure. Treatment of the metabolic acidosis of chronic renal failure is discussed in Chapter 11. The use of HCO_3 therapy in patients with lactic acidosis is controversial (27,28). In patients with malignancy-related acidosis, alkali therapy will normalize the serum HCO_3 concentration in those patients in whom the tumors respond to chemotherapy or are surgically removed (12). In patients with lactic acidosis due to tissue anoxia, the primary effort should be directed at correcting the underlying problem (improving cardiac function, reversing hypotension, treating sepsis, etc). Even though raising the plasma pH and HCO_3 do not lead to any change in systemic hemodynamics or in mortality (28), we agree with Narins and Cohen (29) that, in patients with severe acidemia (pH < 7.2, HCO_3 < 8 mEq/L), alkali therapy to bring the serum HCO_3 to 10 mEq/L should be used to buy sufficient time to eliminate the cause of the acidosis. Dichloroacetate, 50 mg/kg body weight, given intravenously as a bolus at 2-hr intervals, has been shown to lower serum lactate level in a small number of elderly patients. Further study, however, failed to demonstrate any meaningful advantage of this form of treatment over conventional management (30,30a).

The acidosis associated with alcoholic and starvation ketosis is generally mild and responds to dextrose administration. In diabetic ketoacidosis, alkali therapy is indicated only initially and when the acidosis is severe (31).

We use the same guidelines outlined earlier (Chapter 2) to manage the acidotic elderly with gastrointestinal losses of alkali, since these patients are generally hypernatremic and severely volume contracted. Volume expansion should be accomplished with a solution continuing both HCO_3 and chloride.

Drug intoxications (ethylene glycol or methanol) are best treated by ethanol infusion and HCO_3 hemodialysis.

Patients with RTA should be treated with oral alkali as outlined in Chapter 11.

B. Respiratory Acidosis

1. Etiology

Respiratory acidosis was the third most common variety of acid–base abnormality seen in our elderly patients and was usually secondary to either chronic obstructive pulmonary disease (COPD) or chest wall deformity such as kyphoscoliosis. Central nervous system depression related to drugs as well as other disease states such as Guillain-Barré syndrome, polymyositis, obesity, and hypoventilation syndrome were rare causes in this age group.

2. Clinical Manifestations and Pathogenesis

Dyspnea, cough, and a respiratory tract infection are the most common clinical manifestations in these patients. On physical examination, cyanosis, tachypnea, use of the accessory respiratory muscles, increased anteroposterior diameter of the thoracic cage, severe chest deformity (in the kyphoscoliotic patient), and clubbing of the fingers may be found. The retention of CO_2 is responsible for the acidemia through generation of H_2CO_3 which dissociates to H + HCO_3. The H enters the cell in exchange for K and Na and is buffered by cellular proteins. The HCO_3 remains in the extracellular fluid (ECF). In addition, some of the CO_2 enters the red blood cell and undergoes hydration in the presence of CA. The H thus formed is buffered by hemoglobin, whereas the HCO_3 moves into the ECF in exchange for Cl. These changes occur acutely and the HCO_3 gain by the ECF by this mechanism is rather modest, approximately 4–5 mEq/L. During chronic respiratory acidosis the kidneys are primarily responsible for maintaining the more significant elevation of the plasma HCO_3 concentration than that seen during the acute phase by generation of new HCO_3 and increasing proximal tubule and collecting-duct HCO_3 reabsorption (32,33).

Clinical observations in humans with acute or chronic respiratory acidosis have indicated a highly predictable relationship between the degree of hypercapnia and HCO_3 level following the physiological adaptions referred to above. In acute respiratory acidosis, HCO_3 increases 1 mEq/L for every 10-mmHg increase in pCO_2. In chronic respiratory acidosis, HCO_3 increases 3.5 mEq/L for every 10-mmHg increase in pCO_2. A deviation from this predictable pattern of response should suggest the presence of an additional acid–base disturbances.

3. *Treatment*

During acute exacerbations, treatment is directed toward maintaining adequate oxygenation while attempts are made to correct or control the precipitating event (infection, heart failure, drugs). The total management of the patient with COPD is beyond the scope of this discussion.

C. Metabolic Alkalosis

1. *Etiology*

Based on the urinary Cl concentration, metabolic alkalosis is usually classified into Cl responsive (urinary Cl < 10 mEq/L except in the presence of severe K depletion, in which urinary Cl may be greater than 10 mEq/L) and Cl resistant (urinary Cl > 20 mEq/L). The former, by far more common in the elderly, is associated with gastric fluid losses, diuretic therapy, and posthypercapnia. The latter occurs in hyperglucocorticoidism, following the use of mineralocorticoid-like agents (licorice, carbenoxolone) and in primary aldosteronism.

2. *Clinical Manifestations and Pathogenesis*

The clinical manifestations of metabolic alkalosis are usually those of the underlying problem, although severe alkalemia (pH > 7.55) may cause mental confusion, muscle cramps, and cardiac arrhythmias (both supraventricular and ventricular), particularly in patients requiring ventilatory support. Independent of origin, the development of metabolic alkalosis can be divided into a generation phase and a maintenance phase (34).

a. Chloride-Responsive Alkalosis. The generation of metabolic alkalosis during vomiting is related to HCl losses resulting in ECF gain of HCO_3. The latter obligates the renal excretion of Na as an accompanying cation, as well as K (see Chapter 3). If the renal Na and gastric Cl losses are not replaced, volume contraction ensues.

With diuretics such as furosemide, bumetanide, torsemide, or chlorothiazide, which act by blocking NaCl reabsorption in the thick ascending limb of Henle or distal convoluted tubule, alkalosis is a consequence of the increased delivery of Na to the cortical collecting tubule, where it is partially reabsorbed, associated with an increase in the secretion of H and K, leading to an enhancement of NAE and kaliuresis. Since the capacity of this nephron segment to reabsorb Na is limited, ECF volume contraction will develop. If the patient is still on the diuretic, the urine chloride will be greater than 20 mEq/L despite the presence of volume contraction.

The compensatory increase in serum HCO_3 which occurs during respiratory acidosis is also accompanied by a transient increase in NAE and Cl losses. Once the pCO_2 is returned to normal, the excess HCO_3 will be excreted if Cl is available. If the patient has a deficit of NaCl, however, the elevated serum HCO_3 will persist, leading to metabolic alkalosis.

The maintenance of metabolic alkalosis is a consequence of the inability of the kidneys to excrete HCO_3. Several mechanisms are responsible: (a) a decrease in the filtered load of HCO_3 due to a lower GFR as a result of either volume contraction or activation of the tubuloglomerular feedback; (b) K depletion, which stimulates HCO_3 reabsorption in the proximal tubule; and (c) an increase in NAE, since K depletion increases NH_3 synthesis and produces intracellular acidosis. The hyperaldosteronism associated with volume contraction might also participate in the increase in NAE.

b. Chloride-Resistant Alkalosis. The generation and maintenance of metabolic alkalosis in the Cl-resistant form depends on the persistence of a mineralocorticoid excess despite ECF volume expansion. As a consequence, distal H secretion is increased, resulting in an increase in NAE. The mineralocorticoid excess also stimulates K secretion with ensuing hypokalemia. Hypokalemia then contributes to the increase in NAE and proximal HCO_3 reabsorption.

The respiratory compensation pattern seen in patients with pure metabolic alkalosis is erratic. In general, the pCO_2 increases 0.6 mmHg for each 1-mEq/L increase in serum HCO_3; however, a lesser degree of compensation has also been suggested in which $pCO_2 = 0.9\ (HCO_3) + 9$ (37). Significant deviations from this relationships suggest a mixed acid–base disturbance.

3. *Treatment*

In Cl-responsive metabolic alkalosis, both Cl and potassium should be replaced. The rate of replacement will depend on the severity of the ECF depletion. In the presence of hypotension and tachycardia, 0.9% NaCl is the solution of choice. Once the hemodynamics stabilize, the switch can be made to either a 0.45% or 0.33% NaCl with added K. In patients who are on nasogastric suction, the daily losses should be replaced. We also add an H_2-receptor antagonist in an effort to attenuate gastric HCl losses (35).

For treatment of Cl-resistant alkalosis, see Chapters 3 and 12. In patients receiving a saline infusion and pharmacological doses of glucocorticoid, management should include salt restriction and K replacement.

A significant number of our elderly patients with metabolic alkalosis also had associated acute renal failure. Since volume contraction was responsible for the renal failure in most of these patients, recovery was rapid following volume expansion. For patients with acute renal failure who do not respond to fluids, dialysis (preferably continuous arterio-venous hemofiltration with dialysis using NaCl as the replacement solution) may be necessary, since renal failure impairs renal HCO_3 excretion.

In intractable cases (which we have not seen in the elderly), 0.15 N HCl can be infused into a central vein as an isotonic solution, not to exceed 2 L/day. The amount required should be calculated from the HCO_3 space (50% of body weight) (36).

D. Respiratory Alkalosis

Respiratory alkalosis was diagnosed in 12% of our patients. This probably represents an underestimate, since a large number of hospitalized patients with this abnormality go unnoticed (blood gas determination not performed).

1. Etiology

Respiratory alkalosis can occur in any situation in which the depth or rate of respiration increases. The hyperventilation in our elderly patients was caused by hypoxia associated with pulmonary or heart disease, sepsis, liver disease, fever, or artificially by overbreathing while on a respirator. Anxiety, analeptic overdoses, and hyperthyroidism may also be associated with hyperventilation.

2. Clinical Manifestations and Pathogenesis

The patient with respiratory alkalosis might complain of light-headedness and peri-oral numbness and parasthesias of the extremities, presumably due to a decrease in ionized calcium, the altered pH, and, perhaps, to the vasoconstrictive effect of a low pCO_2 on the cerebral vasculature. The mechanisms responsible for the hyperventilation associated with sepsis and fever are not completely understood, but could represent stimulation of the respiratory center both directly and through peripheral baroreceptors. With drugs such as salicylate, the stimulation is direct. The respiratory alkalosis of liver disease may be related to changes in hormonal balance (estrogen and progesterone).

The diagnosis of pure acute respiratory alkalosis can be made if there is a 2-mEq/L decrease in HCO_3 for each 10-mmHg decrease in pCO_2. In the chronic form, HCO_3 decreases 5 mEq/L for each 10-mmHg fall in pCO_2. In the early phase, approximately two-thirds of the decrease in plasma HCO_3 is due to tissue buffering and one-third is due to blood buffering. When the process extends beyond 24 hr, the kidneys respond by decreasing NAE, which leads to the greater decrease in HCO_3.

3. *Treatment*

The treatment for respiratory alkalosis is that of the underlying clinical problem.

E. Mixed Acid–Base Disorders

Mixed acid–base disorders were present in 23% of our elderly patients who had arterial blood gas determinations. The abnormalities encountered were metabolic acidosis/respiratory alkalosis, respiratory and metabolic acidosis, metabolic alkalosis/respiratory acidosis, and respiratory and metabolic alkalosis. A deviation from the expected respiratory compensation for simple metabolic acid–base disturbance (see appropriate section) and/or disproportionate changes in the anion gap and the HCO_3 level should lead one to suspect the presence of a mixed acid–base disorder (37,38). For example, if the ratio between the change in anion gap and the change in serum HCO_3 is less than 0.7, a mixed metabolic acidosis and respiratory alkalosis should be suspected; whereas a value greater than 1.2 suggests a mixed metabolic and respiratory acidosis or a metabolic acidosis and alkalosis. It should be cautioned, however, that these guidelines should be used only as added information to the history and physical examination in assessing the elderly patient in whom a mixed acid–base problem is suspected (39). A mixed metabolic acidosis and respiratory alkalosis was seen with septic shock, pulmonary edema and tissue hypoxia related to low cardiac output, severe liver failure, and drug intoxication (salicylate). Most of the patients were in the intensive care unit with multiple organ failure. Mortality in these patients was close to 100%.

Mixed respiratory and metabolic acidosis was found in patients with COPD admitted with sepsis (generally secondary to pulmonary infection) or with congestive heart failure. In some patients, renal insufficiency was also present. The mortality rate in this group was also extremely high.

Mixed metabolic alkalosis and respiratory acidosis was noted in patients with COPD with associated heart disease or hypertension who were on salt restriction in the hospital and continued on a diuretic. Some of our COPD patients developed metabolic alkalosis while receiving saline expansion, large doses of steroids, and cancer chemotherapeutic drugs.

Mixed respiratory and metabolic alkalosis was found in patients who had undergone abdominal surgery and required nasogastric suction while receiving excessive mechanical ventilation or who had sepsis, severe pain, or sustained neurological damage.

The management of the elderly with these mixed disorders requires a therapeutic approach that attempts to treat both acid–base abnormalities simultaneously (see appropriate sections).

REFERENCES

1. Toto RD. Metabolic acid-base disorders. In: Kokko JP, Tannen RL, eds. fluids and Electrolytes. Philadelphia: Saunders, 1990:301–390.
2. Cogan MG. Regulation and control of bicarbonate absorption in the proximal tubule. Sem Nephrol 1990;10:115–121.
3. Good DW. Bicarbonate absorption by the thick ascending limb of Henle's loop. Sem Nephrol 1990;10:132–138.
4. Schuster VL. Bicarbonate reabsorption, and secretion in the cortical and outer medullary collecting duct. Sem Nephrol 1990;10:139–147.
5. Wall SM, Knepper MA. Acid-base transport in the inner medullary collecting duct. Sem Nephrol 1990;10:148–158
6. Paillard M, Bichara M. Peptide hormone control of urinary acidification and acid-base balance: PTH, ADH and glucagon. Am J Physiol 1989;256:F973–F985.
7. Knepper MA, Packer R, Good DW. Ammonium transport in the kidney. Physiol Rev 1989;69:179–249.
8. Simpson DP. Control of hydrogen ion homeostasis and renal acidosis. Medicine 1971;50:503–541.
9. Garry PJ, et al. Clinical chemistry reference intervals for healthy elderly subjects. Am J Clin Nutr 1989;50:1219–1230.
10. Hidgkins JE, Soeprono FF, Chan DM. Incidence of metabolic alkalemia in hospitalized patients. Crit Care Med 1980;8:725–728.
11. Arieff AI, Graf H. Pathophysiology of type A hypoxic lactic acidosis in dogs. Am J Physiol 1987;253:E271–E276.
12. Doolittle GC, et al. Malignancy-induced lactic acidosis. South Med J 1988;81:533–536.
13. Kreisberg RA. Pathogenesis and management of lactic acidosis. Ann Rev Med 1984;35:181–193.
14. Hood VL, Tannen RL. Lactic acidosis. Kidney 1989;22:1–6.

14a. Sulkin TV, Bosman D, Krentz AJ. Contraindications to metformin therapy in patients with NIDDM. Diabetes Care 1997;20:925–928.

14b. Lalau JD, et al. Role of metformin accumulation in metformin-associated lactic acidosis. Diabetes Care 1995;18:779–784.

14c. Jurovich MR, Woolridge JD, Force RW. Metformin-associated non-ketotic metabolic acidosis. Ann Pharmacother 1997;31:53–55.

14d. Dachman AH, Rotter A. New contraindication to intravascular iodinated contrast material. Radiology 1995;197:545–546.

15. Sejersted OM, et al. Formate concentrations in plasma from patients poisoned with methanol. Acta Med Scand 1983;213:105–110.
16. Jacobson D, Ostby N, Bredesen JE. Studies on ethylene glycol poisoning. Acta Med Scand 1982;212:11–15.
17. Brier LS, Pitts WH, Gonick HC. Metabolic acidosis occurring during paraldehyde intoxication. Ann Intern Med 1963;58:155–158.
18. Gray TA, Buckley BM, Vale JA. Hyperlactataemia and metabolic acidosis following paracetamol overdose. Quart J Med 1987;65:811–821.
19. Paul BN. Salicylate poisoning in the elderly: diagnostic pitfalls. J Am Geriatr Soc 1972;20:387–390.

20. Hill JB. Salicylate intoxication. N Engl J Med 1973;288:1110–1113.
21. Brenner BE, Simon RR. Management of salicylate intoxication. Drugs 1982;24: 335–340.
22. Heller I, et al. Significant metabolic acidosis induced by acetazolamide. Not a rare complication. Arch Intern Med 1985;145:1815–1817.
23. Chapron DJ, Gomolin JH, Sweeney KR. Azetazolamide blood concentrations are excessive in the elderly: propensity for acidosis and relationship to renal function. J Clin Pharmacol 1989;29:348–353.
24. Caruana RJ, Buckalew VM Jr. The syndrome of distal (type I) renal tubular acidosis. Clinical and laboratory findings in 58 cases. Medicine 1988;67:84–99.
25. Adrogué HJ, et al. Plasma acid-base patterns in diabetic ketoacidosis. N Engl J Med 1982;307:1603–1610.
26. Oh MS, Carroll HJ, Uribarri J. Mechanisms of normochloremic and hyperchloremic acidosis in diabetic ketoacidosis. Nephron 1990;54:1–6.
27. Stackpoole PW. Lactic acidosis: the case against bicarbonate therapy. Ann Intern Med 1986;105:276–279.
28. Cooper JD, et al. Bicarbonate does not improve hemodynamics in critically ill patients who have lactic acidosis. Ann Intern Med 1990;112:492–498.
29. Narins RG, Cohen JJ. Bicarbonate theapy for organic acidosis: the case for its continued use. Ann Intern Med 1987;106:615–618.
30. Stackpoole PW, et al. Dichloracetate in the treatment of lactic acidosis. Ann Intern Med 1988;108:58–63.
30a. Stacpoole PW, et al. A controlled clinical trial of dichloracetate for treatment of lactic acidosis in adults. N Engl J Med 1992;327:1564–1569.
31. Hale PJ, Crase J, Nattrass M. Metabolic effects of bicarbonate in the treatment of diabetic ketoacidosis. Br Med J 1984;289:1035–1038.
32. Cogan M. Chronic hypercapnia stimulates proximal bicarbonate reabsorption in the rat. J Clin Invest 1984;74:1942–1947.
33. McKinney TD, Davidson KK. Effects of respiratory acidosis on HCO_3 transport by rabbit collecting tubules. Am J Physiol 1988;255:F656–F665.
34. Galla JH, Luke RG. Pathophysiology of metabolic alkalosis. Hosp Pract 1987;24: 123–145.
35. Barton CH, et al. Cimetidine in the management of metabolic alkalosis induced by nasogastric drainage. Arch Surg 1979;114:70–74.
36. Williams DB, Lyons JH Jr. Treatment of severe metabolic alkalosis with intravenous infusion of hydrochloric acid. Surg Gynecol Obstet 1980;150:315–321.
37. Narins RG, Emmett M. Simple and mixed acid-base disorders: a practical approach. Medicine 1980;59:161–187.
38. Oster JR, Perez GO, Materson BJ. Use of the anion gap in clinical medicine. South Med J 1988;81:225–237.
39. DiNubile MJ: The increment in the anion gap: overextension of a concept. Lancet 1988;2:951–953.

5

Disorders of Calcium, Phosphorus, and Magnesium Metabolism

I. CALCIUM METABOLISM

A. Normal Physiology

The serum calcium is maintained in the narrow range of 8.5–10.5 mg/dl by the interaction of several hormonal systems, including parathyroid hormone (PTH), calcitonin, and vitamin D. The total serum calcium measured routinely consists of three fractions: ionized, which constitutes 41% of the total and is the physiologically active fraction; protein bound (albumin and globulin) (40%); and complexed (13%), bound to multiple organic and inorganic anions (1). Physiologically significant changes in the level of ionized calcium can occur without corresponding changes in total serum calcium; e.g., a rapid increase in pH can decrease and PTH can increase the ionized calcium with only a modest or no change in total calcium. Since changes in serum phosphate can affect serum calcium by binding with free calcium, these two elements should always be measured concurrently.

The concentration of ionized calcium in the blood is the most important factor responsible for the regulation of the PTH secretion, with its release stimulated directly by hypocalcemia and suppressed by hypercalcemia (2–4). The PTH response to extracellular calcium (Ca) is regulated by calcium-ion sensing receptors located in the parathyroid glands (5). In addition to the extracellular calcium concentration, vitamin D, beta-adrenergic agonists, and histamine (H_2 receptors) have been shown to modulate PTH release (6,7). With the exception of vitamin D, however, their physiological importance remains to be determined.

The synthesis of PTH starts as preproPTH in polyribosomes located within the parathyroid cell matrix. The preproPTH is converted to proPTH by enzymatic activity in or near the reticular membrane. ProPTH is converted to PTH in the Golgi apparatus. The intact hormone, which contains 84 amino acids, gains access to the extracellular fluid by exocytosis. It is metabolized by the liver (and to a lesser extent by the kidneys) into an amino and a carboxy fragment. The amino-terminal fragment is the biologically active segment and has a half-life in the circulation of less than 5 min. The carboxy-terminal fragment has a half-life of approximately 30–40 min. The latter is significantly increased in patients with renal insufficiency, since filtration and excretion by the kidney is the only route of removal of this fragment from the circulation. The amino-terminal fragment is also (to a lesser extent) removed by the kidney, by both glomerular filtration and tubular uptake and secretion. The principal action of PTH is to raise extracellular fluid calcium by increasing renal tubular reabsorption of calcium, mobilizing calcium from bone and increasing intestinal calcium absorption (8).

PTH enhances calcium reabsorption in the cortical thick ascending limb of Henle's loop as well as in the distal tubule by binding to receptors located in the basal membranes of cells in these nephron segments and stimulating adenylate cyclase activity (9). PTH, through its amino fragment, can activate osteocytes, osteoblasts, and their precursors (10). It can have either an anabolic (at low concentration) or a catabolic effect (at high concentration). These functions are also initiated through the activation of cyclic AMP.

Besides its direct action on the renal tubule and bone, PTH participates in calcium absorption by the gut through vitamin D activation. Vitamin D is made available in the diet (D_2, D_3), with absorption taking place in the upper part of the small intestine. It then enters the circulation primarily through the thoracic duct in the chylomicron fraction (11). Vitamin D is also made available through photosynthesis (ultraviolet light) in the skin, where previtamin D_3 is formed from 7-dehydrocholesterol. The previtamin D_3 so formed undergoes isomerization, resulting in vitamin D_3 formation. The latter is subsequently transferred to the circulation (12). Vitamin D_3, through carrier proteins, is transported to the liver and undergoes 25-hydroxylation, a reaction catalyzed by both mitochondrial and microsomal enzymes collectively designated vitamin D_3-25 hydroxylase. The synthesis of 25-hydroxyvitamin D_3 [25 $(OH)D_3$] can be inhibited by 1,25-dihydroxyvitamin D_3 [1,25$(OH)_2D_3$] through an increase in hepatocyte cytosolic calcium (13,14). In the kidney, 25$(OH)D_3$ undergoes further hydroxylation by the mitochondrial enzymes, 25-hydroxyvitamin D_3-1 hydroxylase to form 1,25$(OH)_2D_3$ and 25-hydroxyvitamin D_3-24 hydroxylase to form 24,25$(OH)_2D_3$. This process takes place in the proximal tubule. 1,25$(OH)_2D_3$ affects active calcium transport throughout the intestinal tract, with the ileum being the major site adapting to changes in dietary calcium (15). In the enterocyte, the effect of 1,25$(OH)_2D_3$ depends on its binding to a protein receptor, located primarily in the nucleus, resulting in an increased synthesis of messenger RNA for a calcium-binding protein within the intestinal cell. In addition, 1,25$(OH)_2D_3$ increases the uptake of calcium at the brush border of the intestinal cell, facilitating its movement into the cell (16). 1,25$(OH)_2D_3$ is also involved in the mobilization of calcium from bone, an action that is dependent, in part, on the presence of PTH (17). Finally, 1,25$(OH)_2D_3$, through receptors located on parathyroid cells (18), exerts a direct inhibitory effect on PTH synthesis, probably by inhibiting PTH gene transcription (19).

The current view of calcium homeostasis in the normal adult provides a minimal role for bone in the physiological maintenance of plasma calcium, which is determined primarily by the relationship between the rate of calcium absorption from the gut (a vitamin D-dependent phenomenon) and the renal threshold for calcium (a largely PTH-dependent phenomenon) (20).

Calcitonin (CT) is a 32-amino acid hormone derived from a larger polypeptide. This hormone is synthesized by the C cells located throughout the thyroid gland. Its action results from binding to specific membrane receptors of target cells (osteoblasts and perhaps osteocytes) with subsequent stimulation of cyclic AMP. CT synthesis correlates positively with changes in plasma calcium (21). Male subjects usually have a greater secretory capacity for CT than females. CT levels do not change with age (22). The physiological importance of CT as a plasma calcium regulator in humans remains to be defined.

B. Changes in the Calcium-PTH-Vitamin D_3 Axis with Age

Serum calcium (total and ionized fractions) does not generally change with age. In some studies, however, younger subjects were found to have a significantly higher total serum calcium than their older counterparts (23,24). This might be due to the fact that the serum albumin level decreases with age (25). PTH increases gradually with age, and in subjects past the age of 60 may reach values two times the level observed in younger adults (23,24,26–28). As seen in Fig. 1, the variation among patients is rather wide, however. The parathyroid glands undergo involutional changes with aging, manifested by an increase in oxyphil compared with chief cells. Furthermore, the oxyphil cells become hyperplastic and, given the capacity to synthesize and secrete PTH, these changes could account, in part, for the age-related increase in circulating PTH (29). The gradual decrease in GFR seen with age may also explain the elevated PTH, since in most studies where creatinine clearance was measured, an inverse correlation was found between these two parameters (24,27). Besides the structural changes to the parathyroid glands and the lower GFR, the decrease in intestinal calcium absorption seen with aging may also play a role (30). After

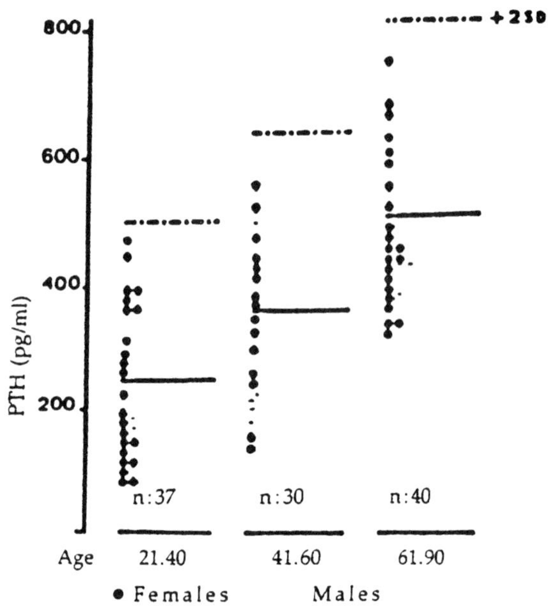

Figure 1 Distribution of individual serum PTH concentrations in 107 normal subjects aged 21 to 90 years. One normal subject, 75 years old, with the highest PTH value (1700 pg/ml) was omitted in the scattergram. (From Chapuy MC, Durr F, Chapuy P. Age-related changes in parathyroid hormone and 25-hydroxycholecalciferol levels. J Gerontol 1983; 38:19–22).

the oral administration of pharmacological doses of $25(OH)D_3$, PTH decreases significantly in the elderly (31).

The reason that intestinal calcium absorption decreases in the elderly is not fully understood, but is of clinical importance since an increase in calcium absorption is the principal mechanism preventing negative calcium balance when dietary calcium intake is decreased (32). This adaptation is impaired in the elderly (33), which explains why the amount of calcium required to prevent negative calcium balance increases with age (34). A possible explanation for the decreased calcium absorption in the elderly is a decrease in plasma $1,25(OH)_2D_3$ levels (30,35–37), as shown in Fig. 2. As noted above, calcium absorption and $1,25(OH)_2D_3$ levels increase in these patients after administration of a pharmacological dose of $25(OH)D_3$ (31). It should be emphasized, however, that the decreased $1,25(OH)_2D_3$ has not been a universal finding (27), but may be of clinical significance in approximately one-third of elderly subjects (38). Moreover, in one study the

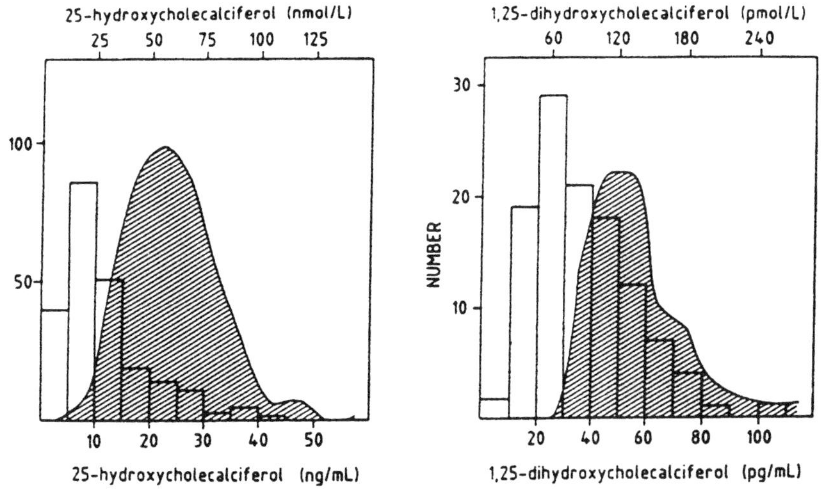

Figure 2 Histogram of the concentration of 25-hydroxycholecalciferol and 1,25-dihydroxycholecalciferol in elderly patients. Conversion of SI to traditional units: for 25-hydroxycholecalciferol, 1 nmol/liter ≈ 0.4 pg/ml. (From Bouillon RA, Subverx JH, Lissens WD, Pelemans WK. Vitamin D status in the elderly: seasonal substrate deficiency causes 1,25-dihydroxycholecalciferol deficiency. Am J Clin Nutr 1987;45: 755–763.

change in calcium absorption did not correlate with the change in plasma $1,25(OH)_2D_3$ (31). In the elderly with low $1,25(OH)_2D_3$,factors such as a decrease in the sensitivity of the enzyme 1 alpha-hydroxylase to PTH and/or an increase in the catabolic rate of $1,25(OH)_2D_3$ might be operative (30,39–42). The plasma $25(OH)D_3$ level is frequently low in the elderly (38,43,44). This finding is more common in European countries than in the United States, in house-bound and institutionalized elderly (45,46), and during the winter months (36). In parts of the world where sunlight is more available and where milk is routinely fortified with vitamin D, this tendency is less common (47). The problem is also compounded by the fact that the skin in the elderly has a greatly diminished capacity to produce previtamin D_3 (48). A summary of the interactions among serum calcium, PTH, and vitamin D is provided in Fig. 3.

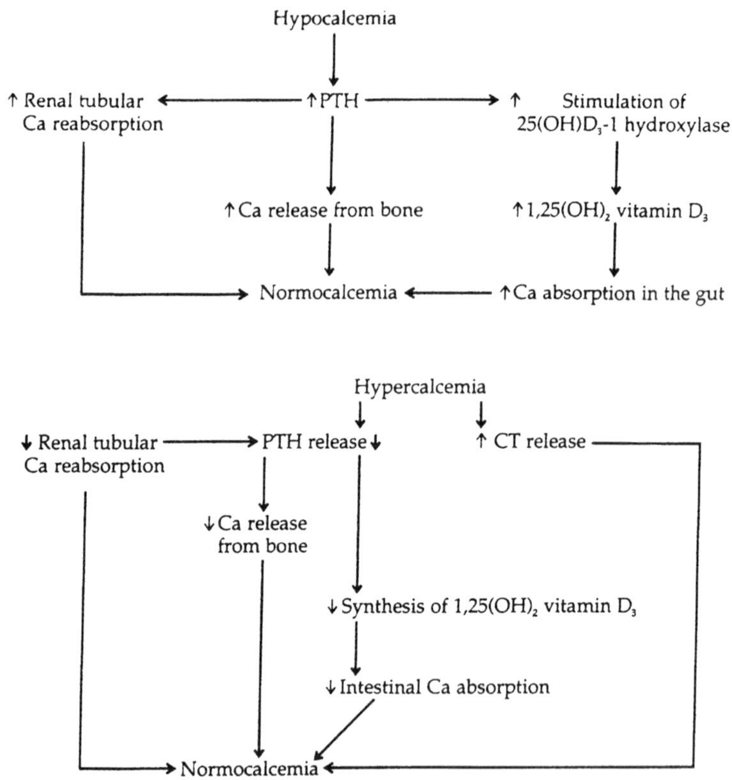

Figure 3 Summary of the relationships between serum calcium, PTH, and vitamin D. CT = calcitonin.

II. HYPERCALCEMIA

A. Incidence and Prevalence

In a screening of 15,903 subjects, Christenson et al. (49) found 95 (0.60%) who had hypercalcemia, with 28 (29%) over the age of 60. A marked female preponderance (25 versus 3) was noted. Two to three percent of elderly patients admitted to long-term facilities were found to be hypercalcemic, 60% of whom were females (50,51). We found hypercalcemia in 12 (3.0%) (9 females, 3 males) of 400 consecutive elderly patients admitted to our hospital for a variety of reasons in whom a serum calcium determination was available.

B. Etiology

The most common causes of hypercalcemia in the elderly are similar to those noted in younger subjects, with primary hyperparathyroidism, malignancy, and drug toxicity (thiazides, vitamin A and D) accounting for well over 80% of the cases. Other etiologies include increased production and/or sensitivity to $1,25(OH)_2D_3$, benign familial hypercalcemia, adrenal insufficiency, hyperthyroidism, and patients in the recovery phase of acute renal failure secondary to rhabdomyolysis.

C. Clinical Manifestations and Pathogenesis

Since calcium plays an important role in the metabolism of every cell, it is not surprising that symptoms produced by hypercalcemia relate to practically every organ. Some of the common symptoms are outlined in Table 1. These symptoms

Table 1 Clinical Manifestations Reported in Association with Hypercalcemia

Central nervous system (very common in the elderly)
Headache
Impaired concentration
Memory defects
Personality changes
Confusion
Lethargy
Renal
Polyuria
Nephrocalcinosis
Acute/chronic renal failure
Gastrointestinal
Anorexia, nausea
Changes in bowel motility: constipation
Pancreatitis
Cardiovascular
Cardiac arrhythmias, heart block
Hypertension
Vascular calcification
Musculo-skeletal
Muscle weakness
Acute arthritis, arthralgia
Ocular
Conjunctival calcification
Band keratopathy

can occur in any combination, with no specific pattern for a specific etiology. In general, the severity of symptoms is proportionate to the level and rate of rise of the serum calcium.

1. Primary Hyperparathyroidism

Primary hyperparathyroidism is the single most common cause of hypercalcemia in the elderly, with the incidence increasing steadily with age, reaching 92 per year per 100,000 males and 188 per year per 100,000 females over the age of 60 at the Mayo Clinic (Fig. 4) (52). An even higher incidence of 250 per year per 100,000 for women over 65 was found by Marx (53). As noted, the disease is more common in the female, with a 7:3 female-to-male ratio. The estimated prevalence has been placed between 1% and 10% in one study involving a relatively small number of elderly males in the United States (54). Evaluating a

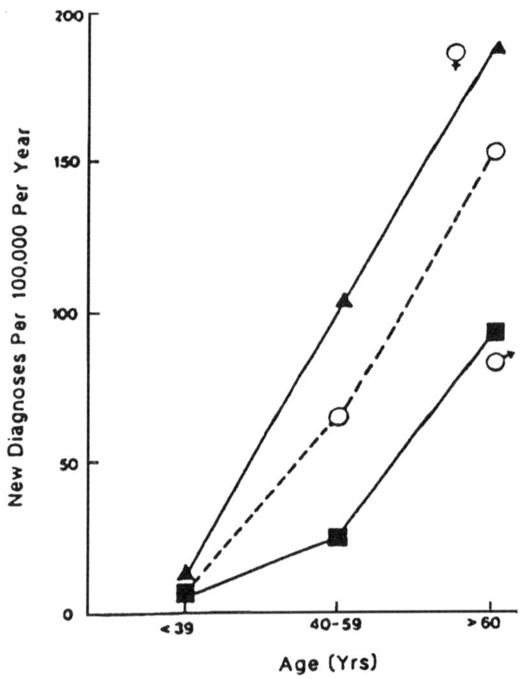

Figure 4 Incidence with which primary hyperparathyroidism is discovered in subjects of various ages in Rochester, Minnesota. The disease is very rare in subjects below age 40 but grows increasingly common thereafter. Dashed line equals average incidence. (From Mallette LE. Review: primary hyperparathyroidism, an update; incidence, etiology, diagnosis and treatment. Am J Med Sci 1987; 293:239–249.)

larger number of elderly patients in Sweden, Tibblin et al. (55) suggested a prevalence of 1.5%. More recently, however, Wermers et al. (55a) noted a decrease in the prevalence of the disease in Rochester, Minnesota. A single adenoma was responsible for the hyperparathyroidism in approximately 90% of the elderly, with multiple adenomas rarely found (56). Hyperplasia accounts for the remaining 10%. Hyperparathyroidism associated with one of the multiple endocrine neoplasias is usually diagnosed at a younger age.

Carcinoma of the parathyroids can also be associated with an elevated parathyroid hormone level and hypercalcemia. It is not clear how often this entity occurs in the elderly. In two earlier reviews, comprising a total of 66 patients reported prior to 1970, only 2 patients (3%) were over the age of 60 (57,58). In more recent reviews, 30% of the reported patients were elderly (59,59a). This change in trend might be due to the fact that more elderly with hypercalcemia undergo extensive clinical evaluation and surgery, rather than a true change in incidence. The etiology of parathyroid adenomas is not known, but it is clear that changes in serum calcium can still influence PTH secretion in most patients, except that the calcium inhibitory set point, defined as the calcium level required to inhibit 50% of PTH release, is shifted toward a higher calcium value (60,61). A lack of complete suppressibility can be found in some adenomas; however, it has also been shown that the abnormal control of PTH secretion might be related to alterations in calcium transport across the plasma membrane of adenomatous cells (62), perhaps as a consequence of decreased sensitivity of the calcium-sensing receptor of the parathyroid gland to extracellular calcium (5,63,64). Once the new set point is achieved in the individual patient, there is then a higher blood–bone calcium equilibrium (65).

For most patients with primary hyperparathyroidism, bone volume is maintained, since the high bone turnover rate results from a parallel increase in both osteoclastic and osteoblastic activity (66). Calcium losses from bone, therefore, play a relatively minor role in the hypercalcemia of hyperparathyroidism. Rather, the hypercalcemia is maintained primarily by an increase in gut absorption and renal distal tubular reabsorption of calcium. In a small number of patients the hypercalcemia may be due to an alteration in the balance between osteoclastic and osteoblastic activity, which also results in overt bone disease (osteitis fibrosa cystica or bone fractures). Interleukin-6 and tumor necrosis factor-α may be involved in the pathogenesis of the bone loss (66a). Interestingly, the plasma $1,25(OH)_2D_3$ level and creatinine clearance have been found to be significantly lower in this group compared to the group in "equilibrium" (37). In approximately 50% of the cases, hyperparathyroidism is discovered by the finding of hypercalcemia during a routine biochemical screening (67).

The clinical manifestations in elderly patients are similar to those of younger patients. The frequency with which they occur in each group varies somewhat, however. As seen in Table 2, neuromuscular complaints (changes in mentation, muscle weakness, asthenia, and fatigue) are the most common clinical manifestation of hyperparathyroidism in the elderly, occurring in 29% compared to 16% in younger patients, in whom renal problems predominate (55,68,69). The prevalence of hyperparathyroidism in a psychogeriatric clinic was found to be approximately 5%, mainly among those with newly diagnosed organic brain syndrome (70). The reason for the increased incidence of central nervous dysfunction in the elderly, which does not necessarily relate to the severity of the hypercalcemia (71), is not clear, but could reflect the compromised cerebral blood supply in the aged. Physical examination in patients complaining of weakness and easy fatigability may reveal proximal muscle weakness, more common in the lower extremities, muscle atrophy, hyperactive deep tendon reflexes, and tongue fasciculations. A neck mass may be palpable, particularly if carcinoma is present. Serum glutamic-oxalacetic transaminase, creatinine phosphokinase, and aldolase levels are, in general, within normal range (72).

Nephrolithiasis and renal insufficiency (due to nephrocalcinosis and/or dehydration) are the most common renal manifestations of hyperparathyroidism. When submitted to a 1000-mg calcium load, patients with a marked elevation of $1,25(OH)_2D_3$, hypercalcuria, and intestinal hyperabsorption are more prone to these renal complications (73). The incidence of nephrocalcinosis and nephrolithiasis is lower in the elderly with hyperparathyroidism compared with younger patients and may be explained by the decreased filtered load of calcium due to a decrease in GFR and decreased levels of $1,25(OH)_2D_3$. It should be noted, however, that the metabolic profile alone does not always distinguish stone-forming from non-stone-forming patients with primary hyperparathy-

Table 2 Presenting Symptoms in Surgically Verified Hyperparathyroidism at Different Ages

Symptoms and signs	< 60 Years of age (%) (n = 74)	> 60 Years of age (%) (n = 112)	≥ 70 Years of age (%) (n = 61)
Neuromuscular	16	31	44
Renal	41	19	10
Hypercalcemia crisis	4	4	3
Gastrointestinal	1	1	2
Skeletal abnormalities	2	1	—
Miscellaneous	3	—	2
Incidental finding of elevated serum Ca	31	42	39

Source: Tibblin S, Palsson N, Rydberg J. Hyperparathyroidism in the elderly. Ann Surg 1983; 197: 135–138.

roidism (74). Therefore, other, as yet unidentified factors are probably playing a role. Hypertension is more common in the elderly with primary hyperparathyroidism than in younger patients when compared with an age-matched control group (75). The hypertension may be corrected after parathyroidectomy (76,77). Although a correlation has been found between blood pressure and PTH level in the elderly (77a), the mechanisms by which an elevated PTH level and hypercalcemia increase the blood pressure have not been completely elucidated (78). Plasma renin and aldosterone have been reported to be either normal (79,80) or elevated (77). Plasma catecholamine levels can be either normal (79) or elevated (81); however, hypertensive hyperparathyroid patients have a more marked response to norepinephrine infusion compared to controls (77,81). The change in sensitivity of vascular smooth muscle cells to the vasoconstrictive effect of circulating catecholamines may be secondary to the modulating effect of the parathyroid hypertensive factor (PHF) on basal intracellular calcium. The chemical structure of PHF, a substance released by the parathyroid gland, has not been determined (81a). Others (82) have found an inverse relationship between blood pressure and serum phosphate level.

Gastrointestinal complaints (peptic ulcer, gastritis, chronic constipation) may bring the patient to medical attention. These symptoms most likely reflect the effect of calcium on gastric acid secretion and on smooth muscle contractility. Hypercalcemic crisis occurs in the elderly (usually in those with some degree of preexisting mild renal insufficiency) who develop a rapid rise in their serum calcium, occasionally as high as 20 mg/dl (83–85). Volume contraction, either from poor intake due to intercurrent illness (infection, etc.) or from increased losses (diarrhea, diuretics, urine concentrating defect), is the triggering factor in the majority of cases. These patients manifest central nervous system symptoms including confusion, stupor, and unresponsiveness, which are reversible with volume expansion but tend to lag beyond the fall in serum calcium. PTH levels are usually very high (20-fold increase) in these patients.

The diagnosis of primary hyperparathyroidism should be confirmed by the measurement of parathyroid hormone. Currently, most laboratories measure the intact parathyroid hormone. There assays are more sensitive than those which measure the mid-region or C-terminal fragment (86–88). An elevated PTH will be found in over 90% of patients with hyperparathyroidism (89). In the remaining 5–7% patients, the PTH value will be in the high-normal range. In these patients, other confirmatory tests might be necessary. Urinary cyclic AMP (expressed as a function of GFR—as long as the latter is above 25 ml/min) is usually elevated in these patients (90). Unfortunately, high levels may also be found in patients with hypercalcemia of malignancy or sarcoidosis, decreasing its diagnostic value substantially (91,92). Other approaches include a variety of noninvasive methods for gland localization, such as high-resolution real-time ultrasonography. This imaging technique, which is very much operator dependant, can detect abnormal glands in 78–86% of cases (93–95). There is a 4–25% false positive and a 6–11% false negative rate. Tumors less than 1 mm in size and those located intrathoracically are usually not detected with this technique. Computed tomography (CT) scanning can identify 40–85% of abnormal parathyroid glands. It is particularly helpful for identifying ectopic glands. It has a false positive rate of 6–38% and a false negative rate of 44% (96–98). The accuracy for both studies combined (ultrasonography and CT) is estimated to be 91% (99). Parathyroid imaging using (^{99m}Tc)-sestamibi (hexakis-2-methoxy-isobutyl isonitrile) has a sensitivity of 85–95% and a false positive rate of 0–15%. It is quite sensitive in detecting single parathyroid adenomas and might detect tumors located in the mediastinum. Its value is somewhat limited when hyperplasia is present. The technique can also be of help in locating glands in patients requiring reexploration of the neck (100,101). Magnetic resonance imaging has also been used, with a sensitivity rate of 57–90%. False positives (9–25%) do occur when enlarged lymph nodes are mistaken for parathyroid adenomas. This diagnostic procedure is particularly useful for detecting parathyroid glands in patients with recurring disease and in those with ectopic glands (102–104).

Primary hyperparathyroidism and nonparathyroid malignancy may be present simultaneously in an elderly patient with hypercalcemia (105,106). If such a patient has superimposed renal insufficiency (as is commonly the case), reaching a definitive diagnosis presents some difficulty. Ljunghall et al. (107,108), attempted to differentiate between these two possibilities by measuring serum calcium and PTH prior to and approximately 8 hr after a single intramuscular injection of 100 IU of calcitonin. This dose of calcitonin is usually associated with a 3–5% decrease in serum calcium, which will result in a 10% or greater increase in serum PTH in patients with hyperparathyroidism (positive response). No significant change in PTH is seen in patients with nonparathyroid hypercalcemia (negative response). A negative response, however, does not necessarily rule out hyperparathyroidism (109). Furthermore, the diagnostic value of this test in patients with hypercalcemia and advanced renal insufficiency (serum creatinine > 5 mg/dl) remains to be determined. In these patients a careful interpretation of all the tests described above is necessary.

a. Normocalcemic Hyperparathyroidism. A small number of elderly patients will have persistently normal to high-normal serum calcium levels despite the presence of hyperparathyroidism. The diagnosis of hyperparathyroidism is usually uncovered in these patients during the investigation for hypophosphatemia. In these patients, the PTH is elevated and the tubular reabsorption of phosphorus is low. $1,25(OH)_2D_3$ is usually normal, as is the urinary calcium excretion. A resistance to the effect of PTH on tubular calcium reabsorption has been postulated as a probable mechanism for the normocalcemia (110).

2. Malignancy

Malignancy is the most common cause for hypercalcemia in the hospitalized elderly, and both our own experience and the literature suggest that it occurs in 8.5–10% of adult patients with cancer (111,112). The pathogenesis of hypercalcemia in malignancy may differ depending on the type of tumor. Mundy and Martin (113) have described three tumor categories: (a) solid tumors with metastasis (most common); (b) solid tumors without metastasis (least common); (c) hematological malignancies.

a. Solid Tumors with Metastasis. The tumors associated with hypercalcemia due primarily to metastases in the elderly is summarized in Table 3, which is derived from our own experience combined with that of Ray and Rao (114). Approximately three-quarters of these patients were known to have bone metastases when hypercalcemia was first noted; however, it should be emphasized that the presence of bone metastases does not necessarily imply a causal relationship between the metastases and the hypercalcemia, since fewer than 30% of patients with bone metastases develop hypercalcemia (115). Furthermore, an inverse, rather than a direct, correlation has been found between the number of bone metastases and serum calcium levels in patients with cancer-related hypercalcemia (116). The hypercalcemia in these patients is primarily the result of increased bone resorption by the tumor through one or more of the following mechanisms: (a) pressure atrophy with subsequent infarction of surrounding bone and calcium release into the extracellular fluid (115); (b) release of prote-

Table 3 Hypercalcemia Associated with Metastatic Carcinoma

Primary tumor site	Number of patients (%)	Patients with known metastatic disease at diagnosis of hypercalcemia (%)
Lungs	11 (29.7)	8 (72.7)
Breasts	8 (21.6)	7 (87.5)
Head/neck	6 (16.2)	4 (66.7)
Renal	5 (13.5)	5 (100.0)
Others:	7 (19.0)	4 (57.1)
(Thyroid, 2)		
(Colon, 2)		
(Genitalia, 3)		

Source: Adapted from Ray AK, Rao DB. Hypercalcemia and malignant disease in the elderly: magnesium sulfate therapy. J Am Geriatr Soc 1974; 22:413–415. Modified to include our own experience.

olytic enzymes (117); (c) stimulation of osteoclastic activity by locally tumor-induced production of prostaglandins and/or other factors such as osteoclastic-activating factor from tumor-derived activated lymphocytes (118).

In 70% of the patients we examined, a decrease in glomerular filtration rate (GFR) was present. The low GFR may contribute to the hypercalcemia by de-

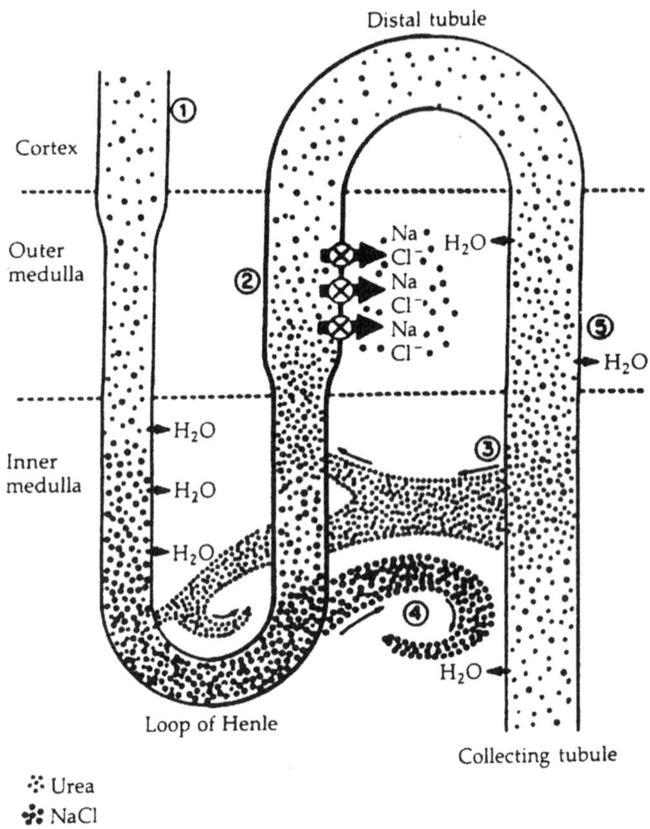

Figure 5 Schematic drawing of the potential sites of action of calcium that alter function of the renal concentrating mechanism. Site 1 = delivery of water and solute to the medulla; site 2 = active sodium chloride transport across the thick ascending limb of Henle; site 3 = urea transport across the medullary collecting duct; site 4 = sodium chloride abstraction across the thin ascending limb of Henle; site 5 = hydroosmotic transfer of water across collecting duct epithelium under the influence of antidiuretic hormone (ADH). (From Goldfarb S, Agus ZS. Mechanism of the polyuria of hypercalcemia. Am J Nephrol 1984; 4:69–76, and modified from Kokko JP. Renal concentrating and diluting mechanisms. Hosp Pract 1979; 14:110–116.)

creasing the filtered calcium load. In the majority of patients, volume contraction due to poor oral intake and the polyuria which frequently accompanies hypercalcemia (119) were responsible for the decrease in GFR, since the BUN and serum creatinine returned to normal after volume expansion and lowering of the serum calcium. Figure 5 diagrams the many ways by which hypercalcemia can alter the renal concentrating mechanism. In the remaining patients, renal insufficiency was secondary either to a direct effect of the elevated calcium on the glomerulus (120), obstructive uropathy, or acute tubular necrosis. PTH, nephrogenic cyclic AMP, and $1,25(OH)_2D_3$ are either low or normal in these patients, so that increased renal or intestinal absorption of calcium do not appear to contribute to the hypercalcemia (121).

b. Solid Tumors Without Metastases. Table 4 summarizes the types of tumors and their relative distribution in 76 elderly hypercalcemic subjects with solid tumors without metastases, also called "humoral hypercalcemia" (122). Increased bone resorption resulting in skeletal calcium loss through systemically released humoral mediators synthesized by the malignant cell is primarily responsible for the hypercalcemia (66). In some patients, besides volume contraction and a direct effect of growth factors to lower the GFR (123,124), there may also be an increase in tubular calcium reabsorption (125,126). Both the site and the mechanism(s) of this increased reabsorption remain to be elucidated. Gut calcium absorption is decreased in this group (127,128). The specific humoral mediators involved in producing the hypercalcemia are described in Table 5 (129) and include transforming growth factor which can stimulate osteoclastic bone resorption and a PTH-related protein (PTHRP). The latter is a protein with significant sequence homology in the NH_2-terminal region of PTH (130,131) and may be elevated in 45–55% of hypercalcemic patients with an associated malignancy

Table 4 Humoral Hypercalcemia

Primary tumor site	Number of patients (%)
Lungs	22 (28.9)
Kidneys	15 (19.7)
Urogenital	15 (19.7)
Gastrointestinal (including liver)	15 (19.7)
Breasts	7 (9.2)
Head/neck	2 (2.8)
Total	76 (100)

Source: Skrabanck P, McPartlin J, Powell D. Tumor hypercalcemia and "ectopic hyperparathyroidism." Medicine 1980; 59:262–282.

Table 5 Pathogenetic Classification of the Hypercalcemia of Cancer

Clinical group	Types of tumors	Bone histological studies	Radiological bone studies	Other laboratory features	Other factors implicated	Local or systemic
Hematological cancers	Myeloma, lymphosarcoma, Burkitt's lymphoma, adult T-cell lymphoma	Increase in osteoclastic bone resorption adjacent to neoplastic cells	Mainly osteolytic lesions; occasionally diffuse osteopenia		Osteoclastic-activating factor: 1,25-dihydroxy vitamin D	Local
					PTH[a]-related protein	Systemic
Solid tumors with bone metastases	Breast, lung, pancreatic	Increase in local osteoclastic bone resorption; variable osteoblastic response	Discrete lytic lesions; variable sclerotic response		Prostaglandins: direct erosion by tumor cells	Local
Solid tumors without metastases	Lung, kidney, pancreatic, ovarian, breast	Increased osteoclastic bone resorption; decreased bone formation	No abnormality	Increase in fractional excretion of phosphate; increase in nephrogenous cyclic AMP; decrease in immunoreactive PTH	1. PTH-related protein 2. Prostaglandins 3. Transforming growth factors 4. Colony-stimulating activity 5. PTH	Systemic

[a]PTH = parathyroid hormone.

Source: Mundy GR, et al. The hypercalcemia of cancer: clinical implications and pathogenic mechanisms. N ENgl J Med 1984; 310:1718–1727, with modifications.

(132,133). This protein has been shown to enhance osteoclastic bone resorption in vitro, and its hypercalcemic effect can be averted by using an antiserum capable of neutralizing its activity (134). Concurrent other factors present in the cancer patient, such as tumor growth factor alpha, interleukin-1, and tumor necrosis factor, most likely play a modifying role as far as the hypercalcemic response to PTHRP is concerned (135).

c. Hematological Malignancies. Multiple myeloma is the most common hematological malignancy associated with hypercalcemia. These patients have increased bone resorption, the result of locally produced cytokines (lymphotoxin) secreted by the malignant cells (136). Other bone-resorbing factors such as interleukin-1, found in monocytic malignancy (137), and $1,25(OH)_2D3$ have been reported in some patients with lymphomas (138,139) (Table 5). In addition to the release of Ca from bone in patients with multiple myeloma, the hypercalcemia is frequently augmented by the presence of a decreased GFR (140). Several factors may be responsible for the renal insufficiency associated with multiple myeloma: (a) direct effects of the tumor, including myeloma kidney, amyloidosis, light-chain nephropathy, and hyperviscosity; (b) nephrotoxicity due to antibiotic treatment or radiographic contrast media; (c) hypercalcemia and hyperuricemia (rare); (d) severe volume contraction; or (e) sepsis.

In addition to the clinical manifestations of hypercalcemia described earlier, bone pain (due to direct lysis of bone or pathological fracture) may be the primary reason a patient with hypercalcemia due to metatastic disease seeks medical attention.

3. Drug-Induced Hypercalcemia

In our experience, thiazide diuretics are the most common cause of drug-induced hypercalcemia. In a minority of patients the increase is mild (serum calcium of 10.5–10.8 mg/dl), and since the ionized calcium is normal, the hypercalcemia represents an increase in the fraction bound to the elevated serum albumin secondary to volume contraction. In most patients, however, the ionized calcium is increased (141). Since the normal negative correlation between ionized calcium and PTH is well maintained, the drug appears to exert its effect directly on calcium metabolism. Indeed, thiazides enhance distal tubular calcium reabsorption (142), but this effect is not essential for the development of hypercalcemia, since it may occur in patients on hemodialysis (143). It has been shown that thiazides directly stimulate calcium release from bone (144). Patients with thiazide-induced hypercalcemia are usually elderly, asymptomatic females taking the drug for hypertension. The hypercalcemia may be seen early or up to 15 years after the institution of therapy. Since this complication occurs most frequently in the elderly female, an age at which primary hyperparathyroidism is also most prevalent, the latter should be ruled out, particularly if hypercalcemia persists despite discontinuing the diuretic (145).

Excess of vitamins A and D can also produce hypercalcemia. It is not clear how often hypercalcemia due to vitamin A intoxication occurs in the elderly. In general, reported patients have been younger (146). The diagnosis can be confirmed by history and measurement of the serum vitamin A level. Hypercalcemia may develop in patients taking large doses of vitamin D, over 20,000 units/day. A greater than 10-fold increase in $25(OH)D_3$ is seen in these patients; $1,25(OH)_2D_3$ may also be increased. The hypercalcemia probably represents a direct effect of the high levels of $25(OH)D_3$ on $1,25(OH)_2D_3$ receptors (147). There may be an additional effect of the 1,25 analog itself, when elevated.

4. Hypercalcemia Due to Increased Production and/or Sensitivity to $1,25(OH)_2D_3$

Patients with granulomatous disorders such as sarcoidosis, tuberculosis, fungal diseases, leprosy, and berylliosis may develop hypercalcemia. Clinical manifestations are usually those of the underlying disease, with an occasional patient presenting with urolithiasis secondary to hypercalciuria (particularly with sarcoidosis). $1,25(OH)_2D_3$ has been found to be increased in these hypercalcemic patients, most likely as a consequence of increased hydroxylation of available $25(OH)D_3$ by 1-hydroxylase produced by the granulomas macrophages (148). An increase in bone resorption and intestinal calcium absorption due to the elevated $1,25(OH)_2D_3$ are probably responsible for the hypercalcemia (149).

5. Benign Familial Hypercalcemia

A small number of patients (7–10%) with benign familial hypercalcemia will be 60 years or older at the time hypercalcemia is discovered (150). The disease is inherited as an autosomal dominant disorder with greater than 90% penetrance and is associated with a mutation in the human calcium-sensing receptor gene (151). Complaints similar to those found in hyperparathyroidism, such as fatigue, weakness, and mental changes, are more frequently reported in these patients. Chondrocalcinosis is common. A positive family history, a tendency toward hypermagnesemia, hypocalciuria (calcium:creatinine clearance ratio < 0.018), and the absence of parathyroid gland enlargement with high-resolution parathyroid ultrasonography and other imaging techniques helps differentiate this syndrome from hyperparathyroidism (152,153), particularly in the occasional patient who exhibits some degree of hypophosphatemia. Because of the defect in the calcium-sensing gene, patients have a mild to moderate resistance to the inhibitory effect of extracellular calcium on PTH secretion; their calciuric response to hypercalcemia is blunted, as well as their homeostatic response to a low calcium diet (154).

6. Other Causes of Hypercalcemia

In recent years the milk-alkali syndrome has been reported with increasing frequency in elderly females ingesting a large quantity (4–12 g) of calcium and alkali (calcium carbonate) as prophylaxis for osteoporosis (154a). The typical patient presents with hypercalcemia and metabolic alkalosis. Serum calcium as high as 22 mg/dl has been reported; the serum bicarbonate is usually greater than 28 mEq/L. Renal insufficiency of varying severity is a universal finding. Serum PTH is generally appropriately suppressed. Since calcium carbonate can be purchased over the counter, patients should be asked specifically about its use (154a).

Hypercalcemia may be seen in association with pheochromocytoma (due to parathyroid hyperplasia) or may be present as part of the multiple endocrine neoplasia syndromes, which, as noted earlier, are rarely initially diagnosed in the elderly. In patients with adrenal insufficiency, hypercalcemia is not uncommon and is, for the most part, secondary to hemoconcentration. The hypercalcemia seen with hyperthyroidism is generally mild. It results from a direct effect of thyroid hormone on bone mobilization. Serum PTH and 1,25(OH)D_3 are suppressed and serum phosphate is elevated (155). The urinary excretion of hydroxyproline and calcium are increased (156).

D. Treatment of Hypercalcemia in the Elderly

The therapy of hypercalcemia can be divided into two stages: (a) emergency therapy, and (b) specific therapy.

1. Emergency Therapy

In general, no correlation exists between the severity of symptomatology and the level of hypercalcemia, so every symptomatic patient, independent of the calcium level, and any patient with a serum calcium greater than 13 mg/dl, should receive emergency treatment.

a. Fluids. As noted earlier, patients with hypercalcemia very often have poor fluid intake, which, when associated with a urinary concentration defect, is a perfect setup for profound dehydration. We usually start fluid replacement with an infusion of normal saline, 200 ml per hour, with constant monitoring of urinary output, particularly in patients with an elevated serum creatinine. Naturally, signs of fluid overload should be looked for. Since calcium reabsorption in the proximal tubule is significantly linked to sodium reabsorption, the natriuresis accompanying volume expansion will also induce a calciuresis. Attention should be paid to the loss of other electrolytes such as Mg and K.

b. Loop Diuretics. Intravenous furosemide (100 mg every 2 hr) has been used with volume expansion to treat hypercalcemia (157). By abolishing the lumen positive charge in the thick ascending limb, furosemide interferes indirectly with calcium reabsorption, which potentiates the effect of saline expansion (158). This combination requires even more careful fluid monitoring, since larger urinary losses than these accompanying saline expansion alone must be replaced.

c. Calcitonin. Calcitonin lowers the serum calcium by inhibiting bone resorption and by decreasing renal tubular reabsorption (159). The resulting hypercalciuria can occur as early as 30 min after administration of the drug and last up to 3 hr (160). The exact tubular site of action has not yet been identified. It should be noted that calcitonin at physiological levels does the opposite; i.e., it increases renal tubular calcium and magnesium reabsorption (160a). The drug can be administered either intramuscularly or intravenously at 4–8 IU/kg/day, given every 12 hr, A decrease in serum calcium is usually noted within 6–8 hr, Bone resorption can be inhibited up to 72 hr by calcitonin but returns to pretreatment status despite continuous administration of the drug because of down-regulation of calcitonin receptors on bone cells (161). This "escape" phenomenon can be delayed by concomitant administration of the equivalent of 100 mg of hydrocortisone every 6 hr, with gradual tapering (162). The mechanism of action of glucocorticoids in lowering serum calcium in this situation is not well understood (163).

d. Biphosphonates. Biphosphonates act by decreasing bone resorption and are associated with a decrease in the number of osteoclasts found in active bone turnover sites. Two preparations are currently available, etidronate and pamidronate. Etidronate is administered intravenously at the dose of 7.5 mg/kg of body weight. It is recommended that the drug be diluted in 250 ml of normal saline and administered over a minimum of 2 hr daily for 3–5 days. Etidronate disodium is very effective in treating the hypercalcemia of malignancy (164). Pamidronate is used at the dose of 1–1.5lmg/kg (60–90 mg) infused over 24 hr one time. It is more potent than etidronate (165) and the same given dose can be used in patients with varying degrees of renal insufficiency (166).

e. Plicamycin. Plicamycin is not recommended for the emergency treatment of hypercalcemia because it does not produce a decline in serum calcium for 24–36 hr. A dose of 15–25 mg/kg is given intravenously during a period of 4–24 hr. It should not be used in patients with renal insufficiency. This drug acts by reducing bone resorption and renal tubular calcium reabsorption (167,168).

Phosphates and sulfates have also been used in the emergency treatment of hypercalcemia. They are not in wide use in the United States at the present time.

2. *Specific Therapy*

After the serum calcium is acutely lowered, strategies for more chronic or definitive therapy can be planned.

a. Hyperparathyroidism. The surgical excision of the adenomatous gland is the treatment of choice for hyperparathyroidism, with normocalcemia achieved in over 95% of the patients. Persistent hypercalcemia in the remaining patients can be attributed to an inexperienced surgeon who failed to perform bilateral cervical exploration, abnormal localization of the tumor, or multiglandular disease (169,170). Patients who remain hypercalcemic require further localization studies prior to re-exploration of the neck. Besides the noninvasive procedures described earlier, selective angiography with venous sampling for parathyroid hormone is available and has a yield of 77%, comparable to that of the sestamibi scan and MRI (169,171). It is our belief that the former should be performed only in experienced centers (96,103). In patients with multiple hyperplastic glands, an intraoperative decrease of urinary cyclic AMP to normal levels has been shown to be helpful in determining the amount of parathyroid tissue to be removed (172). Postoperative hypocalcemia is the most commonly encountered problem. Its duration depends primarily on the extent of bone disease present at the time. This transient complication can be corrected early with the intravenous administration of calcium with regular monitoring of serum calcium. The addition of oral $1,25(OH)_2D_3$ will probably not shorten the time required to correct the hypocalcemia (173).

In 7% of patients, hypertension will persist postsurgery (174). In 14% of those with preexisting renal insufficiency, kidney function can actually worsen. In the remaining 86%, GFR either remains stable or improves (174). The rate of stone formation has been found to decrease from 0.36 to 0.02 per patient per year after surgery (175). In a small number of elderly patients with primary hyperparathyroidism, carcinoma is found. Evidence of local invasion of contiguous structures such as the thyroid, neck muscles, or esophagus is usually present. The characteristic histopathological picture is that of fibrous trabeculae, mitotic figures, and capsular or vascular invasion. Over 5 years of disease-free survival following surgery for parathyroid carcinoma is possible in 30% of elderly patients. Local recurrence or distant metastases (liver, lung, bone) occur in the remaining 70% (57–59a,176–186).

Although most clinicians agree that the presence of complications related to the hypercalcemic state, such as marked hypercalciuria (urinary calcium > 400 mg/g/creatinine), nephrocalcinosis (with or without associated renal insufficiency), bone disease (reduced cortical bone density, osteitis fibrosa), or a serum Ca > 12 mg/dl is an indication for surgery, controversy exists as to the best way of approaching the patient with mild asymptomatic hypercalcemia (serum calcium equal to or less than 11 mg/dl) or normocalcemia (67,179–186). Specific criteria are not available to predict which asymptomatic patient will subsequently develop complications. Our approach is based on the following factors: (a) 30–40% of patients observed over a long period of time will develop complications related to the hypercalcemic state, with no way to predict which patients will (181,187); (b) parathyroid surgery in the elderly performed by an experienced surgeon has a low morbidity and mortality rate, similar to that found in younger patients, and is also curative in a very high proportion of patients (68,188–191); (c) there is a high prevalence of metabolic bone disease (osteoporosis) as well as the risk that PTH will accelerate the rate of loss of appendicular bone in the elderly female (192–194). Therefore, we generally recommend surgery in all of our elderly patients with an established diagnosis of primary hyperparathyroidism unless other serious diseases associated with a limited life expectancy exist (e.g., unrelated malignancy, advanced cardiovascular disease) (195). Patients who refuse or are judged unsuitable candidates for surgery should be followed closely, even though some of these patients will have a relatively benign long-term course (196,197). Close follow-up should include periodic measurement of the serum calcium, urinary calcium excretion, kidney function, and bone densitometry (particularly in females). Emphasis should be placed on maintaining adequate hydration at all times. For those who have or develop symptoms or complications of the disease, medical therapy can be offered (198,199).

In the elderly female with hyperparathyroidism, conjugated estrogens (0.625–to 2.6 mg/day) can be used. These drugs lower serum calcium by acting directly on bone resorption through receptors located on the osteoblasts and on the parathyroid glands, reducing their response to a hypocalcemic stimulus (200). Serum concentrations of calcitonin and free $1,25(OH)_2D_3$ are not affected by this treatment (201,202). Patients with an intact uterus should receive medroxyprogesterone acetate, 10 mg/dl for 7–10 days every 2–3 months, in addition to estrogens, and undergo regular gynecological follow-up (203). Instead of the combination therapy referred to above, good results can be obtained by using norethindrone, 5 mg/day (202,204). This drug might be preferable in the elderly, since it has the added advantage of not producing undesirable effects on the uterus or blood clotting. Since both estradiol and progesterone can stimulate PTH release, there is a potential for worsening of the bone disease on a long-term basis (205). For inoperable males and females who fail to respond to either the estrogen and intermittent progesterone combination or norethindrone, the equivalent of 1500 mg of elemental phosphorus in four divided doses should be tried (206). The serum calcium, fasting Ca excretion, and urinary hydroxyproline may decrease with this therapy, whereas PTH either increases or remains unchanged. Since approximately 65% of the administered phosphorus is reabsorbed, this form of therapy is probably not safe to use in patients with preexisting renal insufficiency and in those with a serum calcium above 11.5 mg/dl. Oral diphosphonates represent another alternative to controlling hypercalcemia in hyperparathyroidism. Further studies are required to confirm their long-term benefits (196,207). Gallium nitrate has been found to lower serum calcium in patients with refractory hypercalcemia associated with parathyroid carcinoma (208). This drug acts by antagonizing the effect of PTH on bone resorptive activity.

b. Hypercalcemia of Malignancy. In addition to specific chemotherapeutic agents aimed at controlling the primary tumor, the patient should be encouraged to eat a regular salt diet (unless contraindicated) and take adequate fluids in order to maintain a normal extracellular fluid volume. Radiation therapy should be tried if bone pain and localized lesions are present. Gallium nitrate can be used either subcutaneously or intravenously. The recommended dosage is 200 mg/m^2 over a 5-day period. If the serum calcium is lowered in less than 5 days, the drug can be discontinued. It acts by increasing net bone formation and decreasing bone resorption. Excretion is entirely renal and should not be used if the serum creatinine is over 2 mg/dl (209). Several oral agents which lower serum calcium are available and can be added to the patient's therapeutic regimen, if necessary. Oral phosphate, 1–3 g daily, in three divided doses, can be used for patients with normal kidney function (209a). Magnesium sulfate, 15 g twice a day, has proved effective in one study involving a small number of elderly patients (114). Diarrhea is the most common side effect. The serum Mg level should be monitored in patients with renal insufficiency. Prednisone, 20–40 mg/day, is helpful in patients with hypercalcemia associated with lymphoproliferative disorders (myeloma, lymphomas producing 1,25$(OH)_2D_3$). Etidronate disodium, 20 mg/kg/day, by mouth is also available. Long-term studies of its efficacy, however, are lacking (210).

c. *Other.* Drug-induced hypercalcemia is best managed by discontinuing the offending agent. Short-term corticosteroid therapy might hasten recovery in patients with vitamin D intoxication. In hypercalcemia associated with tuberculosis and fungal infections or endocrinopathies, adequate therapy of the underlying disease is usually curative. Prednisone (40–60 mg with subsequent tapering) is used in sarcoidosis. The hypercalcemia of benign familial hypercalcemia can be managed conservatively, since complications related to the elevated calcium per se are rare.

The treatment of hypercalcemia in patients with the milk-alkali syndrome is fairly straightforward and includes discontinuation of the calcium carbonate and volume expansion if the hypercalcemia is associated with symptoms. The patients may become hypocalcemic, which can then be treated with lower amounts of calcium than used previously, without an alkalinizing component (184a).

III. HYPOCALCEMIA

A. Incidence and Prevalence

In 485 consecutive patients admitted to a geriatric unit for long-term care, Sorva et al. (51) found hypocalcemia (serum calcium less than 8.5 mg/dl) in 10 (2%), similar to the 2.8% rate seen in the elderly at our own institution.

B. Etiology

Chronic renal insufficiency and/or hypoalbuminemia account for over 60% of the patients with hypocalcemia seen in our elderly hospital population. Other causes, in decreasing order of frequency, include hypomagnesemia, acute pancreatitis, hypoparathyroidism, malabsorption syndrome, acute renal failure, alkalosis, and osteoblastic metastatic malignancy.

C. Clinical Manifestations and Pathogenesis

In most patients, the clinical manifestations are those of the underlying diseases rather than the hypocalcemia per se. Nevertheless, hypocalcemia may be associated with a variety of neurological or neuromuscular disturbances, including apprehension, depression, irritability, anxiety, and parathesis of the hands and feet, increased muscle irritability, carpopedal and laryngeal spasm, and tetany. In addition, patients may have nonspecific gastrointestinal complaints or abdominal pain.

1. Hypocalcemia of Chronic Renal Insufficiency

See section on chronic renal insufficiency.

2. Hypocalcemia of Hypoalbuminemia

Since the calcium measured in most hospital and/or commercial laboratories is the total calcium, including that portion bound to albumin, hypocalcemia is often seen with hypoalbuminemia. In general, the lower the serum albumin, the lower is the serum calcium. Ionized calcium, the physiologically important fraction, is usually normal in these patients, and the hypocalcemia is usually asymptomatic. In others, however, the ionized fraction is also low. Such a group is made up of patients who are acutely ill with sepsis and various other complications (211). The hypocalcemia in this setting is multifactorial and results from parathyroid insufficiency, renal 1 alpha-hydroxylase, or vitamin D deficiency (212). The mortality rate is quite high in this group.

3. Hypocalcemia of Hypomagnesemia

Hypocalcemia develops when the serum magnesium decreases to below 0.3 mmol/L (0.7 mg/dl). The hypocalcemia reflects an inappropriate response of the parathyroid gland to the low calcium (213), as well as a direct effect of hypomagnesemia on bone metabolism, resulting in a relative reduction of calcium release (214). In addition, hypomagnesemia can interfere with the metabolism of vitamin D, since magnesium is required for its hepatic 25-hydroxylation (215). Hypophosphatemia is found in about one-third of patients. Symptoms and signs of hypocalcemia occur in 30–40% of these patients.

4. Hypocalcemia of Acute Pancreatitis

During acute pancreatitis, large amounts of calcium may deposit in areas of fat necrosis. Those patients in whom hypocalcemia develops have been found to have an inadequate parathyroid hormone response to the hypocalcemia (216). The serum Mg and albumin should also be measured, particularly in those patients with alcohol-induced pancreatitis. Clinical manifestations are those of acute pancreatitis, with a small number of patients showing evidence of increased muscle irritability (217).

5. *Hypocalcemia of Hypoparathyroidism*

In 64% of elderly patients with hypoparathyroidism it is secondary to surgical removal of the glands during thyroid surgery. In the remaining 36%, no specific reason for the gland's inability to produce enough PTH to maintain normal extracellular calcium is found (218,219). Often the patient present with symptoms related to the hypocalcemia (see above), and Trousseau and Chvostek's signs will be elicited on physical examination. In these patients the hypocalcemia is frequently associated with hyperphosphatemia; the $25(OH)D_3$ level is usually normal and $1,25(OH)_2D_3$ is low (219).

6. *Hypocalcemia of Malabsorption*

In the elderly with malabsorption and related hypocalcemia, the clinical manifestations are those of the underlying gastrointestinal disease. The hypocalcemia is due to a decrease in both calcium and vitamin D absorption. The unabsorbed free fatty acids form insoluble calcium soaps in the intestinal lumen, making fewer calcium ions available for absorption. Vitamin D, being fat soluble, cannot be absorbed adequately due to the unavailability of bile salts. Plasma levels of phosphorus and $25(OH)D_3$ are decreased. PTH and alkaline phosphatase are increased and $1,25(OH)_2D_3$ is usually normal. Clinical and/or radiological evidence of osteomalacia may be seen in a small number of patients.

7. *Hypocalcemia of Acute Renal Failure*

The hypocalcemia of acute renal failure is rarely clinically significant. Its pathogenesis is the same as in chronic renal insufficiency (see appropriate section). The hypocalcemia tends to be more severe in acute renal failure accompanying rhabdomyolysis, due to metastatic calcification in the traumatized muscle and a decrease in the serum concentration of $1,25(OH)_2D_3$ (220).

8. *Hypocalcemia of Alkalosis*

Hypocalcemia due to a decrease in the ionized serum calcium fraction, severe enough to cause symptoms, can occur occasionally in the elderly subjected to a rapid rise in blood pH.

9. *Hypocalcemia in Patients with Osteoblastic Metastatic Malignancy*

Patients with osteoblastic metastatic tumors from prostate or breast will occasionally present with hypocalcemia. In addition to bone pain due to extensive metastases, patients may (rarely) present with manifestations of hypocalcemia (221). They differ from those with oncogenic osteomalacia (see section on hypophosphatemia) in that their serum phosphorus is either normal or elevated. Hypomagnesemia may occasionally be present. An elevated alkaline phosphatase is universally found. This syndrome may represent an inability of PTH (usually elevated) to maintain an adequate serum calcium level in response to excessive bone calcium accretion. The role of the various forms of vitamin D or a humoral substance produced by the tumor is unclear and deserves further study (222).

D. Treatment and Prognosis

1. Emergency Therapy

The symptomatic patient should receive parenteral therapy in the form of calcium gluconate. This can be used either intermittently or continuously, with the dose adjusted according to the clinical response and serum calcium level.

2. Specific Therapy

As noted, hypocalcemia is the consequence of another disease process except in the case of hypoparathyroidism. Therefore, the prognosis and treatment are those of the underlying disease. In the hypoparathyroid elderly with mild hypocalcemia (Ca 7.5–8.5 mEq/dl), chlorthalidone (50 mg daily), a thiazide diuretic, together with a low-sodium diet (50–100 mEq/day) will raise both total and ionized calcium (223). This results from a direct action of the drug on calcium release by the bone (144) and a decrease in urinary calcium excretion (142). In more severe hypocalcemia, both oral calcium and vitamin D supplementation will be needed. There are several preparations available, but the authors prefer calcium carbonate because of its high concentration of elemental calcium (40%) per tablet. We usually start with 250 mg three times a day with meals in order to lower the serum phosphorus as well (which is usually elevated), by binding ingested phosphate and making it unavailable for absorption. Twenty-four-hour urine calcium excretion should be monitored so that hypercalciuria may be detected and corrected in order to prevent the formation of stones and/or nephrocalcinosis. The maintenance dose required in the elderly varies between 500 and 1000 mg/day. Vitamin D supplementation can be provided either as 1-alpha(OH)D_3 (0.5–1.0 ug/day) or 1-alpha, 25$(OH)_2D_3$ (0.25–1.0 ug/day). Both act by increasing calcium absorption from the gut, although a direct effect on bone is quite probable. They are, in general, well tolerated and relatively safe. The serum calcium should be monitored regularly during therapy, since hypercalcemia is not uncommon when vitamin D and oral calcium supplementation are used (218,224). A synthetic form of human PTH which contains the biologically active region of the intact hormone has been used with success over a short period of time in the elderly (224a). The major drawback is that the drug has to be given daily by subcutaneous injection. This therapeutic modality might be necessary for the patient who is prone to hypercalciuria, stone formation, and/or nephrocalcinosis.

IV. PHOSPHORUS METABOLISM

A. Normal Physiology

Ninety percent of the total body phosphorus serves as a structural component of bone and teeth. The remaining 10% is found intracellularly in soft tissues and body fluids in the form of organic phosphate compounds that contribute to the formation of phospholipids, nucleic acids, and phosphoprotein macromolecules. The phosphate ion is essential for carbohydrate, lipid, and protein metabolism, serves as a cofactor in a variety of enzyme systems, and plays an important role in acid–base metabolism, both intracellularly and in blood.

The serum phosphorus concentration is maintained in the range of 2.8–4.5 mg/dl, with 90% in the free form, complexed with mono- and divalent anions. The remaining 10% is protein bound. That serum pool is in dynamic equilibrium with phosphorus entry and exit from the gastrointestinal tract, bone, kidneys, and soft tissue. Two-thirds of the 1000–1500 mg of daily phosphorus ingested is absorbed in the duodenum and jejunum, a process which is active, sodium dependent, and stimulated by vitamin D. The remaining third is excreted in the stool (225).

Since 90% of the serum phosphorus is in its free form, the kidneys play an important role in phosphorus homeostasis through filtration and reabsorption. Eighty to ninety percent of the filtered load is reabsorbed in the proximal tubule, with the distal convoluted tubule accounting for another 5–10%. It is not clear whether the cortical collecting tubule and the medullary collecting duct participate in phosphorus reabsorption in humans. Several factors, both intrinsic and extrinsic to the tubules, can modulate the rate of phosphorus reabsorption (226). The renal tubule has an intrinsic ability to respond to phosphate availability independent of any extrarenal influences. The exact mechanism by which this adaptive phenomenon takes place is not entirely known, but small changes in the intracellular phosphate availability might play a role (227). PTH is the most important of the extrinsic factors known to regulate tubular phosphorus transport. It acts by blocking the reabsorption of phosphorus in the proximal tubule as well as in the distal portions of the nephron (228,229). It also modulates the phosphaturia seen with volume expansion. If PTH is absent during volume expansion, most of the phosphorus which escapes reabsorption in the proximal tubule is reabsorbed in the distal tubule so that only a small amount appears in the urine. On the other hand, in the presence of PTH distal phosphorus reabsorption is decreased and significant phosphaturia ensues (230). Other hormones (glucocorticoids, growth hormone, thyrocalcitonin), vitamin D, beta-adrenergic receptors, acid–base balance, and the serum concentration of divalent ions (calcium and magnesium) have also been implicated in the regulation of phosphate excretion by the kidneys (226,231).

Serum phosphorus changes with aging, decreasing in the male and increasing in the female (232). The decrease in serum phosphorus in the male is associated with a 14% drop in total body phosphorus from the third to the sixth and a 10% drop from the sixth to the seventh decade of life (233). In normal individuals the kidney maintains the serum phosphorus concentration at a value close to the tubular phosphorus threshold (called the TmP/GFR*) (235), so that the latter also decreases in the male, suggesting a progressive tubular defect in phosphorus reabsorption with age. This defect might be secondary to the increase in PTH in the elderly and/or a decrease in the number or turnover rate of the phosphate carriers located in the proximal tubule (236,237). Age-related biochemical and biophysical alterations in the luminal brush-border membrane involving an impairment in the expression of one of the Na-Pi cotransporter proteins has also been reported (238,239). The mean TmP/GFR seen in 10 elderly men at our institution was 2.9 ± 0.7 mg/dl (range 2.2–4.0 mg/dl), compared with 3.7 ± 0.6 mg/dl (range 2.5–4.2 mg/dl) in 10 males under 50 years of age. In females there is an 18% drop in total body phosphate from the third to the fifth decade; in contrast to males, however, serum phosphorus increases by 3% from the fifth to the sixth decade and by 8–9% from the sixth to the eighth decade (233). The mechanism for this increase in total body phosphorus is not clear, but a positive association has been found with the serum $1,25(OH)_2D_3$ level (240), an unexpected finding since phosphate retention inhibits 1α-hydroxylase (16). As might be expected, the TmP/GFR tends to be higher in postmenopausal women (range 2.8–4.5 mg/dl) compared with their younger counterparts (range 2.5–4.2 mg/dl). Plasma phosphorus as well as TmP/GFR can be lowered to the level seen in males after administration of estrogen (241). Therefore, the hypoestrogenemia which accompanies menopause very likely contributes to the phosphorus retention (242).

V. HYPERPHOSPHATEMIA

A. Incidence and Prevalence

Hyperphosphatemia is found in 3–4% of elderly patients admitted to our hospital. The incidence in a given general hospital population encompassing all age groups is 2.8% (243).

B. Etiology

Renal insufficiency, both acute and chronic, is responsible for 50% of the hyperphosphatemia in elderly patients. Other, less common causes, in decreasing fre-

*TmP/GFR expresses phosphorus reabsorption as a function of both serum phosphorus concentration and glomerular filtration. It is a better index of expressing renal tubular phosphorus reabsorption as long as GFR is above 40 ml/min. A nomogram is available allowing the calculation of the TmP/GFR from a simultaneous determination of creatinine and phosphorus concentrations in both serum and urine (234).

quency, include pseudohyperphosphatemia, hypoparathyroidism, neoplastic diseases, and phosphate enemas.

C. Clinical Manifestations and Pathogenesis

The clinical manifestations associated with hyperphosphatemia are generally those of the underlying disease process.

1. Acute and Chronic Renal Failure

See the appropriate chapters.

2. Pseudohyperphosphatemia

A diagnosis of pseudohyperphosphatemia should be suspected in any elderly patient presenting with hyperphosphatemia (range 10–20 mg/dl) who is otherwise well and has a normal serum calcium and normal kidney function. Two processes may be responsible for the hyperphosphatemia. The first is hemolysis, in which intracellular phosphate is released from destroyed red cells and is measured as inorganic phosphorus. A concomitantly elevated serum K might help in making this diagnosis. The second is the presence of a paraprotein in the serum which spuriously raises phosphorus, if the colorimetric assay is used prior to removal of serum proteins (244). Since hyperglobulinemia is not invariably associated with hyperphosphatemia, it is quite possible that unique physicochemical characteristics of the specific (abnormal) globulin may also account for the spurious hyperphosphatemia (245). A low anion gap, which is often found in these patients, should alert the clinician to the probability of a paraprotein. The diagnosis can be confirmed by serum protein electrophoresis, immunoelectrophoresis, and/or repeating the phosphorus measurement after the serum specimen has been deproteinated (246).

3. Hypoparathyroidism

The clinical manifestations associated with hypoparathyroidism are those of hypocalcemia (see previous section). The hyperphosphatemia is usually mild to moderate (6.0–9.0 mg/dl) and secondary to a decrease in the renal tubular reabsorption of phosphorous.

4. Neoplastic Diseases

Tumor lysis syndrome following chemotherapy for highly responsive tumors is characterized by the development of severe hyperphosphatemia (10–20 mg/dl), with or without symptomatic hypocalcemia, hyperuricemia, hyperkalemia, and acute renal failure. This syndrome, although more prevalent in younger patients, does occur in the elderly and is due to rapid release of intracellular phosphate into the extracellular fluid (247,248) and decreased excretion if volume contraction and/or acute renal failure is present.

5. *Phosphate Enemas*

Hyperphosphatemia can develop in elderly patients who abuse sodium phosphate-containing enemas. Preexisting renal insufficiency is usually present. Volume contraction, symptomatic hypocalcemia (tetany, carpopedal spasm) associated with hypokalemia, and a non-anion gap metabolic acidosis (due to K and HCO_3 losses through the gastrointestinal tract) suggest this diagnosis (249,250). The hyperphosphatemia is due to increased absorption of phosphate from the gastrointestinal tract (108 ml of enema contains 19 g of sodium biphosphate and 7 g of sodium phosphate), together with decreased excretion due to the presence of renal insufficiency. In addition, by suppressing intracellular phosphorylation, the accompanying acidosis may be responsible for a transcellular shift of the ion from the intra- to the extracellular space (251,252).

D. Treatment and Prognosis

The treatment and prognosis of hyperphosphatemia are basically those of the underlying disease. Phosphate binders should be used in patients with renal failure (see Chapter 10), as well as in those with hypoparathyroidism. Hyperphosphatemia secondary to tumor lysis can be prevented by judicious volume expansion and control of the serum uric acid level with allopurinol to prevent development of acute renal failure. Volume expansion, correction of the acidosis, and calcium infusion for control of symptoms (care should be used not to raise the serum calcium level too high to avoid inducing metastatic calcification) are used in overabusers of phosphate enemas in addition to discontinuing the enemas. Dialysis may be indicated in the presence of superimposed acute renal failure.

VI. HYPOPHOSPHATEMIA

A. Incidence and Prevalence

Hypophosphatemia occurs in 4% of elderly hospitalized patients, similar to the 3.2–4.7% rate reported by different groups for the general population (253,254). Mild hypophosphatemia (1.6–2.4 mg/dl) is most common, present in 67% of patients, followed by moderate hypophosphatemia (1.1–1.5 mg/dl) in 20%. The remaining 13% have a phosphorus level of less than 1.0 mg/dl (255,256).

B. Etiology

The different causes of hypophosphatemia in the elderly population in decreasing frequency include dextrose infusion and refeeding after starvation, alcohol withdrawal, treatment for diabetic ketoacidosis, phosphate binders, respiratory alkalosis, and oncogenic osteomalacia. It should be noted, however, that in most patients with severe hypophosphatemia, more than one of these factors is usually present.

C. Clinical Manifestations and Pathogenesis

Patients with mild to moderate hypophosphatemia are usually asymptomatic. In patients with a serum phosphorus of less than 1 mg/dl, CNS dysfunction, ranging from irritability to coma and death, muscle weakness, rhabdomyolysis, elevated creatine phosphokinase (CPK), hemolysis, and white blood cell and platelet dysfunction may be seen (257).

Apart from an increase in CPK found in 10–15% of elderly patients with a serum phosphorus of less than 1 mg/dl, the other manifestations have been rather rare in our experience, an observation also made by others (258).

1. During Dextrose Infusion and Refeeding After Starvation

In these patients, who are generally admitted to the hospital with multiple organ failure and starvation, either enteral or parenteral feeding is usually initiated. Hypophosphatemia frequently ensues as phosphorus is used for tissue repair in a previously phosphorous-depleted patient, particularly when phosphate supplementation is insufficient.

2. Alcohol Withdrawal

The clinical picture here is primarily that of alcohol withdrawal. Hypophosphatemia in the alcoholic depends on several factors, including poor intake, use of antacids (for those with accompanying gastritis), alcoholic ketoacidosis, respiratory alkalosis, and a low TmP/GFR suggestive of a renal leak that is apparently related to hypomagnesemia (259). This group of patients is prone to develop rhabdomyolysis. CPK should be monitored and, if found to be elevated, good hydration should be maintained and the urine alkalinized to prevent the development of myoglobinuric acute renal failure.

3. During Therapy for Diabetic Ketoacidosis

Patients with diabetic ketoacidosis often are found to have a normal phosphorus level on admission despite a decrease in total body phosphorus. As insulin therapy is initiated and the acidosis corrected, the extracellular phosphate ion moves with glucose and potassium intracellularly, unmasking the hypophosphatemia (260). Urinary losses that occur during the osmotic diuresis that accompanies glycosuria also play a role.

4. Phosphate Binders

Phosphate binders are most commonly encountered in patients using either aluminum- or calcium-containing antacids. Hypophosphatemia results from phosphate binding in the gut by these cations.

5. Respiratory Alkalosis

Respiratory alkalosis develops during prolonged and intense hyperventilation, and hypophosphatemia is due, in part, to a shift of phosphorous from the blood to skeletal muscle cells. This shift results from an increase in muscle glycolytic activity (261). Factors which increase muscle glycolysis, such as dextrose administration, may increase the severity of the hypophosphatemia.

6. Oncogenic Osteomalacia

Although oncogenic osteomalacia is more common in younger patients, it has been described in the elderly (262). These patients present with bone and muscle pain and weakness involving mainly the proximal musculature. Besides mild to moderate hypophosphatemia and a low TmP/GFR suggestive of renal phosphate wasting, $1,25(OH)_2D_3$ is also decreased and serum calcium is normal or mildly decreased. PTH and $25(OH)D_3$ are normal. Looser zones, which consist of bands crossing the bones and representing microfractures or pseudofractures, can be found on X-ray. Bone biopsy after tetracycline labeling reveals changes compatible with osteomalacia. Vascular (hemangiopericytoma), prostatic, and lung tumors have been associated with the syndrome (263–266). It is postulated that a factor(s) produced by the tumor blocks either the activity or the synthesis of 25-hydroxy-1α-hydroxylase, accounting for the low $1,25(OH)_2D_3$. A decrease in the tubular transport of phosphate by this factor(s) could also account for the phosphate leak (267). The nephron site where this transport inhibition takes place is not yet known. It should be noted that in patients with prostatic cancer on estrogen therapy, the latter, rather than oncogenic osteomalacia, may be responsible for the hypophosphatemia (268). A normal $1,25(OH)_2D_3$ should help differentiate between these two possibilities.

D. Treatment and Prognosis

Once the diagnosis of hypophosphatemia has been made, a specific etiology should be sought and adequate corrective measures taken. In patients with oncogenic osteomalacia, pharmacological amounts of vitamin D result in only partial improvement of the bone disease. Removal of the tumor may be followed by a lasting remission. Phosphate supplementation should be reserved for patients with severe hypophosphatemia (serum phosphorus $\leq$ 1.0 mg/dl) or for those with any degree of hypophosphatemia and respiratory failure. In these patients the hypophosphatemia may be contributing to respiratory muscle weakness, rendering weaning from mechanical ventilation rather difficult (254). In our elderly patients the approach suggested by Vannatta et al. (269) has been used, in which 4 ml of intravenous phosphate (in the form of potassium phosphate with 2 mmol of phosphorus and 3 mmol of K per milliliter) is infused every 12 hr; serum phosphorus is monitored before each dose. This treatment has worked well in all of our patients within 72 hr. An oral preparation (K-Phos), which provides 125.6 mg of phosphorus, 44.5 mg of potassium, and 67 mg of sodium per tablet, is also available for chronic use.

VII. MAGNESIUM METABOLISM

A. Normal Physiology

Magnesium (Mg) is mainly an intracellular cation. Sixty-five percent of magnesium is found in the skeleton, 34% is intracellular in other tissues, and only 1% is found in the extracellular fluid (270). The skeletal Mg pool has a very low turnover rate, and the small extracellular pool has a rapid turnover. The intracellular pool has a turnover rate about half that of the extracellular pool.

The average diet contains 20–30 mEq of Mg per day (240–360 mg), of which 25–65% is normally absorbed (271), mainly in the small intestine. In certain circumstances, such as in disorders of the small intestine and during enema administration, the colon can also absorb Mg (272). The exact mechanism of transcellular intestinal transport is controversial; however, there is some indirect evidence suggesting that the intestine can absorb Mg against an electrochemical gradient (273). The proportion of Mg absorbed by the gut varies directly with its content in the diet. Mg absorption decreases in subjects with renal insufficiency, most likely as a result of the deficiency in $1,25(OH)_2D_3$ and the increase in intra- and extracellular Mg (274). During Mg-depletion states, Mg absorption varies inversely with the calcium content of the diet.

Normally, the serum Mg level is 1.5–3.0 mg/dl. Seventy-five to eighty percent of Mg exists in the ionic and complexed form and therefore is freely filtered at the glomerulus. The remaining 20–25% is protein bound. Only 3–5% of the filtered Mg appears in the urine (275). During magnesium deprivation or hypomagnesemia, urinary Mg excretion decreases to less than 1 mEq/24 hr (12 mg). In contrast, during parenteral Mg infusion or with a high Mg intake, urinary excretion of Mg is increased. In normal subjects the Tm Mg has been found to be 1.4 mg/dl GFR/1.73 m^2 for the ionized portion, or 2.0 mg/dl GFR/1.73 m^2 for total Mg (276). The average daily Mg excretion is 100 mg/day in men and 90 mg/day in women (range 50–225 mg).

The proximal tubule reabsorbs 20–30% of the filtered Mg. The exact mechanism is not known, but the reabsorption depends on Na and water transport and the intraluminal Mg concentration. Fifty to sixty percent of Mg is reabsorbed in the loop of Henle by a mechanism which is voltage dependent and secondary to active chloride transport. This portion of the nephron is also the major segment where various hormones such as PTH, calcitonin, glucagon, and ADH modulate Mg reabsorption. Only a small portion of the remaining filtered Mg (approximately 20%) is reabsorbed by the distal tubule. Extracellular fluid volume expansion, osmotic diuresis, diuretic therapy, hypercalcemia, and alcohol ingestion are known to decrease tubular reabsorption of Mg (277).

B. Changes in Magnesium Metabolism in the Elderly

The plasma Mg level tends to decrease with age, as shown by Hollifield (278). This concurs with our own observation involving a small number of elderly of both sexes. In the 60–69 age group the serum Mg was 1.6–2.2 mg/dl, in the 70–79 year age group the serum Mg was 1.5–2.1 mg/dl, and in the 80–89 age group it was 1.5–1.9 mg/dl. A decreased dietary intake has been implicated as a possible cause for the decrease with age (279). These findings have not been universal, as some authors have not found an age-related decrease (280), and still others have found a significant increase in serum Mg in postmenopausal women associated with an increase in urinary excretion, which is reversible by estrogen administration (281). The exact mechanism by which estrogen exerts its effect is unclear. Further studies dealing with Mg absorption, total body Mg, and Tm Mg/GFR in a large number of elderly subjects (both male and female) are needed before any definite conclusion can be reached as to what happens to this cation with aging.

VIII. HYPERMAGNESEMIA

The incidence of hypermagnesemia in the elderly is not known. Since clinical manifestations associated with an elevated Mg level are not unique and do not constitute a syndrome that is readily recognizable, the serum Mg is not usually measured. In a survey of 621 patients of different ages, hypermagnesemia was found in 9.3% (282). A somewhat lower incidence of 5.6% was found in another study (283). Increased intake in the presence of renal insufficiency accounts for practically all the instances of hypermagnesemia seen in the elderly at our hospital. Magnesium-containing antacids have been responsible for most of the cases, although on occasion we have seen hypermagnesemia in cathartic abusers (284). Mild hypermagnesemia has also been reported in patients with hypocalciuric familial hypercalcemia (see the section on hypercalcemia). Patients with hypermagnesemia are usually asymptomatic except when severe (Mg > 6 mg/dl), at which point hypotension, bradycardia, changes in mentation, respiratory failure, and hypocalcemia have been described (285,286). Treatment in these patients should include calcium chloride infusion and other supportive measures, including dialysis.

IX. HYPOMAGNESEMIA

A. Incidence and Prevalence

Since serum Mg is not routinely measured, the true incidence of hypomagnesemia in the elderly is not known. In the same study noted above, where Mg was determined in 621 randomly selected subjects, hypomagnesia was present in 11% (282). The incidence in Whang's study (283) was 6.9%. Nineteen percent of elderly patients evaluated by Martin and Milligan (287) had a serum Mg of 1.6 mg/dl or less. A serum Mg of less than 1 mg/dl was found in 10.7% of 1576 consecutive elderly patients at the time of hospital admission by Martin et al. (288). In our experience in which serum magnesium was measured in 40 elderly patients, hypomagnesemia (< 1.5 mg/100 ml) was found in 4 (10%). These findings very likely underestimate the problem in terms of total body Mg, because significant Mg depletion can be present despite a normal serum Mg level.

B. Etiology

Hypomagnesemia in the elderly is generally due to: (a) increased urinary losses due to diuretics or other drugs; (b) increased gastrointestinal losses associated with malabsorption or laxative abuse; (c) a combination of factors (vide infra) such as the hypomagnesemia of alcoholism; (d) endocrine disturbances including hyperthyroidism, hyperaldosteronism, and diabetes mellitus. In one study of 35 patients aged 21–79 years, alcoholism was present in 34% and cisplatin administration in 31% (288a).

C. Clinical Manifestations and Pathogenesis

Mg, being the second most prevalent intracellular cation, is involved in the activation of various enzyme systems that play key roles in intermediary metabolism and phosphorylation. Therefore, it is not surprising that symptoms of hypomagnesemia may involve several organ systems. When the serum Mg is < 1 mg/dl, a variety of symptoms may be seen, including difficulty with concentration, confusion, disorientation, hallucinations, neuromuscular irritability, tingling, numbness, tremor, twitching, anorexia, diarrhea, abdominal pain, and constipation. In addition, cardiac arrhythmias (mainly ventricular), hypotension, and sudden cardiac death may ensue.

Obviously, most of those symptoms can very easily be attributed to the accompanying disease state rather than the hypomagnesemia per se. Therefore, it is advisable that Mg be measured in patients at risk (see etiology above), as well as in those with acute respiratory failure, hypokalemia, hypophosphatemia, hyponatremia, and hypocalcemia, since these abnormalities have been found to be associated with a significantly high incidence of hypomagnesemia (288a–290). Since the correlation between extracellular fluid Mg and intracellular Mg stores is poor, we suggest that urinary Mg be measured in those patients at risk of developing hypomagnesemia but with a normal serum Mg level. A value of less than 12 mg/24 hr should be taken as evidence of depletion.

1. Drug-Induced Hypomagnesemia

a. Diuretics. Thirty to forty-eight percent of elderly patients on diuretics develop hypomagnesemia (278,291). Diuretic-induced renal losses are responsible for 75% of the hypomagnesemia seen in the elderly (278,287,288). Both thiazide and loop diuretics interfere with distal nephron Mg reabsorption. As might be expected, the losses are more significant with loop diuretics. Hypokalemia, which may be correctable only after magnesium repletion, is also common in these patients. It is postulated that Mg deficiency alters cell membrane permeability to K, either directly or through a decrease in activation of the Na-K ATPase (292). Magnesium-depleted patients are also at risk for the development of cardiac arrhythmias (extrasystole, torsade de pointes), particularly if they are receiving digitalis concomitantly (293). The exact mechanisms for this complication are not known, but it is possible that Mg deficiency leads to an alteration in the response of myocardial cells to digitalis (294). Also, K depletion very likely potentiates the arrhythmogenic effect of Mg depletion.

b. Other Drugs. Hypomagnesemia may be seen in the elderly patient taking cisplatin (usually women who are being treated for ovarian cancer), due to a decrease in renal tubular Mg reabsorption (295). A large percentage of these patients are brought to medical attention because of the development of symptoms and signs of increased muscle irritability due, in part, to hypocalcemia (see earlier section on hypocalcemia of hypomagnesemia). The development of hypomagnesemia depends on the cumulative dose of cisplatin used (296).

Twenty-five percent of patients on aminoglycoside antibiotics develop hypomagnesemia, which occurs early during therapy (average of 2.8 ± 0.5 days) and is due to a decreased tubular reabsorption of Mg, since urinary Mg excretion is elevated (297). Hypocalcemia may also be present. The concomitant presence of hypophosphatemia, hypokalemia, and hypouricemia in some patients suggests that the defect is located in the proximal tubule, most likely a result of direct toxicity of the aminoglycoside (298). An indirect effect, through hyperaldosteronism, has also been postulated (299). Hypomagnesemia and hypokalemia due to renal losses have been reported with amphotericin B (300).

2. *Malabsorption*

Severe hypomagnesemia can occur in patients with malabsorption syndrome as well as in those abusing laxatives. The hypomagnesemia is secondary to the formation of Mg soaps and their subsequent loss in the stool. Urinary magnesium is low in these patients and should be measured since it is an earlier and more reliable indicator of evolving Mg deficiency (301).

3. *Alcoholism*

Hypomagnesemia in alcoholics is multifactorial and results from decreased intake, decreased intestinal absorption (diarrhea, pancreatic insufficiency), starvation ketosis, and increased urinary losses, either secondary to a direct suppressive effect of ethanol on the renal tubule or through binding of luminal Mg with lactate (288a,302), making it unavailable for reabsorption.

4. *Endocrine Disorders*

Hypomagnesemia can occur in patients with thyrotoxicosis, although the mechanism is not known (303). In those with hyperaldosteronism, the hypomagnesemia is due to an increase in Mg excretion. It is not clear whether this represents a direct effect of aldosterone on Mg reabsorption or a reflection of some degree of volume expansion with the resulting increase in the delivery of Na and Mg to the distal tubule, where mineralocorticoids may enhance sodium reabsorption without affecting Mg transport (304). The hypomagnesemia of hyperaldosteronism is reversed by spironolactone (Aldactone) administration. In uncontrolled diabetes mellitus, urinary Mg losses occur because of the osmotic diuresis associated with glycosuria. In these patients, serum Mg may be normal despite severe deficiency; however, during insulin therapy the extracellular Mg enters the cell, causing a subsequent drop in serum Mg.

D. Treatment and Prognosis

Since part of the decrease in serum Mg with age reflects poor dietary intake, any elderly person who is at increased risk of developing hypomagnesemia should be encouraged to consume foods that are rich in Mg, such as vegetables, cereals, seafood, etc. In symptomatic patients and in those with severe hypomagnesemia, therapy can be started with a loading dose of 3–4 g (25–32.4 mEq) of a 10% solution of magnesium sulfate ($MgSO_4$) administered intravenously over a 20- to 80-min period (301,305). Deep tendons reflexes should be followed during treatment and the infusion stopped if they decrease in intensity. Repeated doses of 1 g can be given hourly for a maximum 8 g. Despite cellular depletion, only approximately 50% of each administered dose of $MgSO_4$ is retained, so oral therapy in the form of magnesium oxide, 300 mg (24.7 mEq) every 6 hr, should be continued, generally for 4–5 days or longer if the reason for the hypomagnesemia persists (306)—for example, cisplatin-induced hypomagnesemia might persist long after the drug has been discontinued. Diarrhea, which is the most common side effect, can be controlled by lowering the dose. Magnesium chloride (Slow-Mag) tablets, which provide 64 mg of elemental Mg per tablet, are an even better alternative. For those patients who require continuous diuretic treatment, consideration should be given to adding either amiloride, 5 mg/day, or triamterene, 50–100 mg/day, because Mg sparing has been reported for both those agents (307,308). The hypomagnesemia which occurs during therapy for diabetic ketoacidosis is usually mild and of short duration. It rarely requires therapy.

REFERENCES

1. Moore EW. Ionized calcium in normal serum, ultrafiltrates and whole blood determined by ion-exchange electrodes. J Clin Invest 1970;49:318–334.
2. Sherwood LM, et al. Regulation of parathyroid hormone secretion: proportional control by calcium, lack of effect of phosphate. Endocrinology 1968;83:1043–1051.
3. Yamamoto M, et al. Hypocalcemia increases and hypercalcemia decreases the steady-state level of parathyroid hormone messenger RNA in the rat. J Clin Invest 1989;83:1053–1056.

4. Fuleihan GEH, et al. Calcium dependent release of N-terminal fragments and intact immunoreactive parathyroid hormone by human pathological parathyroid tissue in vitro. J Clin Endocrinol Metab 1989;69:860–867.
5. Brown EM, et al. Calcium-ion-sensing cell-surface receptors. N Engl J Med 1995;333:234–240.
6. Naveh-Many T, et al. Calcium regulates PTH messenger ribonucleic acid (mRNA) but not calcitonin mRNA in vivo in the rat. Dominant role of 1,25-dihydroxyvitamin D. Endocrinol 1979;125:275–280.
7. Brown EM. Regulation of synthesis, metabolism and actions of parathyroid hormone. In: Contemporary Issues in Nephrology. Vol II. New York: Churchill, Livingstone, 1983:151–188.
8. Habener JF, Rosenblatt M, Potts JT Jr. Parathyroid hormone: biochemical aspects of biosynthesis, secretion, action and metabolism. Physiol Rev 1984;64:985–1053.
9. Morel F. Sites of hormone action in the mammalian nephron. Am J Physiol 1981; 240:F159–F164.
10. Martin KJ, et al. Selective uptake of the synthetic aminoterminal fragment of bovine parathyroid hormone by isolated perfused bone. J Clin Invest 1978;62:256–261.
11. Hollander D, Muralidhara KS, Zimmerman A. Vitamin D_3 intestinal absorption in vivo: influence of fatty acids, bile salts and perfusate pH on absorption. Gut 1978; 19:267–272.
12. Holick MF, et al. Photosynthesis of previtamin D_3 in human skin and the physiologic consequences. Science 1980;210:203–205.
13. Bell NH, Shaw S, Turner RT. Evidence that 1,25-dihydroxyvitamin D_3 inhibits the hepatic production of 25-hydroxyvitamin D in man. J Clin Invest 1984;74: 1540–1544.
14. Baran DT, Milne ML. 1,25-dihydroxyvitamin D increases hepatocyte cytosolic calcium levels. A potential regulator of vitamin D-25 hydroxylase. J Clin Invest 1986;77:1622–1626.
15. Norman DA, et al. Jejunal and ileal adaptation to alterations in dietary calcium. Changes in calcium and magnesium absorption and pathogenetic role of parathyroid hormone and 1,25-dihydroxyvitamin D. J Clin Invest 1981;67:1599–1603.
16. Audran M, Kumar R. The physiology and pathophysiology of vitamin D. Mayo Clin Proc 1985;60:851–866.
17. Tanaka Y, DeLuca HF. Bone mineral mobilization activity of 1,25-dihydroxycholecalciferol, a metabolite of vitamin D. Arch Biochem Biophys 1971;146:574–578.
18. Hughes MR, Haussler MR. 1,25 dihydroxycholecalciferol receptors in parathyroid glands. J Biol Chem 1978;253:1065–1069.
19. Silver J, et al. Regulation by vitamin D metabolites of messenger ribonucleic acid for preproparathyroid hormone in isolated bovine parathyroid cells. Proc Natl Acad Sci USA 1985;82:4270–4273.
20. Peacock M, Robertson WG, Nordin BEC. Relation between serum and urinary calcium with particular reference to parathyroid activity. Lancet 1969;1:384–388.
21. Heath H IV, Sizemore GW. Plasma calcitonin in normal man. Differences between men and women. J Clin Invest 1977;60:1135–1140.
22. Torring O, Bucht E, Sjöberg HE. Plasma calcitonin response to a calcium clamp. Influence of sex and age. Horm Metab Res 1985;17:536–539.

23. Chapuy MC, Durr F, Chapuy P. Age-related changes in parathyroid hormone and 25-hydroxycholecalciferol levels. J Gerontol 1983;38:19–22.
24. Marcus R, Madirg P, Young G. Age-related changes in parathyroid hormone and parathyroid hormone action in normal humans. J Clin Endocrinol Metab 1984;58: 223–230.
25. Greenblatt DJ. Reduced serum albumin concentration in the elderly: a report from the Boston Collaborative Drug Surveillance Program. J Am Geriatr Soc 1979;27: 20–22.
26. Wiske PS, et al. Increase in immunoreactive parathyroid hormone with age. N Engl J Med 1979;300:1419–1421.
27. Orwoll ES, Meier D. Alterations in calcium, vitamin D and parathyroid hormone physiology in normal man with aging: relationship to the development of senile osteopenia. J Clin Endocrinol Metab 1986;63:1262–1269.
28. Endras DB, et al. Age-related changes in serum immunoreactive parathyroid hormone and its biological action in healthy men and women. J Clin Endocrinol Metab 1979;65:724–736.
29. Blumenthal HT, Perlstein IB. The biopathology of aging of the endocrine system: the parathyroid glands. J Am Geriatr Soc 1993;41:1116–1129.
30. Gallagher JC, et al. Intestinal calcium absorption and serum vitamin D metabolites in normal subjects and osteoporotic patients. J Clin Invest 1979;64:729–736.
31. Francis RM, et al. Calcium malabsorption in the elderly: the effect of treatment with oral 25-hydroxyvitamin D_3. Eur J Clin Invest 1983;13:391–396.
32. Malm OJ. Calcium requirement and adaptation in adult men. Scand J Clin Lab Invest 1958;10(suppl 36):1–289.
33. Ireland P, Fordtran JS. Effect of dietary calcium and age on jejunal calcium absorption in humans studied by intestinal perfusion. J Clin Invest 1973;52:2672–2681.
34. Gallagher JC, Riggs LB. Current concepts in nutrition. Nutrition and bone disease. N Engl J Med 1978;298:193–195.
35. Paillard M, Patron P, Gardin JP. Determinants of circulating levels of 1,25-dihydroxyvitamin D_3 in primary hyperparathyroidism (PHPT). Min Electrol Metab 1985;11:334, A79.
36. Bouillon RA, et al. Vitamin D status in the elderly: seasonal substrate deficiency causes 1,25 dihydroxycholecalciferol deficiency. Am J Clin Nutr 1987;45:755–763.
37. Mori S, et al. Bone fracture in elderly female with primary hyperparathyroidism: relationship among renal function, vitamin D status and fracture risk. Horm Metabol Res 1097;19:183–185.
38. Komar L, et al. Calcium homeostatis of an elderly population upon admission to a nursing home. J Am Geriatr Soc 1993;41:1057–1064.
39. Armbrecht HJ, Forte LR, Halloran BP. Effect of aging and dietary calcium on renal 25-hydroxyvitamin D metabolism, serum $1,25(OH)_2D$ and PTH. Am J Physiol 1984;246:E266–E270.
40. Armbrecht HJ, Forte LR, Wongsurawat N. Forskolin increases 1,25-dihydroxyvitamin D_3 production by rat renal slices in vitro. Endocrinology 1984;114:644–649.
41. Ishida M, et al. Hydroxylation of 25-hydroxyvitamin D_3 by renal mitochondria from rats of different ages. Endocrinology 1987;121:443–448.

42. Silverberg SJ, et al. Abnormalities in parathyroid hormone secretion and 1,25-dihydroxyvitamin D_3 formation in women with osteoporosis. N Engl J Med 1989;320:277–289.
43. Editorial: Vitamin D supplementation in the elderly. Lancet 1987;1:306–307.
44. O'Dowd KJ, et al. Exogenous calciferol (vit D) and vitamin D endocrine status among elderly nursing home residents in the New York area. J Am Geriatr Soc 1993;41:414–421.
45. Toss G, Sörbo B. Serum concentrations of 25-hydroxyvitamin D and vitamin D-binding protein in elderly people. Acta Med Scand 1986;220:273–277.
46. Goldray D, et al. Vitamin D deficiency in elderly patients in a general hospital. J Am Geriatr Soc 1989;37:589–592.
47. Sommerville PJ, Lien JWK, Kaye M. The calcium and vitamin D status in an elderly female population and their response to administered supplemental vitamin D_3. J Gerontol 1977;32:659-663.
48. Maclaughlin J, Holick MF. Aging decreases the capacity of human skin to produce vitamin D_3. J Clin Invest 1985;76:1536–1538.
49. Christensson T, et al. Prevalence of hypercalcemia in a health screening in Stockholm. Acta Med Scand 1976;200:131–137.
50. Grero PS, Hodkinson HM. Hypercalcemia in elderly hospital in-patients: values of discriminant analysis in differential diagnosis. Age & Ageing 1977;6:14–20.
51. Sorva A, Tilvis R. Survival and calcemic status of geriatric inpatients. Lancet 1987; 1:799.
52. Mallette LE. Review: primary hyperparathyroidism, an update: incidence, etiology, diagnosis and treatment. Am J Med Sci 1987;293:239–249.
53. Marx SJ. New insights into primary hyperparathyroidism. Hosp Pract 1984;19:55-63.
54. Taffet GE, et al. Elevated parathyroid hormone in elderly males. J Am Geriat Soc 1986;34:906A.
55. Tibblin S, Pälsson N, Rydberg J. Hyperparathyroidism in the elderly. Ann Surg 1983;197:135–138.
55a. Wermers Ra, et al. The rise and fall of primary hyperparathyroidism. A population-based study in Rochester, Minnesota 1965–1992. Ann Intern Med 1997;125: 433–440.
56. Carnevale N, Samson R, Bennett BP. Multiple parathyroid adenomas. JAMA 1981; 246:1332–1333.
57. Black BK. Carcinoma of the parathyroid. Ann Surg 1954;139:355-363.
58. Holmes EC, Morton DL, Ketcham AS. Parathyroid carcinoma: a collective review. Ann Surg 1969;169:631–640.
59. Shane E, Bilezikian JP. Parathyroid carcinoma: a review of 62 patients. Endocrine Rev 1982;3:218–226.
59a. Wynne AG, et al. Parathyroid carcinoma: clinical and pathologic features in 43 patients. Medicine 1992;71:197–205.
60. Murray TM, et al. Non-autonomy of hormone secretion in primary hyperparathyroidism. Clin Endocrinol 1972;1:235–239.
61. Brown EM, et al. Dispersed cells from human parathyroid glands: distinct calcium sensitivity of adenomas vs primary hyperplasia. J Clin Endocrinol Metab 1978; 46:267–275.

62. Dietel M, et al. Abnormal calcium distribution in human parathyroid adenomas as possible cause of primary hyperparathyroidism. Horm Metab Res 1987;19:177–181.
63. Bellorin-Font E, et al. Altered adenylate cyclase kinetics in hyperfunctioning human parathyroid glands. J Clin Endocrinol Metab 1981;52:499–507.
64. Juhlin C, et al. Monoclonal antiparathyroid antibodies revealing defect expression of a calcium receptor mechanism in hyperparathyroidism. World J Surg 1988;12: 552–558.
65. Parfitt AM. Equilibrium and disequilibrium hypercalcemia. New light on an old concept. Metab Bone Dis 1979;1:279–283.
66. Stewart AF. Is there a role for parathyroid hormone in humoral hypercalcemia of malignancy? Min Electrol Metab 1982;8:215–226.
66a. Grey A, et al. Circulating levels of interleukin-6 and tumor necrosis factor-α are elevated in primary hyperparathyroidism and correlates with markers of bone resorption. J Clin Endocrinol Metab 1996;81:3450–3454.
67. Silverberg SJ, Bilezikian JP. Evaluation and management of primary hyperparathyroidism. J Clin Endocrinol Metab 1996;81:2036–2040.
68. Heath DA, et al. Surgical treatment of hyperparathyroidism in the elderly. Br Med J 1980;280:1406–1408.
69. Brothers TA, Thompson NW. Surgical treatment of primary hyperparathyroidism in elderly patients. Acta Clin Scand 1987;153:175–178.
70. Joborn C, et al. Primary hyperparathyroidism in patients with organic brain syndrome. Acta Med Scand 1986;219:91–98.
71. Joborn C, et al. Psychiatric morbidity in primary hyperparathyroidism. World J Surg 1988;12:476–481.
72. Patten BM, et al. Neuromuscular disease in primary hyperparathyroidism. Ann Intern Med 1974;80:182–193.
73. Broadus AE, et al. The importance of circulating 1,25-dihydroxyvitamin D in the pathogenesis of hypercalciuria and renal stone formation in primary hyperparathyroidism. N Engl J Med 1980;302:421–426.
74. Pak CYC, et al. A lack of unique pathophysiologic background for nephrolithiasis of primary hyperparathyroidism. J Clin Endocrinol Metab 1981;53:536–542.
75. Lafferty FW. Primary hyperparathyroidism. Changing clinical spectrum, prevelance of hypertension and discriminant analysis of laboratory tests. Arch Intern Med 1981;141:1761–1766.
76. Diamond TW, et al. Parathyroid hypertension. A reversible disorder. Arch Intern Med 1986;146:1709–1712.
77. Gennari C, Nami R, Gonnelli S. Hypertension and primary hyperparathyroidism the role of adrenergic and renin-angiotensin-aldosterone systems. Miner Electrol Metab 1995;21:77–81.
77a. Morfis L, Smerdely P, Howes LG. Relationship between serum PTH levels in the elderly and 24 hours ambulatory blood pressures. J Hypertens 1997;15:1271–1276.
78. Salahudeen AK, et al. Hypertension and renal dysfunction in primary hyperparathyroidism: effect of parathyroidectomy. Clin Sci 1989;76:289–296.
79. Ganguly A, et al. The renin-angiotensin system and hypertension in primary hyperparathyroidism. Metabolism 1982;31:595–600.

80. Richards AM, et al. Hormone, calcium and blood pressure relationship in primary hyperparathyroidism. J Hypertens 1980;6:747–752.
81. Vlachakis ND, et al. Sympathetic system function and vascular reactivity in hypercalciuric patients. Hypertens 1982;4:452–458.
81a. Pang PKT et al. Parathyroid hypertensive factor and intracellular calcium regulation. J Hypertens 1996;14:1053–1060.
82. Daniels J, Goodman DA. Hypertension and hyperparathyroidism. Inverse relation of serum phosphate level and blood pressure. Am J Med 1983;75:17–23.
83. Payne RL Jr, Fitchett CW. Hyperparathyroid crisis. A survey of the literature and a report of two additional cass. Ann Surg 1965;161:737–747.
84. Mundy GR, Cove DH, Fisken R. Primary hyperparathyroidism: changes in the pattern of clinical presentation. Lancet 1980;1:1317–1320.
85. Fitzpatrick LA, Bilezikian JP. Acute primary hyperparathyroidism. Am J Med 1987; 82:275–282.
86. Lufkin EG, Kao PC, Heath H III. Parathyroid hormone radioimmunoassays in the differential diagnosis of hypercalcemia due to primary hyperparathyroidism or malignancy. Ann Intern Med 1987;106:559–560.
87. Martin KJ, et al. Clinical utility of radioimmunoassay for parathyroid hormone. Min Electr Metab 1980;3:283–290.
88. Mallette LE, et al. Radioimmunoassay for the middle region of human parathyroid hormone using an homologous antiserum with a carboxyterminal fragment of bovine PTH as radioligand. J Clin Endocrinol Metab 1982;54:1017–1024.
89. Nussbaum SR, et al. Highly sensitive two-site immunoradiometric assay of parathyrin and its clinical utility in evaluating patients with hypercalcemia. Clin Chem 1987;33:1364–1367.
90. Broadus AE, Rasmussen H. Clinical evaluation of parathyroid function. Am J Med 1981;70:475–478.
91. Rude RK, et al. Urinary and nephrogenous adenosine 3'5'-monophosphate in the hypercalcemia of malignancy. J Clin Endocrinol Metab 1981;52:765–771.
92. Torring O, et al. Urinary cyclic AMP corrected for glomerular filtration rate in the differential diagnosis of hypercalcemia. Acta Med Scand 1982;211:401–405.
93. Sample WF, Mitchell SP, Bledsoe RC. Parathyroid ultrasonography. Radiol 1978;127:485–490.
94. Gatekunst R, et al. Parathyroid localization. J Clin Endocrinol Metab 1986;63: 1390–1393.
95. Mazzeo S, et al. Comparison among sonography, double tracer substraction scintigraphy and double-phase scintigraphy in the detection of parathyroid lesions. Am J Roentgenol 1996;166:1465–1470.
96. Krudy AG, et al. The detection of mediastinal parathyroid glands by computed tomography, selective arteriography and venous sampling. Radiology 1981;140:739–744.
97. Kovarik J, et al. The value of computed tomography as a noninvasive method for preoperative localization of parathyroid adenomas of the neck in primary hyperparathyroidism. Min Electrol Metab 1981;5:228–232.
98. Cates JD, et al. CT evaluation of parathyroid adenomas. Diagnostic criteria and pitfalls. J Comp Ass Tomogr 1988;12:626–629.

99. Clark OH, et al. Localization studies in patients with persistent or recurrent hyperparthyroidism. Surgery 1985;98:1083–1094.
100. Turton DB, Miller DL. Recent advances in parathyroid imaging. Trends Endocrinol Metab 1996;7:163–168.
101. McHenry CR, et al. Parathyroid localization with technetium-99m-Sestamibi: a prospective evaluation. J Am Coll Surg 1996;183:25–30.
102. McDermott VG, et al. Preoperative MR imaging in hyperparathyroidism; results and factors affecting parathyroid detection. Am J Roentgenol 1996;166:705–710.
103. Abboud B, et al. Role of selective venous catheterization with assay of PTH 1–84 in the treatment of persistent hyperparathyroidism. Ann Chir 1997;51:130–135.
104. Aufferman W, et al. Diagnosis of recurrent hyperparathyroidism: comparison of MR imaging and other imaging techniques. Am J Roentgenol 1988;150: 1027–1033.
105. Farr HW. Hyperparathyroidism and cancer. CA 1976;26:66–74.
106. Wajngot A, et al. Occurrence of pituitary adenomas and other neoplastic diseases in primary hyperparathyroidism. Surgery Gyn and Obstet 1980;151:401–403.
107. Ljunghall S, et al. Dynamic tests of parathyroid function for diagnosis of primary hyperparathyroidism in malignancy. Clin Endocrinol 1987;27:163–170.
108. Ljunghall S, et al. Improved differential diagnosis of hypercalcemia by hypocalcemic stimulation of parathyroid hormone. World J Surg 1988;12:496–502.
109. Bensen L, et al. A stimulation test with calcitonin for differential diagnosis of hypercalcemia. Acta Endocrinol 1984;107:237–244.
110. Gardin JP, Paillard M. Normocalcemic primary hyperparathyroidism: resistance to PTH effect on tubular reabsorption of calcium. Min Electrol Metab 1984;10: 301–308.
111. Myers WPL. Hypercalcemia in neoplastic disease. Arch Surg 1960;80:308–310.
112. Burt ME, Brennan MF. Incidence of hypercalcemia and malignant neoplasm. Arch Surg 1980;115:704–707.
113. Mundy GR, Martin TJ. The hypercalcemia of malignancy: pathogenesis and management. Metabolism 1982;31:1247–1277.
114. Ray AK, Rao DB. Hypercalcemia and malignant disease in the elderly: magnesium sulfate therapy. J Am Geriatr Soc 1974;22:413–415.
115. Levine MM, Kleeman CR. Hypercalcemia: pathophysiology and treatment. Hosp Pract 1987;22:93–110.
116. Ralston S, et al. Hypercalcemia and metastatic bone disease: is there a causal link? Lancet 1982;2:903–905.
117. Eilon G, Mundy GR. Effects of inhibition of microtubule assembly on bone mineral release and enzyme release by human breast cancer cells. J Clin Invest 1981; 67:69–76.
118. Mundy GR, Ibbotson KJ, D'Souza SM. Tumor products and the hypercalcemia of malignancy. J Clin Invest 1985;76:391–394.
119. Goldfarb S, Agus ZS. Mechanism of the polyuria of hypercalcemia. Am J Nephrol 1984;4:69–76.
120. Lins LE. Renal function in hypercalcemia. A clinical and experimental study. Acta Med Scand 1979;632(suppl):1–46.

121. Stewart AF, et al. Biochemical evaluation of patients with cancer-associated hypercalcemia. Evidence for humoral and nonhumoral groups. N Engl J Med 1980; 303:1377–1383.
122. Skrabanek P, McPartlin J, Powell D. Tumor hypercalcemia and "ectopic hyperparathyroidism." Medicine 1980;59:262–289.
123. Harris RC, et al. Evidence for glomerular actions of epidermal growth factor in the rat. J Clin Invest 1988;82:1028–1038.
124. Insogna KL, et al. Native and a synthetic analogue of the malignancy-associated parathyroid-hormone-like protein have in vitro transforming growth factor-like properties. J Clin Invest 1989;83:1057–1060.
125. Ralston SH, et al. Hypercalcemia of malignancy. Evidence for non-parathyroid humoral agent with an effect on renal tubular handling of calcium. Clin Sci 1984;66: 187–197.
126. Tuttle KR, et al. Altered renal calcium handling in hypercalcemia of malignancy. J Am Soc Nephrol 1991;2:191–199.
127. Ralston SH. The pathogenesis of humoral hypercalcemia of malignancy. Lancet 1987;2:1443–1446.
128. Mundy GR. The hypercalcemia of malignancy. Kidney Int 1987;31:142–155.
129. Mundy GR, et al. The hypercalcemia of cancer. Clinical implications and pathogenic mechanisms. N Engl J Med 1984;310:1718–1727.
130. Suva LJ, et al. A parathyroid hormone related protein implicated in malignant hypercalcemia: cloning and expression. Science 1987;237:893–896.
131. Broadus A, et al. Humoral hypercalcemia of cancer. Identification of a novel parathyroid hormone-like peptide. N Engl J Med 1988;319:556–563.
132. Budayr AA, et al. Increased serum levels of parathyroid hormone-like protein in malignancy-associated hypercalcemia. Ann Intern Med 1989;111:807–812.
133. Kao PC, et al. Parathyroid hormone-related peptide in plasma of patients with hypercalcemia and malignant lesions. Mayo Clin Proc 1990;65:1399–1407.
134. Kukreja SC, et al. Antibodies to parathyroid hormone-related protein lower serum calcium in athymic mouse models of malignancy-associated hypercalcemia due to human tumors. J Clin Invest 1988;82:1798–1802.
135. Mundy GR. Hypercalcemia of malignancy revisited. J Clin Invest 1988;82: 1–6.
136. Ross Garrett I, et al. Production of lymphotoxin, a bone-resorbing cytokine by cultured human myeloma cells. N Engl J Med 1987;317:526–532.
137. Gowan M, et al. An interleukin-1 like factor stimulates bone resorption in vitro. Nature 1983;306:378–380.
138. Breslay NA, et al. Hypercalcemia associated with increased serum calcitrol levels in three patients with lymphoma. Ann Intern Med 1984;100:1–7.
139. Zaloga GP, Eil C, Medberry CA. Humoral hypercalcemia in Hodgkin's disease. Arch Intern Med 1985;145:155–157.
140. Mundy GR, Bertolini DR. Bone destruction and hypercalcemia in plasma cell myeloma. Sem Oncol 1986;13:291–299.
141. State RM, et al. Hydrochlorothiazide effects on serum calcium and immunoreactive parathyroid hormone concentrations. Studies in normal subjects. Ann Intern Med 1972;77:587–591.

142. Costanzo LS, Windhagen EE. Calcium and sodium transport by the distal convoluted tubule of the rat. Am J Physiol 1978;235:F492–F506.
143. Koppel JH, et al. Thiazide-induced rise in serum calcium and magnesium in patients on maintenance hemodialysis. Ann Intern Med 1970;72:895–901.
144. Malluche HH, et al. Evidence for a direct effect of thiazide on bone. Min Electrol Metab 1980;4:89–96.
145. Christensson T, Hellström K, Wengle B. Hypercalcemia and primary hyperparathyroidism. Prevalence in patients receiving thiazides as detected in a health screen. Arch Intern Med 1977;137:1138–1142.
146. Frame B, et al. Hypercalcemia and skeletal effects in chronic hypervitaminosis A. Ann Intern Med 1974;80:44–48.
147. Mawber EB, et al. Vitamin D metabolism in patients intoxicated with ergocalciferol. Clin Sci 1985;68:135–141.
148. Reichel H, et al. Regulation of 1,25-dihydroxyvitamin D_3 production by cultured alveolar macrophages from normal human donors and from patients with pulmonary sarcoidosis. J Clin Endocrinol Metab 1987;65:1201–1209.
149. Strewler GJ, Nissenson RA. Nonparathyroid hypercalcemia. Adv Intern Med 1987;32:235–258.
150. Marx SJ, et al. The hypocalciuric or benign variant of familial hypercalcemia: clinical and biochemical features in fifteen kindreds. Medicine 1981;60:397–412.
151. Aida K, et al. Familial hypocalciuric hypercalcemia associated with mutation in the human calcium sensing receptor gene. J Clin Endocrinol Metab 1995;80: 2594–2598.
152. Marx SJ, et al. Divalent cation metabolism. Familial hypocalciuric hypercalcemia versus typical primary hyperparathyroidism. Am J Med 1978;65:235–242.
153. Law WM Jr, et al. High-resolution parathyroid ultrasonograhy in familial benign hypercalcemia (familial hypocalciuric hypercalcemia). Mayo Clin Proc 1984;59: 153–155.
154. Chattopadhyay N, Mithal A, Brown EM. The calcium-sensing receptor: a window into the physiology and pathophysiology of mineral ion metabolism. Endocr Rev 1996;17:289–307.
154a. Beall DP, Scofield RH. Milk-alkali syndrome associated with calcium carbonate consumption. Medicine 1995;74:89–96.
155. Bouillon R, Muls E, DeMoor P. Influence of thyroid function on the serum concentration of 1,25-dihydroxyvitamin D_3. J Clin Endocrinol Metab 1980;51:793–797.
156. Mosekilde L, Christensen MS. Decreased parathyroid function in hyperthyroidism: interrelationships between serum parathyroid hormone, calcium-phosphorous metabolism and thyroid function. Acta Endocrinol 1977;84:566–575.
157. Suki WN, et al. Acute treatment of hypercalcemia with furosemide. N Engl J Med 1970;283:836–840.
158. Edwards BR, et al. Micropuncture study of diuretic effects on sodium and calcium reabsorption in the dog nephron. J Clin Invest 1978;52:2418–2427.
159. Ralston SH, et al. Comparison of amino hydoroxypropylidene, diphosphonate, mitramycin and corticosteroid calcitonin in treatment of cancer-associated hypercalcemia. Lancet 1985;2:907–910.

160. Malatino LS, et al. Acute effects of salmon calcitonin in man include stimulation of the renin-angiotensin-aldosterone system. Min Electrol Metab 1987;13:316–322.
160a. Carney SL. Calcitonin and human renal calcium and electrolytes transport. Min Electrol Metab 1997;23:43–47.
161. Wener JA, Gorton SJ, Raisz LG. Escape from inhibition of resorption in cultures of fetal bone treated with calcitonin and parathyroid hormone. Endocrinol 1972;90: 752–759.
162. Binstock ML, Mundy GR. Effect of calcitonin and glucocorticoids in combination in malignant hypercalcemia. Ann Intern Med 1980;93:269–272.
163. Suda T, Testa NG, Allen TD. Effects of hydrocortisone on osteoclasts generated in cat bone marrow cultures. Calcif Tissue Intern 1983;35:82–86.
164. Singer FR, et al. Treatment of hypercalcemia of malignancy. Arch Intern Med 1991;151:471–476.
165. Gucalp R, et al. Comparative study of pamidronate disodium and etidronate disodium in the treatment of cancer related hypercalcemia. J Clin Oncol 1992;10:134.
166. Machado CE, Flombaum CD. Safety of pamidronate in patients with renal failure and hypercalcemia. Clin Nephrol 1996;45:175–179.
167. Evans RA. Hypercalcemia, what does it signify? Drugs 1986;31:64–74.
168. Singer FR, Fernandez M. Therapy of hypercalcemia of malignancy. Am J Med 1987;82(suppl 2A):34–41.
169. Bruining HA, et al. Causes of failure in operations for hyperparathyroidism. Surgery 1987;101:562–565.
170. Shen W, et al. Reoperation for persistent or recurrent primary hyperparathyroidism. Arch Surg 1996;131:861–867.
171. Numerow LM, et al. Persistent, recurrent hyperparathyroidism. A comparison of sestamibi scintigraphy, MRI and ultrasonography, J Magn Reson Imaging 1995;5: 702–708.
172. Spiegel AM, et al. Intraoperative measurements of urinary cyclic AMP to guide surgery for primary hyperparathyroidism. N Engl J Med 1980;303:1457–1460.
173. Gonzalez-Villapando C, et al. Vitamin D metabolism during recovery from severe osteitis fibrosa cystica of primary hyperparathyroidism. J Clin Endocrinol Metab 1980;51:1180–1183.
174. Niederle B, et al. Successful parathyroidectomy in primary hyperparthyroidism: a clinical follow-up study of 212 consecutive patients. Surgery 1987;102:903–909.
175. Deaconson TF, Wilson SD, Lemann J Jr. The effect of parathyroidectomy on the recurrence of nephrolithiasis. Surgery 1987;102:910–913.
176. Schatz A, Castleman B. Parathyroid carcinoma: a study of 70 cases. Cancer 1973; 31:600–605.
177. McCance DR, et al. Parathyroid carcinoma: a review. J R Soc Med 1987; 80:505–514.
178. Hakaim AG, Esselstyn CB Jr. Parathyroid carcinoma: 50 year experience at the Cleveland Clinic Foundation. Cleveland Clin J Med 1993;60:331–335.
179. Heath H III, Hodgson SF, Kennedy MA. Primary hyperparathyroidism: incidence, morbidity and potential economic impact in a community. N Engl J Med 1980;302: 189–193.

180. Coe FL, Favus MJ. Does mild, asymptomatic hyperparathyroidism require surgery? N Engl J Med 1980;302:224–225.
181. Scholz DA, Purnell DC. Asymptomatic primary hyperparathyroidism. Ten year prospective study. Mayo Clin Proc 1981;56:473–378.
182. Hodgson SF, Heath H III. Asymptomatic primary hyperparathyroidism: treat or follow? Mayo Clin Proc 1981;56:521–522.
183. Lueg MC. Asymptomatic primary hyperparathyroidism. Hosp Prac 1982;17:29–39.
184. Amorosa LF, Amorosa JK. Hyperparathyroidism with asymptomatic hypercalcemia. Hosp Prac 1983;18:223–246.
185. Pearson MW. Asymptomatic primary hyperparathyroidism in the elderly. Age & Ageing 1984;13:1–5.
186. Van't Hoff W, Ballardi FW, Bicknell EJ. Primary hyperparathyroidism: the case for medical management. Br Med J 1983;287:1605–1608.
187. Corlew DS, et al. Observations on the course of untreated primary hyperparathyroidism. Surgery 1985;98:1064–1070.
188. Alveryd AS, et al. Indication for surgery in the elderly patient with primary hyperparathyroidism. Acta Chir Scand 1976;142:491–494.
189. Lifschitz BM, Barzel US. Parathyroid surgery in the aged. J Gerontol 1981;36: 573–575.
190. Peskin GW, Greenberg GA, Salk RP. Expanding indications for early parathyroidectomy in the elderly female. Am J Surg 1978;136:45–48.
191. Brothers TE, Thompson NW. Surgical treatment of primary hyperparathyroidism in elderly patients. Acta Chir Scand 1987;153:175–178.
192. Kochersberger G, et al. What is the clinical significance of bone loss in primary hyperparathyroidism? Arch Intern Med 1987;147:1951–1953.
193. Wilson RJ, et al. Mild asymptomatic primary hyperparathyroidism is not a risk factor for vertebral fractures. Ann Intern Med 1988;109:959–962.
194. Block MA, Daily GE III, Muchmore DE. Bone demineralization, a factor of increasing significance in the management of primary hyperparathyroidism. Surgery 1989;106:1063–1069.
195. Block MA, Xavier A, Brush BE. Management of primary hyperparathyroidism in the elderly. J Am Geriatr Soc 1975;23:385–389.
196. Sampson MJ, Van't Hoff W, Bicknell EJ. The conservative management of primary hyperparathyroidism. Quart J Med 1987;65:1009–1014.
197. Silverberg SJ, et al. Longitudinal measurements of bone density and biochemical indices in untreated primary hyperparathyroidism. J Clin Endocrinol Metab 1995; 80:723–728.
198. Bilezikian JP. The medical management of primary hyperparathyroidism. Ann Intern Med 1982;96:198–202.
199. Editorial: Medical management of primary hyperparathyroidism. Lancet 1984;2: 727–728.
200. Eriksen EF, et al. Evidence of estrogen receptors in normal human osteoblast-like cells. Science 1988;241:84–86.
201. Marcus R, et al. Conjugated estrogens in the treatment of postmenopausal women with hyperparathyroidism. Ann Intern Med 1984;100:633–640.

202. Selby PL, Peacock M. Ethinyl estradiol and norethindrone in the treatment of primary hyperparathyroidism in postmenopausal women. N Engl J Med 1986;314: 1481–1485.
203. Judd HL, et al. Estrogen replacement therapy. Obstet Gynecol 1981;58:267–275.
204. Horowitz M, et al. Treatment of postmenopausal hyperparathyroidism with norethindrone. Effects on biochemistry and forearm mineral density. Arch Intern Med 1987;147:681–685.
205. Duarte B, Hargis GK, KuKreja SC. Effects of estradiol and progesterone on parathyroid tissue. J Clin Endocrinol Metab 1988;66:584–587.
206. Broadus AE, et al. A detailed evaluation of oral phosphate therapy in selected patients with primary hyperparathyroidism. J Clin Endocrinol Metab 1983;56: 953–961.
207. Shane E, Baquiran DC, Bilezikian JP. Effects of dichloromethylene diphosphonate on serum and urinary calcium in primary hyperparathyroidism. Ann Intern Med 1981;95:23–27.
208. Warrell RP Jr, et al. Gallium nitrate for treatment of refractory hypercalcemia from parathyroid carcinoma. Ann Intern Med 1987;107:683–686.
209. Leyland-Jones B. Gallium nitrate for treatment of cancer-related hypercalcemia. Pharm and Therapeutics 1996;21:370–384.
209a. Ringenberg QS, Ritch PS. Efficacy of oral administration of etidronate disodium in maintaining normal serum calcium levels in previously hypercalcemic cancer patients. Clin Ther 1987;9:1–8.
210. Van-Holten-Verzantvoort A Th, et al. Reduced morbidity from skeletal metastases in breast cancer patients during long term biphosphonate (APD) treatment. Lancet 1987;2:983–985.
211. Desai TK, Carlson RW, Gehab MA. Prevalence and clinical implications of hypocalcemia in acutely ill patients in a medical intensive setting. Am J Med 1988;84: 209–214.
212. Zaloga GP, Chernow B. The multifactorial basis for hypocalcemia during sepsis. Studies of the parathyroid hormone-vitamin D axis. Ann Intern Med 1987;107: 36–41.
213. Chase LR, Slatopolsky E. Secretion and metabolic efficacy of parathyroid hormone in patients with severe hypomagnesemia. J Clin Endocrinol Metab 1974;38:363–371.
214. Rude RK, Oldham SB, Singer FR. Functional hyperparathyroidism and parathyroid hormone end-organ resistance in human magnesium deficiency. Clin Endocrinol 1976;5:209–224.
215. Rosler A, Rabinowitz D. Magnesium-induced reversal of vitamin D resistance in hyperparathyroidism. Lancet 1973;1:803.
216. Robertson GM Jr, et al. Inadequate parathyroid response in acute pancreatitis. N Engl J Med 1976;294:512–516.
217. Haldeman B, et al. Renal function and blood levels of divalent ions in acute pancreatitis. Min Electrol Metab 1980;3:190–199.
218. Breslau NA, Pak CYC. Hypoparathyroidism. Metabolism 1979;28:1261–1276.
219. Fourman P, et al. Parathyroid insufficiency after thyroidectomy. Review of 46 cases with the study of the effects of hypocalcemia on the electroencephalogram. Br J Surg 1963;50:608–619.

220. LLach F, Felsenfeld AJ, Haussler MR. The pathophysiology of altered calcium metabolism in rhabdomyolysis induced acute renal failure. N Engl J Med 1981;305: 117–123.
221. Riancho JA, et al. The clinical spectrum of hypocalcemia associated with bone metastases. J Intern Med 1989;226:449–452.
222. Smallbridge RC, Wray HL, Schaef M. Hypocalcemia with osteoblastic metastases in a patient with prostate carcinoma. A cause of secondary hyperparathyroidism. Am J Med 1981;71:184–188.
223. Porter RH, et al. Treatment of hypoparathyroid patients with chlorthalidone. N Engl J Med 1978;298:577–581.
224. Davies M, et al. 1,25 Dihydroxycholecalciferol in hyperparathyroidism. Lancet 1977;1:55–59.
224a. Winer KK, Yanouski JA, Cutler GB. Synthetic human parathyroid hormone 1–34 vs calcitriol and calcium in the treatment of hyperparathyroidism. JAMA 1996; 276:631–636.
225. Wasserman RH. Intestinal absorption of calcium and phosphorus. Fed Proc 1981; 40:68–72.
226. Mizgala CL, Quamme GA. Renal handling of phosphate. Physiol Rev 1985;65: 431–466.
227. Mühlbauer RC, Bonjour JP, Fleisch H. Tubular localization of adaptation to dietary phosphate in rats. Am J Physiol 1977;233:F342–F348.
228. Dennis VW, Bello-Reuss E, Robinson R. Response of phosphate transport to parathyroid hormone in segments of rabbit nephron. Am J Physiol 1977;233:F28–F38.
229. Pastoriza-Muñoz E, et al. Effect of parathyroid hormone on phosphate reabsorption in rat distal convolution. Am J Physiol 1978;235:321–330.
230. Beck LH, Goldberg M. Mechanism of the blunted phosphaturia in saline-loaded thyroparathyroidectomized dogs. Kidney Int 1974;6:18–23.
231. Tucker RR, et al. Propranolol blocks the hypophosphaturia of acute respiratory alkalosis in human subjects. J Lab Clin Med 1996;128:423–428.
232. Garry PJ, et al. Clinical chemistry reference intervals for healthy elderly subjects. Am J Clin Nutr 1989;50:1219–1230.
233. Cohen SH, et al. Changes in body chemical composition with age measured by total-body neutron activation. Metabolism 1976;25:85–95.
234. Bijvoet OLM. Relation of plasma phosphate concentration to renal tubular reabsorption of phosphate. Clin Sci 1969;37:23–36.
235. Walton RJ, Bijvoet OLM. Normogram for derivation of renal threshold phosphate concentration. Lancet 1975;2:309–310.
236. Halloran BP, Lonergan ET, Portale AA. Aging and renal responsiveness to parathyroid hormone in healthy men. J. Clin Endocrinol Metab 1996;81:2192–2197.
237. Kiebzak GM, Saktor B. Effect of age on renal conservation of phosphate in the rat. Am J Physiol 1986;251:F399–F407.
238. Levi M, Jameson DM, Van Der Meer WB. Role of brush border membrane lipid composition and fluidity in impaired renal P_i transport in aged rats. Am J Physiol 1989;256:F85–F94.
239. Sorribas V, et al. Cellular mechanisms of the age-related decrease in renal phosphate reabsorption. Kidney Int 1996;50:855–863.

240. Aloia JF, et al. Total body phosphorus in postmenopausal women. Mineral Electrol Metab 1984;10:73–76.
241. Young MM, Nordin BEC. Some effects of ethinyl oestradiol on calcium and phosphorus metabolism in osteoporosis. Clin Sci 1968;34:411–417.
242. Tschöpe W, et al. Decreased plasma phosphate under hormonal contraceptives. Min Electrol Metab 1984;10:88–91.
243. Betro MG, Pain RW. Hypophosphatemia and hyperphosphatemia in a hospital population. Br Med J 1972;1:273–276.
244. Busse JC, et al. Pseudohyperphosphatemia and dysproteinemia. Arch Intern Med 1987;147:2045–2046.
245. Adler SG, et al. Hyperglobulinemia may seriously elevate measured serum inorganic phosphate levels. Am J Kidney Dis 1988;II:260–263.
246. Weinberg J, Adler AJ. Spurious hyperphosphatemia in patients with dysglobulinemia. Min Electrol Metab 1989;15:185–186.
247. Muggia FM, Chia GA, Mickley DA. Hyperphosphatemia and hypocalcemia in neoplastic disorders. N Engl J Med 1974;290:857–858.
248. Tsokos GC, et al. Renal and metabolic complications of undifferentiated and lymphoblastic lymphomas. Medicine 1981;60:218–229.
249. Goldfinger P. Hypokalemic metabolic acidosis and hypocalcemic tetany in a patient taking laxatives. J Mt Sinai Hosp 1969;36:113–116.
250. Korzets A, et al. Life-threatening hyperphosphatemia and hypercalcemic tetany following the use of Fleet enemas. J Am Geriatr Soc 1992;40:620–621.
251. Pitts RF, et al. The renal regulation of acid-base balance in man. I. The nature of the mechanism of acidifying the urine. J Clin Invest 1948;27:48–61.
252. Barsotti G, et al. The role of metabolic acidosis in causing uremic hyperphosphatemia. Min Electrol Metab 1986;12:103–106.
253. Larsson L, Sörbo B. Hypophosphatemia: a neglected electrolyte disturbance. Min Electrol Metab 1981;6:249A.
254. Gravelyn TR, et al. Hypophosphatemia-associated respiratory muscle weakness in a general inpatient population. Am J Med 1988;84:870–876.
255. Juan D, Elrazak MA. Hypophosphatemia in hospitalized patients. JAMA 1979; 242:163–164.
256. Larsson L, Rebel K, Sörbo B. Severe hypophosphatemia. A hospital survey. Acta Med Scand 1983;214:221–223.
257. Knochel JP. Hypophosphatemia. Clin Nephrol 1977;7:131–137.
258. King AL, et al. Severe hypophosphatemia in a general hospital population. South Med J 1987;80:831–835.
259. Adler AJ, Gudis S, Berlyne GM. Reduced renal phosphate threshold concentration in alcoholic cirrhosis. Min Electrol Metab 1984;10:63–66.
260. Kebler R, McDonald FD, Cadnapaphornchai P. Dynamic changes in serum phosphorus levels in diabetic ketoacidosis. Am J Med 1985;79:571–576.
261. Brautbar N, Leibovici H, Massry SG. On the mechanism of hypophasphatemia during hyperventilation: evidence for increased muscle glycolysis. Min Electrol Metab 1983;9:45–50.
262. Ryan EA, Reiss E. Oncogenous osteomalacia. Review of the world literature of 42 cases and report of 2 new cases. Am J Med 1984;77:501–512.

263. Lyles KW, et al. Hypophosphatemic osteomalacia: association with prostatic carcinoma. Ann Intern Med 1980;93:275–278.
264. Taylor HC, Fallon MD, Velasco ME. Oncogenic osteomalacia and inappropriate antidiuretic hormone secretion due to oat-cell carcinoma. Ann Intern Med 1984; 101:786–788.
265. McClure J, Smith PS. Oncogenic osteomalacia. J Clin Pathol 1987;40:466–453.
266. McMurtry CT, et al. Oncogenic osteomalacia associated with metastatic prostate carcinoma: case report and review of the literature. J Am Geriatr Soc 1993;41: 983–985.
267. Mirjauchi A, et al. Hemangiopericytoma-induced osteomalacia: tumor transplantation in nude mice causes hypophasphatemia and tumor extract inhibit renal 25(OH)D 1alpha-hydroxylase activity. J Clin Endocrinol Metab 1988;67:53.
268. Citrin DL, et al. Decreased serum phosphate levels after high dose estrogens in metastatic prostate cancer. Possible implications. Am J Med 1984;76:787–793.
269. Vannatta JB, Whang R, Papper S. Efficacy of intravenous phosphorus therapy in the severly hypophasphatemic patient. Arch Intern Med 1981;141:885–887.
270. Levine BS, Cobern JW. Magnesium, the mimic/antagonist of calcium. N Engl J Med 1984;310:1253–1254.
271. Wacker WEC, Parisi AF. Magnesium metabolism. N Engl J Med 1968;278:658–663, 712–717, 772–776.
272. Seelig MS. Perspectives in nutrition. The requirement of magnesium by the normal adult. Am J Clin Nutr 1964;14:342–390.
273. Brannan PG, et al. Magnesium absorption in the human small intestine. Results in normal subjects, patients with chronic renal disease and patients with absorptive hypercalciuria. J Clin Invest 1976;57:1412–1418.
274. Spencer H, et al. Magnesium absorption and metabolism in patients with chronic renal failure and in patients with normal renal function. Gastroenterology 1980;79:26–34.
275. Massry SG. Pharmacology of magnesium. Ann Rev Pharmacol Toxicol 1977;17: 67–82.
276. Rude RK, Bethume JF, Singer FR. Renal tubular maximum for magnesium in normal, hyperparathyroid and hypoparathyroid man. J Clin Endocrinol Metab 1980; 51:1425–1431.
277. DeRouffignac C, Quamme G. Renal magnesium handling and its hormonal control. Physiol Rev 1994;74:305–322.
278. Hollifield JW. Magnesium depletion, diuretics and arrhythmias. Am J Med 1987; 82(suppl 3A):30–37.
279. Lindsay R, Hart DM, Forrest C. Effect of a natural and artificial menopause on serum, urinary and erythrocyte magnesium. Clin Sci 1980;58:255–257.
280. Keating RF Jr, et al. The relation of age and sex to distribution of values in healthy adults of serum calcium, inorganic phosphorus, magnesium, alkaline phosphatase, total proteins, albumin and blood urea. J Lab Clin Med 1969;73:825–834.
281. McNair P, Christiansen C, Transbol IB. Effect of menopause and estrogen substitutional therapy on magnesium metabolism. Min Electrol Metab 1984;10:84–87.
282. Wong ET, et al. A high prevalence of hypomagnesemia and hypermagnesemia in hospitalized patients. Am J Clin Pathol 1983;79:348–352.

283. Whang R. Magnesium deficiency: pathogenesis, prevalence and clinical implications. Am J Med 1987;82(suppl 3A):24–29.
284. Smilkstein MJ, et al. Severe hypermagnesemia due to multiple-dose cathartic therapy. West Med 1988;148:208–210.
285. Mordes JP, Swartz R, Arky RA. Extreme hypermagnesemia as a cause of refractory hypotension. Ann Intern Med 1975;83:657–658.
286. Fassler CA, et al. Mg toxicity as a cause of hypotension and hypoventilation. Occurence in patients with normal renal function. Arch Intern Med 1987;147:1768–1771.
287. Martin BJ, Milligan K. Diuretic-associated hypomagnesemia in the elderly. Arch Intern Med 1987;147:1768–1771.
288. Martin BJ, et al. Hypomagnesemia in elderly hospital admissions: a study of clinical significance. Quart J Med 1991;286:177–184.
288a. Elisaf M, Milionis H, Siamopoulos KC. Hypomagnesemic hypokalemia and hypocalcemia: clinical and laboratory characteristics. Min Electrol Metab 1997; 23:105–112.
289. Fiaccadori E, et al. Muscle and serum magnesium in pulmonary intensive care unit patients. Crit Care Med 1988;16:751–760.
290. Whang R, et al. Predictors of clinical hypomagnesemia. Hypokalemia, hypophosphatemia, hyponatremia and hypocalcemia. Arch Intern Med 1985;145:1086–1089.
291. Petri M, Cumber P, Grimes L. The metabolic effects of thiazide therapy in the elderly: a population study. Age & Ageing 1986;15:151–155.
292. Whang R, et al. Magnesium depletion as a cause of refractory potassium repletion. Arch Intern Med 1985;145:1086–1089.
293. Dyckner T, Wester P. Relation between potassium and magnesium in cardiac arrhythmias. Acta Med Scand 1981;647(suppl):163–169.
294. Roden DM, Iansmith DHS. Effects of low potassium or magnesium concentrations on isolated cardiac tissue. Am J Med 1987;82(suppl 3A):18–23.
295. Schilsky RL, Anderson T. Hypomagnesemia and renal magnesium patients receiving cis-platin. Ann Intern Med 1979;90:929–931.
296. Buckley JE, et al. Hypomagnesemia after cisplatin combination chemotherapy. Arch Intern Med 1984;144:2347–2348.
297. Chernow B, et al. Aminoglycoside induced hypomagnesemia: a prospective study. Clin Res 1982;30:863A.
298. Keating MJ, et al. Hypocalcemia with hypoparathyroidism and renal tubular dysfunction associated with aminoglycoside therapy. Cancer 1977;39:1410–1414.
299. Patel R, Savage A. Symptomatic hypomagnesemia associated with gentamicin therapy. Nephron 1979;23:50–52.
300. Barton CH, et al. Renal magnesium wasting associated with amphotericin B therapy. Am J Med 1984;77:471–474.
301. Fleming CR, et al. The importance of urinary magnesium values in patients with gut failure. Mayo Clin Proc 1996;71:21–24.
302. Sullivan JF, Lankford HG, Robertson P. Renal excretion of lactate and magnesium in alcoholism. Am J Clin Nutr. 1966;18:231–237.

303. Doe RP, Flink EB, Prased AS. Magnesium metabolism in hyperthyroidism. J Lab Clin Med 1959;54:805–810.
304. Horton R, Biglieri EG. Effect of aldosterone on the metabolism of magnesium. J Clin Endocrinol Metab 1962;22:1187–1192.
305. Oster JR, Epstein M. Management of magnesium depletion. Am J Nephrol 1988; 8:349–354.
306. Elin RJ. Magnesium metabolism in health and disease. DM 1988;34:166–218.
307. Ryan MP. Diuretics and potassium/magnesium depletion. Directions for treatment. Am J Med 1987;82(suppl 3A):38–47.
308. Dyckner T, Wester PO, Widman L. Amiloride prevents thiazide-induced intracellular potassium and magnesium losses. Acta Med Scand 1988;224:25–30.

6

Primary Glomerular Disease

I. THE KIDNEY BIOPSY

The kidney biopsy is the primary method of diagnosing glomerulonephritis and other parenchymal disease of the kidney. This procedure is as safe in the elderly as in younger patients, even though associated conditions such as hypertension and renal insufficiency theoretically increase the risk of complications. In an analysis of over 2000 biopsies performed in subjects 65 years and older, the complication rate varied between 2.2% and 9.8%, similar to the 7% rate reported in younger subjects (1–8). Bleeding (both micro- and macroscopic hematuria, or perirenal hematoma) was the most commonly encountered complication (88%). Indications for kidney biopsy in this age group were nephrotic syndrome (48%), acute renal failure (25%), chronic renal insufficiency (19%), and urinary abnormalities: hematuria or proteinuria less than 3 g (8%).

II. INCIDENCE

Primary glomerular diseases are not uncommon in the elderly. Of 379 patients aged 14 to 89 years diagnosed as having a primary glomerular disease in our hospital during the past 20 years, 67 (18%) were over 60 years old (Fig. 1); this rate is similar to the 11% reported by Davison et al. (9) and Columbo et al. (5) and to

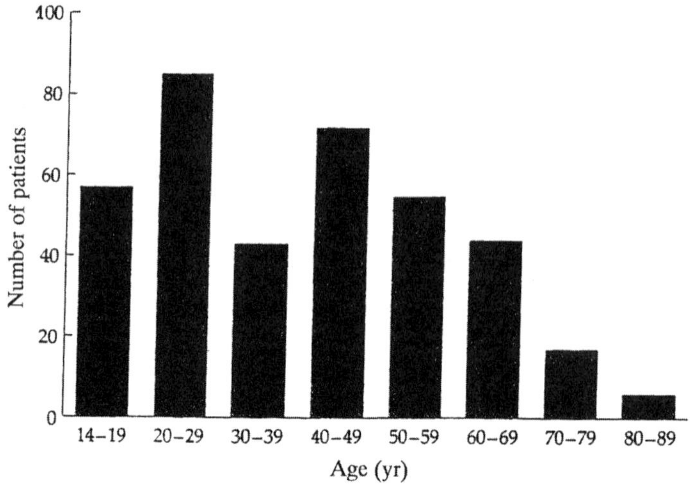

Figure 1 Age distribution of 379 patients with primary glomerular disease seen at the Brookdale Hospital Medical Center (1968–1987).

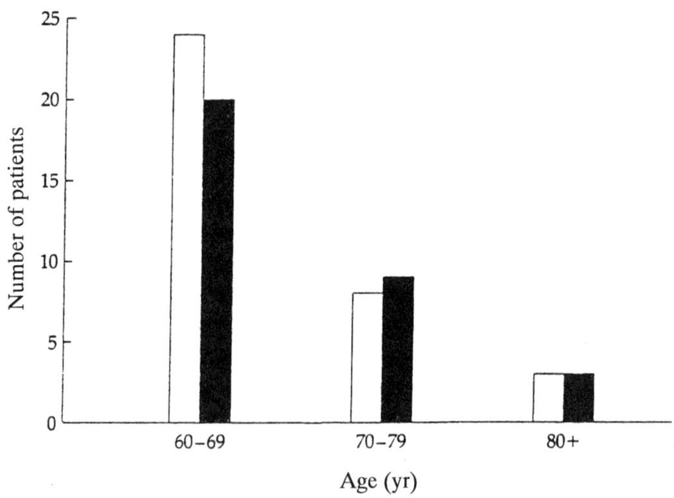

Figure 2 Age and sex distribution of 67 elderly patients with primary glomerular disease. Open bar: male; dark bar: female.

Table 1 Frequency of Associated Arteriosclerosis Among Biopsied Patients (%)

Age (*n*)	10–19 (407)	20–39 (1278)	40–64 (1481)	≥65 (752)
Arterial sclerosis ≥ 2+[a]	7	24	50	77
Arteriolosclerosis	0	0	2	5

[a]On a scale of 0 to 4+.
Source: Falk RJ, Jennette JC. Glomerular disease in the elderly. In: Jacobson HR, Striker GE, Klahr S, eds. The Principles and Practice of Nephrology. 2d ed. St. Louis: Mosby, 1995: 518–523.

the 19% reported by Cameron (10). Figure 2 shows the sex distribution according to age; there were 35 males (52%) and 32 females (48%).

The pathological diagnosis of glomerular diseases in the elderly as derived from the literature and our own experience is similar to that of younger adults with the exception of the increased incidence of associated arterial sclerosis and arterionephrosclerosis (Table 1). The incidence of membranous nephropathy, the most common form of the primary glomerular diseases in the elderly, has been estimated to be 2.5 times higher than in younger subjects. Crescentic glomerulonephritis was 4 times higher and IgA nephropathy approximately one-third as common. The incidence for the other glomerulopathies is identical between the two groups (9,11). Some authors, however, have found minimal change disease to be one-third to one-half as common in the elderly compared to younger adults (4,5,10).

III. HALLMARKS

Proteinuria (with or without the nephrotic syndrome), edema, hypertension, hematuria (gross or microscopic), and renal insufficiency are the clinical hallmarks of primary glomerular disease in the elderly, as in younger adults.

A. Proteinuria

In normal adults, protein excretion is usually less than 150 mg/24 hr. Friedman et al. (12) measured 24-hr urine protein excretion in 21 patients over age 60 and found the same normal range. We examined protein excretion in 40 elderly patients (age 60–90 years), using the single-voided urine sample. A normal protein–creatinine ratio of less than 0.2, as reported by Ginsberg and colleagues (13), was found in all these subjects, who had a serum creatinine of less than 1.5 mg/dl and no evidence of infection, decompensated congestive heart failure, or hypertension. In 29 normotensive nondiabetic subjects 60 years and older studied by Fliser et al. (14), 76% had albuminuria of less than 20 ug/ml, similar to younger subjects.

In experimental studies the following factors have been shown to play a role in the glomerular filtration of protein.

Size. Smaller proteins filter more easily than larger ones. It has been estimated that the normal glomerular capillary wall acts as a membrane that has uniform pores with a radius of approximately 50 Å. Macromolecules that have a molecular radius less than 24 Å have a clearance identical to that of the glomerular filtration rate, whereas molecules greater than 60 Å are completely excluded from the glomerular ultrafiltrate.

Charge. The backbone of the glomerular basement membrane is composed mainly of type IV collagen to which are attached negatively charged glycoproteins and proteoglycans. Electrostatic interactions at the glomerular capillary wall tend to retard the filtration of polyanions such as albumin while enhancing the filtration of polycations, as shown by Rennke et al. (15). Impairment of this electrostatic barrier contributes to the magnitude of albuminuria in the nephrotic syndrome (16).

Hemodynamic factors. Conditions associated with a decrease in glomerular plasma flow such as congestive heart failure are associated with an increase in protein excretion (17). Molecular configuration may also play a role.

With this background, the specific mechanisms responsible for the increased permeability of the glomerular capillary to plasma protein in different forms of glomerulopathy may be examined. Blau and Haas (18), using cytochemical techniques, have shown severe depletion of the fixed negatively charged components of the glomerular capillary wall in virtually all proteinuric disorders of humans. More recently, Meyers and associates (19) have postulated that there is a loss of the fixed negative charge in the glomerular wall in patients with selective proteinuria (excreting mainly albumin). In patients with nonselective proteinuria, the glomerular capillary wall becomes a heteroporous membrane with a bimodal pore size distribution; a large-pore ultrafilter develops that is responsible for the increased filtration of large molecules (such as IgG) of varying charges (20). Therefore, proteinuria in most nephrotic patients results from the combined impairment of barrier charge and size selectivity (20a).

B. Edema

The edema of nephrotic syndrome is due to salt retention, with both extrarenal and renal factors implicated in its pathogenesis.

1. *Extrarenal Factors*

a. Plasma Volume. Patients with the nephrotic syndrome develop hypoalbuminemia due to increased urinary losses of protein and fractional renal catabolic rate. According to the traditional view, hypoalbuminemia, by lowering the plasma oncotic pressure, favors the movement of water from the intravascular to the interstitial space, resulting in a decrease in plasma volume, which then leads to renal salt and water retention. The plasma volume is usually low in patients with severe hypoalbuminemia (serum albumin less than 1.0 g/dl); however, in the majority of patients with nephrotic syndrome, the plasma volume is either normal or increased (21–23). Furthermore, plasma volume expansion with hyperoncotic albumin does not necessarily induce natriuresis (24). Finally, in patients with nephrotic syndrome who undergo water immersion, the urinary excretion of sodium peaks toward the end (third or fourth hour) of immersion, when volume expansion has presumably been present for some time (25,26). It appears that intravascular hypovolemia, per se, is not solely responsible for the salt retention of nephrotic syndrome.

b. Salt-Regulating Hormones. The renin-angiotensin-aldosterone system is frequently activated in patients with nephrotic syndrome; however, it may be normal in a substantial number of patients (27). Moreover, patients with nephrotic syndrome who are placed on a high-salt diet may continue to retain salt despite lowering plasma renin and aldosterone (28). Also, captopril, 50 mg three times a day orally, given to nephrotic patients with elevated plasma aldosterone does not induce a natriuresis despite lowering the aldosterone level (29). Identical results were also reported with infusion of saralasin (an angiotensin II competitive inhibitor that lowers plasma aldosterone) (30).

Many animal studies have documented a role for catecholamines in increasing renal sodium reabsorption (31). Oliver et al. (32) found an increased catecholamine excretion in patients with the nephrotic syndrome. This, however, was not confirmed by Geers and associates (33). The latter measured plasma noradrenalin in normal subjects and in patients with nephrotic syndrome and found it identical in both groups.

Since the kidneys play an important role in the catabolism of atrial natriuretic peptides (ANP) (34), the plasma concentration of these peptides tends to vary in direct proportion to the glomerular filtration rate (GFR). In patients with glomerular disease but normal kidney function, plasma ANP is similar to that in normal controls, whereas in those with renal insufficiency the ANP level is increased (35,36). During the phase of active renal salt retention in nephrotics, a blunted natriuretic response to ANP in the inner medullary collecting duct has been found (37). This altered tubular response to ANP may be due not only to a defect in the number and affinity of its receptor-binding sites, but also to a defect at the level of intracellular cyclic guanosine monophosphate, its second messenger (38). During the maintenance phase of edema or in the nonedematous patient with glomerular disease, the response reverts to normal (39). Renal production of prostaglandin E_2, a natriuretic substance, is suppressed in nephrotic patients (40). The significance of this observation in the salt retention of nephrotic syndrome is not clear, however.

2. *Renal Factors*

The GFR is frequently decreased in patients with nephrotic syndrome (41), due to a lowering of the glomerular ultrafiltration coefficient (42), but a significant number of patients with minimal change disease have a normal GFR despite massive edema. Also, during water immersion, natriuresis may be dissociated from changes in GFR. Using a model of unilateral puromycin aminonucleoside-induced albuminuria in the rat, Ichikawa et al. (43) demonstrated that only the proteinuric kidney retained salt, but the specific mechanism responsible for the salt retention was not defined. Using a variety of methods, most investigators have placed the site of increased salt reabsorption in the distal nephron (44); however, evidence for increased proximal reabsorption has also been provided by Koomans and associates (24).

In summary, the edema and salt retention characteristic of the nephrotic syndrome is the consequence of multiple factors, one or several of which may be present at any time in a given patient. These factors include a decreased plasma volume, the renin-angiotensin-aldosterone system, ANP, other vasoactive hormones, a decrease in GFR, and other, still undefined, renal mechanisms (43).

C. Hypertension

Hypertension is frequently present in patients with glomerular disease. In the majority of these patients renal insufficiency (defined as a serum creatinine greater than 1.5 mg/dl) is present. It has been suggested that the hypertension represents a trade-off necessary for the restoration of sodium balance (45). Other factors such as increased angiotensin II activity and the inhibition of the vasodilatory effect of nitric oxide by circulating endogenous nitric oxyde synthase inhibitors are also involved (46). Although hypertension is secondary to renal disease in most of these patients, some may have essential hypertension. Also, given the prevalence of atheromatous renovascular disease in the elderly, one should always keep in mind the possibility that the hypertension is secondary to renal artery stenosis, and clues to this diagnosis, such as evidence of peripheral vascular disease, an abdominal bruit, or a discrepancy in kidney size, should be looked for carefully.

D. Hematuria

Hematuria, either microscopic (more than 5 red blood cells per high-power field) or macroscopic, is frequently present in patients with glomerular disease. In the elderly, in whom even intermittent hematuria may be due to other serious conditions of the genitourinary tract (46a,47), the decision is whether the red blood cells (RBCs) originate from the glomeruli or from more distal portions of the urinary tract. RBC casts suggest renal hematuria. The red blood cell morphology may also help to determine the origin of the cells. More than 90% of patients with glomerular disease have distorted, dysmorphic red blood cells in their urine, unlike the more uniform red blood cell morphology found in patients with hematuria due to other causes (47–49). To evaluate red cell morphology, a simple Sedicolor staining procedure of the urinary sediment can be used (50). Briefly, 10 ml of fresh clean-voided urine is centrifuged at 1500 rev/min for 5 min. Two drops of the stain are added to the sediment. Examination is done by light microscopy under oil immersion. It should be noted, however, that a close correlation (as reported above) between red cell morphology and diagnosis has not been found by all observers (51). A urine specimen with an osmolality greater than 700 mOsm/kg/H_2O and a pH less than 7 will increase the diagnostic yield of such a test, since both lower osmolality and higher pH could result in lysis of the red blood cells (52). Nevertheless, as a rule, less than 15% of dysmorphic red cells in a sediment makes a renal cause of hematuria quite unlikely (53). When in doubt, lesions of the urinary tract should be adequately ruled out using imaging techniques and cystoscopic examination.

IV. SPECIFIC GLOMERULOPATHIES

A. Membranous Nephropathy

Membranous nephropathy is the most common form of primary glomerular disease in the elderly (Table 2). Of 80 patients with membranous nephropathy seen in our hospital over a period of 15 years, 14, or 17.5%, were over the age of 60. This proportion is similar to the 18% reported by Noel et al. (59), and the 17% reported by Davison et al. (9). Lower (8%) and higher (27%) proportions have also been reported (4,5). There was a slight preponderance of males over females (57% to 43%). In Table 2, an attempt was made to include only patients with the idiopathic variety; however, it should be emphasized that in certain patients, particularly when disease is associated with carcinoma, the nephropathy may develop before the underlying disease becomes apparent.

1. Pathology

a. Light Microscopy. The characteristic finding is thickening of the glomerular capillary wall. In the early stages of the disease, however, the wall may appear normal. By means of special stains (silver, trichrome), the thickening of the basement membrane can be seen to be due to the presence of subepithelial deposits. The mesangium is usually not affected, although in a small percentage of patients mild to moderate cellular proliferation has been described.

b. Electron Microscopy. The capillary wall changes have been divided into four stages by Ehrenreich and Churg (60).

Stage I. Characterized by the presence of small scattered subepithelial electron-dense deposits in the basement membrane.

Table 2 Histopathological Diagnosis in 1416 Elderly Patients with Primary Glomerular Disease

Glomerular disease	Number of patients	Percentage (%)
Membranous nephropathy[a]	398	28
Difuse mesangial or focal glomerulonephritis[b]	337	24
Extracapillary glomerulonephritis	187	13
Minimal change disease	137	10
Focal segmental glomerulonephritis	132	9
Mesangiocapillary glomerulonephritis	112	8
Chronic glomerulonephritis	62	4
Acute endoproliferative glomerulonephritis	51	4
	1,416	(100)

[a]Only patients with idiopathic membranous nephropathy are included.
[b]Including IgA and other mesangial proliferative diseases.
Source: From Refs. 4, 5, 6, 9, 11, 54–58.

Stage II. The deposits are more numerous and are separated by projections arising from and having the appearance of the lamina densa.

Stage III. The spikes fuse over the deposits incorporating them into the basement membrane.

Stage IV. Most of the deposits disappear, leaving an irregularly thickened basement membrane.

It is possible to see more than one stage in the same biopsy specimen.

c. *Fluorescence Microscopy.* Fluorescence microscopy reveals the presence of evenly distributed granular deposits of IgG and C3 along the glomerular capillary wall.

2. *Pathogenesis*

The nature and source of the deposits found in patients diagnosed as having idiopathic membranous nephropathy are not clear and are still a matter of controversy. Two major hypotheses have been proposed: circulating immune complexes and in-situ immune complexes. In the former the complexes are formed by antibodies of low avidity with an overall cationic charge that become entrapped in the subepithelium (61). This may account for the infrequent finding of circulating immune complexes by conventional methods in patients with membranous nephropathy. According to the hypothesis of in-situ immune complexes, subepithelial deposits of IgG and complement result from antibody binding to either a fixed glomerular antigen or a planted antigen, and $C5_b$-9 membrane insertion is required for proteinuria to develop (62). This could explain why some patients with membranous nephropathy have an increased urinary excretion of $C5_b$-9

(62a). Endocytosis of membrane-inserted $C5_b$-9 complexes by glomerular epithelial cells followed by transcellular transport and exocytosis into the urinary space could explain this increase in the urinary excretion of $C5_b$-9. Even though there is considerable experimental evidence in favor of this mechanism, which is also compatible with the general absence of circulatory immune complexes, the nature of the antigens and antibodies responsible for the human disease remains to be determined.

3. *Clinical Manifestations*

Nephrotic syndrome (i.e., proteinuria of more than 3.0–3.5 g/24 hr and hypoalbuminemia) was the initial presentation in 91% of our elderly patients with membranous nephropathy. The remaining 9% had nonnephrotic proteinuria (less than 3.0 g/24 hr). Renal insufficiency, defined as a serum creatinine greater than 1.5 mg/dl or a creatinine clearance less than 50 ml/min, was more commonly present at the time of diagnosis in the elderly compared to younger patients, and present in 40% of the patients. Microscopic hematuria was present in 78%. Hypertension (blood pressure over 160/90) was detected in 49%. There is not enough information in the literature to suggest a specific association between the presence of renal insufficiency and a specific histological appearance; however, our 14 patients with a serum creatinine of over 1.5 mg/dl had either stage II or stage III disease. In general, 56% of the elderly biopsied have either stage II or stage III. Hypertension was found more frequently in patients with renal failure.

4. *Natural History and Treatment*

Because of the varying natural history in patients with idiopathic membranous nephropathy, it has been very difficult to assess the results of therapeutic interventions in this disease. In general, membranous nephropathy in adults has the following natural history independent of age. In approximately 25% the disease undergoes a spontaneous remission. In 25%, proteinuria persists (usually nonnephrotic range) without progressive renal failure. The remaining 50% of patients develop renal insufficiency, usually progressing slowly (reaching end-stage kidney disease in 20 years or more), but with some progressing relatively rapidly and reaching end-stage renal disease in 5–7 years (59,63–65). The rate of progression of the disease is similar in older and younger patients (65a).

Patients with less than 2 g of proteinuria/24 hr tend to do better than those with nephrotic-range proteinuria, and those with more advanced histological stages of the disease do worse. Males generally do worse than females. There are many exceptions, however, so it is not easy to prognosticate. Although there have been suggestions that early glomerular sclerosis, increases in mesangial cellularity, or chronic tubulointerstitial changes may portend a worse prognosis (66), these associations have not been definitely proven. Our approach to the disease in the elderly is similar to that in other adults.

a. Patients with Nonnephrotic Proteinuria. Because these patients usually have a benign course, therapy is recommended only for those in whom the proteinuria subsequently progresses to nephrotic proteinuria or who develop renal failure (approximately 20%) (67).

b. Patients with Nephrotic Syndrome and Normal GFR. Three options are presently available for managing patients in this group: no therapy, prednisone alone, and an alkylating agent with or without prednisone. Recent meta-analysis of previously published studies dealing with therapy of membranous nephropathy reveal that treatment with alkylating agents with or without steroids is associated with a higher incidence of remission than are steroids alone or no treatment (68,68a). Progression to end-stage renal failure, which occurs in 35% of patients after 10 years and 41% after 15 years, is not prevented by these agents; however, steroids alone should probably not be used in the elderly, as suggested by Zent et al. (65a). One regimen consists of 3 consecutive days of pulse (1 g) methylprednisolone followed by oral prednisone (0.5 mg/kg of body weight/day) given in a single dose for 1 month. At the end of the first month, the prednisone is stopped and cyclophosphamide (2 mg/kg/day) is given for 1 month. Each drug is repeated in alternate months for 6 months (63). In another regimen, chlorambucil 0.2 mg/kg/day is substituted for the cyclophosphamide (64,65). With the latter regimen a higher incidence of drug-induced complications (mainly infectious) was found in the elderly compared to younger subjects in one study, forcing the authors to suggest that the dose of chlorambucil be halved in the former (65). Cyclosporine, 4–5 mg/kg/day in two divided doses, has been shown in a relatively small number of adults to be effective in reducing the rate of deterioration of renal function as well as proteinuria, by enhancing the barrier size selectivity (69,69a). Worsening hypertension and a transient rise (> 30%) in serum creatinine are common side effects. In these studies, patients were treated for an average of 3–10 months. It is noteworthy that cyclosporine does not prevent continuing autoantibody formation (69a). Our recommendation is that specific therapeutic intervention be limited to those elderly with severe nephrotic syndrome (proteinuria greater than 5 g, disabling edema), those with a rapid decline in kidney function using either of the two regimen outlined above (69b–70a), and perhaps those with persisting urinary C5b-9 excretion (62a).

c. Patients with Renal Insufficiency. There are no published results of a prospective study in this patient group. A striking finding in our retrospective analysis was that none of the untreated patients had a remission of proteinuria, and in 92% the renal failure was progressive (67). In the treated group, by contrast, 53% had complete or partial remission or improved renal function, whereas renal function became progressively worse in 37%. Based on these findings, our own approach is to treat these patients, alternating prednisone and cyclophosphamide as outlined above. In general, we use only supportive care (Chapter 11) for patients with a serum creatinine greater than 3 mg/dl (70b).

So far we have discussed patients with the idiopathic form of the disease. It should be noted that in 15% of patients with membranous nephropathy, a variety of infections, multisystem diseases, neoplasms, or drugs may be associated with membranous nephropathy; these will be dealt with in another section of this chapter as well as in Chapter 7.

B. Diffuse Mesangial or Focal Proliferative Glomerulonephritis

1. Incidence

Diffuse mesangial or focal proliferative glomerulonephritis was found in 24% patients (Table 2). Mesangial nephritis consists of a heterogeneous group of diseases in which IgA, IgM, or C3 may be seen in the mesangium with a varying degree of electron-dense deposits (71,72). Thirty-one to eighty-six percent of elderly with mesangial nephritis have IgA (3–5,9). This wide variation most likely reflects selection bias as far as kidney biopsy is concerned, since hematuria is the most common manifestation of this disease and it is quite likely that many elderly with IgA nephritis are originally seen and investigated by urologists. Following investigation of the genitourinary tract with IVP and cystoscopy, some of these patients are probably diagnosed as hematuria of unknown etiology and managed accordingly. There is no doubt that IgA nephropathy is the most common form of the disease and the best studied. The following discussion deals primarily with this form of mesangial proliferative nephritis. In most reported biopsy series comparing younger to older patients, IgA is three to five times more common in the younger age group (5,9). Eighty-three percent of elderly patients with IgA nephropathy are males (73–76).

2. Pathology

According to Sinniah (77), the pathology of mesangial nephritis can be classified as follows:

Class I. Minimal lesions, appearing "normal" on light microscopy.

Class II. Minor changes with widening of the mesangium and increased cellularity in groups of up to three cells per mesangial area in the periphery of the glomerulus.

Class III. Focal and segmental glomerulonephritis with less than 50% of the glomeruli showing localized or segmental sclerosis and mesangial cell proliferation, the remaining glomeruli showing minor changes only.

Class IV. Diffuse mesangial cell proliferation. Segmental crescents may be found.

Class V. Diffuse sclerosing glomerulonephritis in which more than 80% of the glomeruli are involved.

Focal interstitial edema with lymphocytic cell infiltrates may also be present, as well as fibrosis, which varies with the severity of the glomerular lesions.

In patients with IgA nephropathy, C_3, IgM, and/or IgG may also be present along the glomerular capillary wall, a finding associated with a rather poor prognosis (78,79).

A modified classification with only three stages of disease has also been published (76):

Class I. Mesangial matrix expansion alone.

Class II. Diffuse or focal segmental mesangial cell proliferation.

Class III. Diffuse or focal segmental mesangial proliferation with or without segmental necrosis, synechiae, sclerosis or crescent formation.

3. Pathogenesis

As with other glomerular diseases, the pathogenesis of IgA nephropathy is still not clear; however, increased levels of IgA, especially the lambda-IgA subclass, have been found in the plasma in a significant number of the patients (80,81). This finding suggests that in these immunologically susceptible patients a specific clone (or clones) of lymphocytes from the bone marrow (82) produces an increased amount of IgA_1 when challenged with an exogenous antigen (e.g., virus or bacteria); the resulting antigen–antibody complexes are then deposited in the mesangium (79,80,83). The nature of the genetic defect and the reason for the mesangial location of the immune complexes are not clear, although factors such as the polymeric nature of IgA, the formation of lambda-IgA complexes, and the anionic charge of IgA have been suggested as possibilities (81,84). Also, there remains the possibility that the entire reaction may be secondary to the formation of in-situ immune complexes in response to planted or "trapped" antigens. The deposition of polymeric lambda-IgA_1 in the mesangium then creates conditions favoring activation of the complement pathway as well as release of inflammatory mediators (various cytokines) and coagulation factors (85), the end point being mesangial cell proliferation, increase in mesangial matrix, and sclerosis.

4. Clinical Manifestations

Indications for kidney biopsy in 70 elderly patients with IgA nephropathy reported in the different series described above were proteinuria or hematuria (92%), with nephrotic syndrome present in 30%, chronic renal insufficiency in 25%, and acute renal failure in 19%. In some patients, the acute renal failure was associated with episodes of macroscopic hematuria (86). Hypertension was present in 66% of the patients at the time of diagnosis (87).

5. Natural History and Treatment

IgA nephropathy is, in general, a benign disease; the vast majority (>80%) of patients maintain stable renal function, with some patients (12%) undergoing complete remission (88). The clinical and pathological features which adversely affect outcome include age of onset, family history of nephritis, nephrotic-range proteinuria, hypertension, increased renal gallium uptake (89), the percentage of glomeruli with segmental or global sclerosis, the degree of tubular atrophy, interstitial fibrosis and/or inflammation, blood vessel thickening, and the intensity of IgA deposition. Most of the factors associated with a poor outcome have been found with a higher frequency in older patients (73–75,86,90–93) at the time of diagnosis. In the patients reported by Caillette et al. (87), approximately half developed end-stage renal failure.

No proven effective therapy is available for managing patients with IgA nephropathy. Phenytoin, dipyridamole, danazole, clyclosporine, and plasma exchange have all been tried with either limited or no success at all (94–100). In patients with nephrotic syndrome or renal insufficiency with or without nephrotic syndrome, it is reasonable to recommend steroid therapy, 120 mg every other day for 12 weeks or longer, depending on the patient's response and tolerance for the drug. The rational for this approach is derived from the fact that in most reported studies to date the best results were observed in those patients receiving steroids, but none of the studies was definitive (101–104). Experience with the use of cytotoxic agents in IgA nephropathy is very limited (101–104).

In patients with rapidly progressive renal failure and crescentic disease on biopsy, pulse steroids should be administered, 1000 mg of methylprednisolone (or its equivalent) intravenously for 3 days, followed by oral steroids, as described above. The ratio of cellular (C) to fibrous (F) crescents has been found to be helpful in predicting the response to steroids (105). Patients with a C:F ratio of >0.25 appear to do better.

In patients who cannot tolerate steroids, particularly those patients with heavy proteinuria, it is probably reasonable to suggest that they receive concentrated fish oil, 12 g daily, (106,106a). The ongoing collaborative study using concentrated fish oil in IgA nephropathy should provide significant new information on this therapeutic modality (101).

IgA deposition is also seen in a variety of glomerular diseases associated with systemic involvement, such as Henoch-Schönlein purpura, systemic lupus erythematosus, liver disease, and HIV infection (Chapter 7).

C. Extracapillary Glomerulonephritis

1. Incidence

Extracapillary or crescentic glomerulonephritis was found in 13% of reported elderly patients with primary glomerular disease (Table 2). Based on immunohistological and serological criteria, extracapillary glomerulonephritis has been divided into three different groups: pauci-immune, found in 79% of the elderly; antiglomerular basement membrane antibodies in 12%; immune complex deposits in 9% (6,107).

2. *Pathology*

The light microscopic findings are identical in all these patients and are characterized by epithelial cell proliferation with mononuclear and polymorphonuclear cell infiltration during the active phase of the disease. These cells eventually disappear as the crescents become fibrous. Tubular degeneration may be present. With electron microscopy, fibrin is seen in Bowman's space or the capillary lumen. The capillary walls may show "breaks" in the areas of crescents or elsewhere, as well as fibrinoid necrosis. On occasion, translucent deposits may occupy the lamina rara interna. Frequently, no deposits are seen with immunofluorescent microscopy, but linear capillary wall staining with IgA and C_3 may be present in those patients with antiglomerular basement membrane antibodies. In the immune complex deposit group there is granular capillary wall or mesangial staining with a variety of immunoglobulins and C_3.

Patients with the latter form of crescentic disease usually have concurrent systemic immune-complex diseases such IgA nephropathy, collagen vascular diseases, or postinfectious glomerulonephritis. The pauci-immune variety of crescentic glomerulonephritis very likely represents a form of systemic disease affecting essentially, but not exclusively, the kidneys. The antineutrophil cytoplasmic autoantibodies (ANCA), which are serological markers for a spectrum of disease characterized by necrotizing vascular inflammation, are positive in 82–92% of these patients (108–110). ANCAs directed against the proteolytic enzymes, such as the neutral serine proteinase 3, are called C-ANCA (PR3), and those directed against the antigen myeloperoxidase are called P-ANCA (MPO). In general, in patients with pauci-immune glomerulonephritis and either negative ANCA or positive P-ANCA (MPO), the disease tends to be limited to the kidneys, whereas in those with positive C-ANCA (PR_3), extrarenal involvement is quite prominent. The majority of patients in this group have Wegener's granulomatosis (111).

3. *Pathogenesis*

In patients with the antiglomerular basement membrane (anti-GBM) form of the disease, antibodies are formed against of an alpha-3 chain of type IV collagen of the glomerular and alveolar basement membrane. The reason for this preferential binding is not clear. Better and greater accessibility and/or greater expression of the alpha-3 chain in these organs remain distinct possibilities. What triggers the immune response, however, remains to be determined.

The proposed hypotheses have been summarized by Lewis and Schwartz (112) and include release into the systemic circulation of cross-reacting endogenous nonrenal antigen (alveolar basement membrane) or exogenous antigen (microorganisms), which elicits an immune response at the glomerular level, or an abnormality (congenital or acquired) in the antigenic structure of the glomerular basement membrane that leads to antibody formation.

Whatever the pathogenic mechanism, there is experimental evidence that complement and leukocytes participate in the clinical manifestations of the disease (113). Leukocyte depletion with irradiation can prevent the decrease in the ultrafiltration coefficient (LpA or Kf) and single-nephron GFR in a rat model of antiglomerular basement membrane antibody nephritis (114). Proinflammatory cytokines (interleukin-1, tumor necrosis factor-α) and locally produced lytic factors have also been found to participate in the damage to the glomerular basement membrane (115,115a).

For those patients with pauci-immune glomerulonephritis, the pathogenesis of disease is even less clear; however, there is experimental evidence suggesting that soluble immune complexes that do not deposit in glomeruli may be primary mediators of damage to the glomeruli (116). Also, as noted by Cohen et al. (117), the absence of deposits at the time of biopsy does not necessarily rule out a pathologic process involving humoral immunity. Indeed, Olsen and associates (118) reported a patient in whom the initial biopsy was free of deposits, but 12 days later a nephrectomy specimen disclosed granular deposits of immunoglobulins and complement. Although the presence of ANCA antibodies has correlated to some extent with disease activity in pauci-immune glomerulonephritis, their potential role in the pathogenesis of this entity remains to be elucidated (119).

4. *Clinical Manifestations*

As noted earlier, the presence of linear deposits on biopsy is less common in the elderly. Of 23 patients reported in the literature, 12 were males and 11 were females. Acute renal failure was the initial presentation in all patients, with pulmonary hemorrhage a less frequent occurrence. All patients had hematuria (microscopic or macroscopic) with red blood cell casts. Protein excretion generally ranged between 500 and 1000 mg per 24 hr. Two patients had a history of hydrocarbon exposure. Glomerular basement membrane (GBM) antibody, determined by radioimmunoassay, was positive in 95% of the patients (117,120–126). A significant number of those patients (30–40%) also have a positive P-ANCA (75%) or C-ANCA (25%) (107,126).

In general, these patients tend to have more systemic manifestations and more frequent relapses than those who are anti-GBM positive but ANCA negative. The association of alveolar hemorrhage and rapidly progressive glomerulonephritis is often referred to as the pulmonary-renal syndrome. Antig-GBM antibody is responsible for only 7–17% of the patients. The majority (50–55%) have pauci-immune glomerulonephritis and alveolar capillaritis. The remaining patients have either Wegner's granulomatosis (8–18%) or unrelated pulmonary and renal diseases (127–129).

Sixty percent of the elderly with pauci-immune glomerulonephritis are males. Clinical manifestations depend on whether the disease process is limited to the kidneys. In that case, complaints are limited to malaise, weight loss, and nausea. Hypertension is present in 57%. Fever, arthralgia, and other systemic manifestations suggest the presence of a vasculitis (Chapter 7). Acute renal failure is the most common renal presentation and occurs in 78% of the patients. All the patients have microscopic or macroscopic hematuria with or without RBC casts. Twenty-two percent have chronic renal failure. Protein excretion ranges between 200 and 3000 mg per 24 hr. P-ANCA, as noted earlier, is positive in most patients (117,120–122,130–135).

5. *Natural History and Treatment*

It is very difficult to decide whether or not treatment is beneficial in the elderly with crescentic disease, because there is still no reported double-blinded prospective study comparing any given therapeutic regimen with no therapy. In general, older do worse than younger patients (136). In most series, therapy has not been uniform. Although the great majority of patients reported received some form of treatment, in those with granular or no deposits 74% either died or were placed on dialysis in a relatively short period of time (weeks to months). The remaining 26% either recovered renal function or had stable chronic renal insufficiency. The outcome appears to be just as severe in patients with linear deposits, although the number of such elderly patients reported is quite small. The presence of oliguria, a high percentage of crescents, interstitial fibrosis on initial renal biopsy, and a high entry serum creatinine level are usually associated with a poor outcome.

Even though there is no proof that therapy alters the course of the disease, most authors suggest early institution of intensive plasma exchange and immunosuppression for patients with anti-GBM antibody disease (linear deposits). Johnson et al. (137) used 4-L exchange with type-specific frozen plasma, together with saline or saline-albumin solution every 3 days. Plasma exchange was continued until the anti-GBM antibody titer was less than 5% binding or the patient required maintenance hemodialysis for longer than 30 days. Alternate-day or daily exchange regimens have also been used. Immunosuppressive treatment usually consists of prednisone, 2 mg/kg daily for 1 week, followed by 1 mg/kg daily for the next 3 weeks, and then tapered to alternate-day therapy for the next 3 months. In addition, cyclophosphamide, 2 mg/kg/day, is frequently added. This regimen is recommended for patients who have a positive ANCA with high-titer anti-GBM antibody or who are dialysis dependent. Patients with low-titer anti-GBM are managed with pulse steroid (vide infra), which is substituted for plasmapheresis (126).

Episodes of pulmonary hemorrhage are best managed with high-dose intravenous prednisone (30 mg/kg to a maximum single dose of 3 g), infused over 20 min on alternate days for three treatments (1 g can also be used on a daily basis for 3 days). Attention should be paid to avoiding volume overload and treating superimposed infection, because these factors have been shown to precipitate hemorrhage (123).

In general, patients who are ANCA positive and have anti-GBM antibodies respond better to therapy (137a).

In patients with pauci-immune glomerulonephritis and negative ANCA, high-dose intravenous methylprednisolone followed by maintenance oral therapy (see regimen described earlier) is the preferred treatment (126,131–133). Cyclophosphamide, started at an initial dose of 2 mg/kg/day and tapered according to the degree of renal impairment, white blood cell count, and platelets response, is added in the ANCA positive patients.

According to our experience, the patients who improve or stabilize do so early during the course of therapy, usually within the first 6–12 weeks. No data are available as to how long treatment should be continued in these patients. We believe the decision should be individualized. For patients who are ANCA positive, monitoring the serial titers might prove useful, since the risk of relapse is increased when the level of ANCA increases or remains persistently elevated (138).

D. Minimal Change Disease (Lipoid Nephrosis)

1. Incidence

Minimal change disease is found in 10% of elderly patients with primary glomerular disease (Table 2).

2. Pathology

On light microscopy the glomeruli appear normal, although the mesangium may be slightly widened, with increased matrix and a mild increase in mesangial cells. Completely sclerosed glomeruli are frequently present and at times may be quite significant (see Chapter 1). The tubules exhibit the usual findings of nephrotic syndrome, i.e., hyaline casts, hyaline droplets in the cytoplasm, and small areas of calcification. On electron microscopy the main finding is the loss or effacement (fusion) of the foot processes of the epithelial cells. This is a nonspecific finding seen in all forms of glomerular disease.

Immunofluorescence microscopy is usually completely negative. On occasion, a small amount of immunoglobulin such as IgM may be found in the mesangium. The significance of these deposits is a matter of controversy. It is not clear whether these patients should be classified as having mesangial nephritis (see section on "Diffuse Mesangial or Focal Proliferative Glomerulonephritis") or considered a special category of minimal change disease with a different and worse prognosis. There are arguments on both sides (139,140).

3. Pathogenesis

Increased suppressor cell function has been found in patients in relapse with minimal change disease (141). The activity of one of the products of the activated suppressor T cell, the lymphokine-soluble immune response suppressor (SIRS), has been found to be increased in the urine of patients with minimal change disease, which disappears after steroid treatment (142). Whether these lymphokines are responsible for the generalized loss of the membrane negative charge reported in patients with minimal change disease (143) is not clear, but there is experimental evidence that lymphocytes may mediate depletion of glomerular polyanion (144). An allergic history is found in 40–70% of patients with minimal change disease (145). Indeed, serum IgE levels are frequently increased in these patients. After exposure to a contact allergen, these patients demonstrate lymphocyte (T- or B-cell?) stimulation, with subsequent production of a lymphokine. The latter has been named the vascular permeability factor; its exact role in modifying the sialo-proteins of the glomerular capillary wall is not known.

In an experimental model of minimal change disease (puromycin-induced proteinuria), GFR was decreased, supposedly secondary to a decrease in the surface areas available for filtration (Kf or LpA) (146). In patients with minimal change disease a strong inverse correlation between GFR and the degree of foot process fusion was found by Bohman et al. (147), lending support to the possibility that in the human disease the decreased GFR may also be due to a decrease in Kf. A similar conclusion has been reached by Bridges and colleagues (148). Since the effective pore size was not changed, these authors concluded that the decreased Kf most likely represents a reduction in the number of pores. Patients with minimal change disease have a reduction in the concentration of fixed negative charges in the glomerular membrane. Therefore, the proteinuria appears to be mainly a consequence of defective electrostatic function of the glomerular barrier to protein filtration (149).

4. *Clinical Manifestations*

In 81 elderly patients reported with minimal change disease, 47 (58%) were males, and all had proteinuria in the nephrotic range (2,55,57,150–155). Microscopic hematuria was seen in 16 (20%), hypertension in 38 (47%), and renal insufficiency in 18 (22%).

5. *Natural History and Treatment*

The prognosis of minimal change disease in the elderly is rather good in terms of progression to end-stage kidney disease. The survival of elderly patients was only 50% at 10 years in the series of Nolasco and colleagues (156); however, only 5 of 15 deaths were related to complications of the nephrotic syndrome per se. From an analysis of the reported cases there is a 9% rate of spontaneous remission. The high incidence of ischemic changes found on biopsy by Cameron et al. (152) in patients 60 years and older did not seem to have any prognostic significance. Moreover, this histological picture has not been universally observed (54,55).

In our experience and that of others, the response to immunosuppressive therapy tends to be slower in the elderly compared with younger patients (156, 157). Eighty-seven percent of patients treated with steroids or cytotoxic agents (cyclophosphamide, azathioprine, chlorambucil) undergo complete remission; however, among these, 35% have one or more relapses at varying intervals (sometimes several years later), which require subsequent courses of therapy, which are generally well tolerated by the elderly. Based on these data, we recommend an 8-week course of prednisone (60 mg daily), followed by tapering over a 4-week period. In those patients who fail to respond to this regimen, we usually continue therapy for at least 4 months. Three daily doses of intravenous pulse methylprednisolone followed by oral prednisolone, 0.5 mg/kg/day, decreasing this dose by 0.1 mg/kg every month for 3 months, has also been used (158). If the patient does not go into remission or manifests severe steroid side effects such as proximal muscle weakness, cyclophosphamide (2 mg/kg per day for 8 weeks) can be used, usually with good results (158). There is not enough experience with azathioprine, chlorambucil, or cyclosporine in the elderly with minimal change disease to recommend their routine use.

E. Focal Segmental Glomerulosclerosis

1. *Incidence*

Focal segmental glomerulosclerosis was present in 9% of elderly patients with primary glomerular disease (Table 2), which is similar to the incidence in younger adults (4,5,9).

2. *Pathology*

Light microscopy is characterized by focal mesangial expansion and collapse of the capillaries. The sclerotic lesions involve only a portion of the glomerular tuft (segmental), most often in the juxtamedullary glomeruli. The areas of sclerosis contain hyaline material, and the sclerotic segment is frequently adherent to Bowman's capsule. The percentage of glomeruli involved varies according to the severity of the disease. Tubular atrophy with interstitial fibrosis and inflammatory cell infiltration are commonly present. On electron microscopy, there is foot process fusion, capillary collapse, areas of epithelial detachment, with formation of subepithelial zones containing fibrillar material. Electron-dense deposits may be found in the mesangium or in the subendothelial or intraluminal space. On immunofluorescence microscopy, most often no immune deposits are found; when present, they are seen in the sclerotic areas and in the mesangium of the affected glomeruli, with IgM and C_3 the most common.

3. *Pathogenesis*

Focal glomerulosclerosis is the most common isolated glomerular disease in intravenous drug users and patients with human immunodeficiency virus (HIV) infections (159). It also is the histological picture seen in patients with nephrotic syndrome associated with reflux nephropathy and various other disorders (160). The remaining patients are usually classified as having the "idiopathic" form of the disease, which is the predominant form of focal glomerulosclerosis in the elderly. The pathogenesis of this disease is unknown; however, the fact that it can reoccur early after renal transplantation suggests that a humoral factor might cause changes in glomerular permeability to albumin, at least in some patients (161,162). Abnormalities of cell-mediated immunity such as increased concanavalin A-induced suppressor cell activity have been described (163). Whether these activated cells secrete a lymphokine capable of injuring the glomerulus is not clear. Overloading of phagocytic mechanisms in the mesangium, with the sclerotic glomerular lesions a consequence of increased glomerular permeability, may also play a role (161), as may genetic factors.

4. *Clinical Manifestations*

In the 85 elderly patients with focal glomerulosclerosis culled from the literature and combined with our own experience, 51 (60%) were males (41,43,139,144). Sixty-three (74%) had hypertension, 47 (55%) had renal insufficiency (serum creatinine greater than 1.5 mg/dl), and 66 (78%) had nephrotic syndrome (3,9,55,57,107,155,164,165). The decrease in GFR in patients with focal glomerulosclerosis has been attributed to a reduction in the filtering surface area. The proteinuria, which consists mainly of albumin, is thought to be secondary to a defect in the electrostatic barrier due to a depletion of glomerular polyanion (166).

5. *Natural History and Treatment*

Age, per se, has been found in one study to affect the prognosis negatively (167), but not in others (168–170). The presence of renal insufficiency, large amounts of proteinuria, and severe tubulo-interstitial changes at the time of diagnosis are usually associated with progressive renal failure (168–171). Seventy-eight percent of the elderly patients with focal glomerulosclerosis referred to above presented with both nephrotic range proteinuria and renal insufficiency and appeared to have a poor prognosis. In the series of Beaufils et al. (172), which included younger patients, the incidence of nephrotic-range proteinuria was 56%, compared with nonnephrotic proteinuria of 44%. These authors noted a 10-year renal survival rate of only 45% in the group with nephrotic syndrome, compared to 91% in those with nonnephrotic proteinuria. Similar data, unfortunately, are not available for the elderly.

Some adult patients with focal segmental glomerulosclerosis and nephrotic proteinuria respond to corticosteroids. Those who respond usually have a significantly more favorable prognosis than nonresponders and patients not treated (164,169,170). Since, at present, there are no clinical or histological grounds on which to predict who will respond, our approach is to administer a short course of prednisone, 120 mg on alternate days for 12 weeks followed by gradual tapering, to every elderly patient with focal glomerulosclerosis and nephrotic proteinuria unless it is absolutely contraindicated. This regimen, as previously noted, is relatively well tolerated. Thirty percent of our patients responded with a decrease in proteinuria below 1 g. In the 17 patients reported by Nagai et al. (164), 7 of the 8 nontreated patients either developed progressive renal failure or were unchanged. One had a decrease in proteinuria from 4 to 1.8 g (partial remission). Of the 7 patients treated with prednisone alone, 4 achieved a complete remission, 1 had a partial remission, 1 reached end-stage renal disease, and 1 had persistent proteinuria. The other 2 patients received prednisone and cyclophosphamide. Both developed progressive renal failure. Their approach is to limit therapy to 3 months in the responders and to 6 months for the others, although a longer course (up to 12 months) is quite an acceptable alternative in the latter group as long as the drug is well tolerated. Various other drugs, including chlorambucil, cyclophosphamide, azathioprine, and cyclosporine, have been tried in patients with focal glomerulosclerosis that is resistant to corticosteroids. Their use in the elderly is rather limited and therefore cannot yet be recommended (173,173a).

Meclofenamate, a nonsteroidal antiinflammatory drug (NSAID), has been tried in 16 patients with focal glomerulosclerosis who had persistent nephrotic syndrome after having received daily prednisone (1 mg/kg body weight) for at least 6 weeks (174). The starting dose was 50 mg orally twice a day, gradually increasing to 50 mg every 6 hr. Eight patients were classified as responders (a 40% or greater decrease in protein excretion) and 6 as nonresponders. Drug side effects, requiring discontinuance of the therapy, developed in the remaining 2 patients. The rationale for using meclofenamate in preference to other nonsteroidal antiinflammatory drugs has been reviewed (175). The drug not only inhibits the synthesis of prostaglandins but also may block the prostaglandin receptors of the effector cells. Furthermore, meclofenamate can block the increase in capillary permeability that usually follows administration of the so-called vascular permeability factor, which has been isolated from these patients.

The experience with this regimen in the elderly is limited. One should remember, however, that the elderly are more susceptible to the serious side effects of NSAIDs than are younger patients and require close follow-up. For those patients who do not respond to steroids and are clinically nephrotic, we opt for other supportive care (vide infra) rather than the use of NSAIDs.

F. Mesangiocapillary (Membranoproliferative) Glomerulonephritis

1. *Incidence*

As shown in Table 2, mesangiocapillary glomerulonephritis was present in 8% of elderly patients with primary glomerular disease.

2. *Pathology*

Mesangiocapillary glomerulonephritis has been divided into three different types.

Type I. Light microscopy reveals the presence of increased mesangial cells and matrix. Polymorphonuclear leukocytes may be present, often in large numbers. One characteristic feature of the disease is the thickening of the capillary wall, which on special stains such as periodic acid-Schiff (PAS) has a "double contour," i.e., two dark lines separated by a pale zone. Crescents are also commonly present. With immunofluorescence microscopy, IgG and C3 may be found. With electron microscopy, one sees increased cells, matrix, and electron-dense deposits in the expanded mesangium. Deposits may also be seen in the subendothelial space.

Type II. This variation is also called "dense deposit disease" because of the presence of electron-dense deposits in the lamina densa of the capillary basement membrane seen with electron microscopy. Deposits may also be seen in the mesangium. With immunofluorescence microscopy, the most constant finding is the extensive deposition of C3 in the mesangium. The light microscopic changes are similar to type I.

Type III. This is a variant of type I and is characterized by the presence of extensive subepithelial deposits with intervening projections of basement membrane-like material in conjunction with the lesions described for type I disease (176). With immunofluorescence microscopy, C3 is almost invariably present in a granular pattern along the capillary wall. Other components of the complement cascade (C1q, C4, C2) may also be present along with immunoglobulins IgG, IgM, or IgA.

There are not enough data in the literature concerning the incidence of type II mesangiocapillary glomerulonephritis in the elderly, although some of the patients described by Cameron and associates (177) were over the age of 55. In any case, type II and type III disease are rare in the elderly, and most (if not all) elderly patients with mesangiocapillary glomerulonephritis have type I disease.

3. *Pathogenesis*

The pathogenesis of mesangiocapillary glomerulonephritis is not known. Since circulating immune complexes have been found in some patients with the disease (178,179), an immune mechanism seems likely. The specific antigen responsible for the activation of the process has not been identified. Whatever the precise mechanism might be, the complement system is probably involved, with activation of both the classic and alternate pathways (180,181).

4. *Clinical Manifestations*

Males are affected more frequently than females (6:4). Proteinuria and hematuria are present in over 90% of the patients. Nephrotic-range proteinuria occurs in 58%. Acute nephritis is the initial presentation in 30%. Chronic renal insufficiency of varying severity is found in 43%. C3 is usually normal and C4 depressed in 22% (1–5,9,154,155,182). Sixty-four percent of the patients are hypertensive.

5. *Natural History and Therapy*

Mesangiocapillary glomerulonephritis usually progresses to end-stage renal failure; however, the clinical course is extremely variable. Therefore, the efficacy of a given therapeutic regimen is difficult to assess unless one is dealing with a well-controlled prospective study involving a large number of patients followed for a long period of time.

At present an effective therapy for idiopathic mesangiocapillary glomerulonephritis has not emerged. Warfarin (at a dose adjusted to keep the prothrombin time 1.5–2 times the control value) and dypiridamole (100 mg 4 times a day) have been used in younger patients. The high incidence of bleeding complications makes this therapy rather risky in the elderly (183). Dipyridamole (75 mg/day) and aspirin (500 mg/day) have been found to have a modest effect on proteinuria but no significant effect on renal survival (184). Higher doses of dipyridamole (75 mg trice daily) and aspirin (325 mg thrice daily) have also been used without any significant long-term benefit (185). Cyclosporine has also been tried in a few patients with mesangiocapillary glomerulonephritis (186), with insufficient experience to recommend it for the elderly.

Although corticosteroids at various doses and schedules have been tried in this disease, there is no clear evidence that they are useful in the elderly. However, we have had a relatively good experience with the use of prednisone (approximately 40–60 mg, as tolerated), every other day, in 11 elderly patients with mesangiocapillary glomerulonephritis.

G. Chronic Glomerulonephritis

Twenty-four patients (4% of reported elderly with glomerular disease) were diagnosed as having nonclassifiable chronic glomerulonephritis (Table 2). This does not represent the true incidence of this entity in the elderly, because patients with the same clinical picture who have small kidneys at the time of diagnosis usually do not undergo biopsy. Histologically, the diagnosis of chronic glomerulonephritis is made when there is so much scarring that the original disease is no longer discernible. The glomeruli are sclerosed and there is extensive tubular atrophy, associated with interstitial fibrosis and lymphocytic infiltration. With electron microscopy, basement membrane wrinkling is usually seen. There is no constant pattern as far as the presence of immunoglobulins and complement are concerned.

1. *Clinical Manifestations*

Renal insufficiency of varying severity and proteinuria (more than 2 g per 24 hr) were present in all our patients at the time of diagnosis. Seventy-five percent were also hypertensive. Hematuria was found in 20%.

2. *Natural History and Treatment*

The disease is usually progressive, and management is identical to that for any patient with chronic renal insufficiency (see Chapter 11).

H. Acute Endoproliferative Glomerulonephritis

1. Incidence

Acute endoproliferative glomerulonephritis accounts for the remaining 4% of elderly patients with primary glomerular disease (Table 2).

2. Pathology

With light microscopy, all glomeruli exhibit endothelial and mesangial cell proliferation. There is also infiltration of polymorphonuclear and mononuclear leukocytes. Crescent formation and adhesions between the capillary loops and Bowman's capsule may be seen. With immunofluorescence microscopy, granular deposits of complement and, frequently, immunoglobulins (IgG) are found. Electron microscopy is characterized by the presence of subepithelial electron-dense humplike deposits in the capillary wall.

3. Pathogenesis

The current evidence strongly suggests that acute endoproliferative glomerulonephritis is an immune-complex disease. Serum complement level is depressed in the majority of the patients, with a pattern suggesting activation of the alternate pathway; C4 is normal in all patients and C3 is depressed in over 85% (187,188). Circulating immune complexes, as measured by C1q-binding activity, have been found in the serum of two-thirds of patients in the first week of the disease (189,190). The antigen responsible for the disease (which is supposedly of bacterial origin) could induce disease by stimulating antibody production, with the resulting antigen–antibody complex deposited in the glomerulus, or the antigen could be planted in the glomerulus, triggering an in-situ immune reaction (191). Factors such as electrical charge could influence the location of the antigen (192).

A role for antiglobulin antibodies has been postulated, but the exact mechanism whereby immunoglobulins become autoantigenic is not clear. Circulating antiimmunoglobulins have been detected in the serum in a large percentage of patients with acute poststreptococcal glomerulonephritis (193).

4. Clinical Manifestations

The clinical manifestations of the disease in the elderly are similar to those seen in other age groups (194,195). A history of antecedent streptococcal infection can be elicited from most patients (83%), with pharyngeal involvement in 50% and skin in 33%. In 17% a nonstreptococcal infection precedes the onset (usually pulmonary). Heart failure is the initial presentation in 43% of the elderly. Renal insufficiency of varying severity is present in more than 71%, and hypertension is present in 83%. Hematuria, either microscopic or macroscopic, is a universal finding, as is proteinuria. The latter varies in degree from nonnephrotic (74%) to nephrotic levels (26%). ASO titer is elevated in only 56% of patients (4,5,155,187,195–200). The relatively low incidence of an elevated ASO titer may be related to the fact that when the streptococcal infection originates in the skin the antibody response may be blunted, and the ASO titer may not rise because of binding of antigen by lipids present in the skin (201). According to Montoliu et al. (202), the immune response to deoxyribonuclease B is more constant and diagnostically helpful. As noted earlier, serum C4 is usually normal, whereas C3 is depressed in more than 85% of patients.

5. *Clinical Course*

Severe renal failure may be seen in elderly patients with acute endocapillary glomerulonephritis, and a significant number may require dialytic intervention, most frequently for control of fluid overload (196–200,203). The course can be protracted, lasting weeks or months; however, the prognosis is usually good, with clinical recovery being the rule, and only a minority of patients are left with mild to moderate impairment of kidney function, particularly those who present initially with nephrotic syndrome (204). Therefore, an aggressive approach should be adopted and dialysis used as necessary in order to sustain these patients through the acute phase of their illness.

If a patient is seen early in the course of the disease or if streptococci are recovered from the throat or skin, penicillin or one of its derivatives should be administered. Antibiotics are not necessary for patients seen late or with negative cultures. Fluid and sodium restriction and bed rest are usually recommend until signs of circulatory overload disappear. Blood pressure and serum potassium must be monitored regularly (particularly if the patient is oliguric), and hypertension and hyperkalemia treated. Corticosteroid therapy is not recommended in the management of patients with acute endocapillary glomerulonephritis.

V. SPECIAL PROBLEMS ASSOCIATED WITH PRIMARY GLOMERULAR DISEASE IN THE ELDERLY

A. Hypoalbuminemia and Edema

In our experience, most elderly patients tolerate moderate hypoalbuminemia as well as younger patients, so our management of these patients is similar to that suggested for nephrotics in general (205). On occasion, some patients may develop severe edema associated with local discomfort or abdominal pain, usually seen when the serum albumin is very low (< 1.5 g/dl). We treat these patients with salt-poor albumin infusion followed by furosemide. The dose of furosemide in this setting is higher than usual. In nephrotic syndrome, there is a reduced ability of the renal tubule to respond to furosemide, which may be related to its binding to the albumin present within the renal tubule (206). In patients in whom diuresis fails to occur with this regimen, metolazone, a thiazide diuretic capable of potentiating the effect of furosemide, may be added. Weight should be carefully monitored. This approach is continued until the patient is comfortable.

The majority of patients do well on salt restriction (2–3 g/day) with or without an oral diuretic. When needed, our preference is to use furosemide, administered on an alternate-day basis. Attention should be paid to potassium balance, particularly in patients receiving concomitant digitalis. We also recommend a diet with moderate protein restriction of high biological value, approximately 0.8–1.0 g/kg of ideal body weight, plus urinary losses for proteinuria if more than 5 g/24 hr. Protein restriction, per se, is associated with an increase in serum albumin, as well as a decrease in albuminuria, by inducing a decrease in glomerular capillary pressure and subsequent improvement in the size selective defect in glomerular permselectivity (207,208).

Despite those measures, a small number of elderly (10% in our experience) continue to be incapacitated by edema and hypoalbuminemia. In these patients, angiotensin-converting enzyme inhibitors can be tried. These agents reduce proteinuria by decreasing the GFR as well as by restoring the barrier size selectivity of the glomerular basement membrane (209). Their antiproteinuric effect peaks after 4–8 weeks of treatment. Furthermore, their effect on proteinuria might be additive to that of protein restriction (210). NSAIDs (e.g., indomethacin, meclofenamate) exert a similar effect on protein excretion through similar mechanisms (211,212). Given the high incidence of side effects associated with NSAIDs in the elderly (as noted earlier), we ordinarily do not recommend their use.

B. Hyperlipidemia

The incidence of hyperlipidemia in the elderly patient with nephrotic syndrome has not been addressed specifically; however, if one can extrapolate from published studies on adult nephrotics in general, it should occur in 50–70% of patients (213,214). Primarily, the plasma cholesterol is elevated, with lesser changes in triglyceride levels. Lipoprotein profiling has revealed that most subjects fall into three groups, type II (IIa, IIb), III, and V (215). Lipoprotein fractionation showed that the cholesterol is mainly in the LDL fraction, with a smaller proportion in VLDL and HDL. Whereas plasma LDL and VLDL were elevated in most of the patients reported by Appel and colleagues (214), HDL was either normal or low. The presence of a normal total HDL, however, does not rule out an abnormality in the metabolism of this lipoprotein. As shown by Short and associates (216), the HDL_3 subfraction of HDL might be elevated in nephrotic patients, whereas the HDL_2 subfraction is reduced. The latter is probably the one most closely associated with decreasing the risk of ischemic heart disease.

The hyperlipidemia is probably the result of both altered catabolism and enhanced synthesis of lipids and apolipoprotein B (217,218). The stimulus for increased synthesis is mainly the low plasma albumin concentration and oncotic pressure. It is also quite possible that renal losses of macromolecules such as lipoprotein lipase contribute to the altered rate of removal and processing of VLDL (219). The relatively low concentration of HDL might reflect, in part, its loss in the urine through its major protein moiety, apolipoprotein A1 (220,221).

The role of hyperlipidemia on the incidence of atherosclerotic heart disease in nephrotic patients has been a matter of controversy (222,223). However, a recent study with long-term follow-up of nondiabetic nephrotic patients suggests a significantly increased risk of coronary-artery disease compared to matched controls (224). Also, there is experimental evidence that disturbed lipid metabolism, similar to that seen in nephrotic syndrome, may have damaging effects on the kidney (225).

Our approach is to do a complete fasting lipid profile on all nephrotic patients. For those with an elevation of total LDL cholesterol, as well as those with an elevated triglyceride, appropriate dietary changes are recommended (226). If hyperlipidemia is not controlled by diet and if there are associated risk factors such as cigarette smoking, diabetes mellitus, hypertension, or obesity, a more aggressive approach with pharmacological intervention should be undertaken (227).

The HMG-CoA reductase inhibitors (fluvastatin, lovastatin pravastatin, simvastatin, atorvastatin) have become the drugs of choice for treating the hyperlipidemia associated with nephrotic syndrome. They are well tolerated and effective in decreasing total and LDL cholesterol. HDL is usually not affected. Long-term benefits, safety, and efficacy remain to be determined. One major drawback for the elderly is cost, since these drugs are quite expensive. Fluvastatin, 20–40 mg daily, is the most cost effective (228–231), followed by atorvastatin.

C. Calcium and Vitamin D Alterations

The elderly nephrotic is more prone than younger patients to alterations in calcium and vitamin D metabolism. In addition to the increased losses of both $25(OH)D_3$ and $1,25(OH)_2 D_3$ in the urine, attributable to the nephrotic state per se, calcium absorption as well as plasma levels of $1,25(OH)_2 D_3$ are decreased as a function of aging (232–234) (see Chapter 5). Thus, it is not surprising that both osteomalacia and hyperparathyroid bone disease have been found on bone biopsies in these patients, more so in those with superimposed renal insufficiency (235,236). Finally, glucocorticoids, which are commonly used in treating elderly patients with glomerular diseases, decrease intestinal calcium and phosphorus absorption by a mechanism that is not fully elucidated and also increase the rate of bone resorption, exceeding that of bone formation (237). As a consequence, this therapy facilitates either the new development or the exacerbation of preexisting osteoporosis (238,238a). Therefore, it has been our policy to administer vitamin D supplementation to our elderly nephrotics, either in the form of vitamin D (400 IU/day) or calcitriol (0.25–1.0 μ g/day) (239). Elemental calcium supplementation, 500–1000 mg daily, can be added if calcium intake is judged inadequate (240). The 24-hr urine calcium excretion should be monitored, together with plasma Ca and $1,25(OH)_2D_3$ levels.

D. Thromboembolism

The nephrotic syndrome is characterized by a hypercoagulable state caused by several abnormalities of the coagulation cascade and of platelet function. The predisposition to thrombosis in a given patient varies depending on the balance of procoagulant and anticoagulant factors. Plasma concentration of the natural anticoagulant protein C (an inhibitor of both factor V and factor VIII) and its cofactor protein S have been found to be either normal or elevated in proteinuric patients (241,242). The reason for such variability might depend on the type of glomerular disease present or the technique used (bound or unbound fraction measured) (243). In recent studies involving mainly the unbound fraction of this protein, both qualitative (decrease specific activity) and quantitative (decreased plasma level) defects have been found which may contribute to the increased incidence of thrombosis in nephrotics (244). Du et al. (245) have postulated that an increased level of alpha-antiplasmin may increase susceptibility to renal vein thrombosis in nephrotic patients. An increase in platelet aggreability is also present in patients with nephrotic syndrome (246), related to the hypoalbuminemia, the hypercholesterolemia, and the high plasma fibrinogen level that are frequently present (247).

Both arterial and venous thrombosis can occur in nephrotic subjects (248). Even though arterial occlusion can occasionally be seen in adults, its occurrence in the elderly is quite unusual. Apparently, deep leg veins thrombosis, as diagnosed by Doppler ultrasound, is not uncommon in adult nephrotics (249). It is not clear how frequently pulmonary embolism occurs in these patients, but a ventilation-perfusion lung scan suggestive of pulmonary embolism has been reported in 15–25% of nephrotics, although only 5% were symptomatic (250). Comparable data are not available for the elderly.

Renal vein thrombosis is the most common thrombotic complication associated with nephrotic syndrome. In a recent meta-analysis of the literature, it was estimated that renal vein thrombosis occurs in 21% of nephrotic patients, and pulmonary embolism in 14% (251). This complication, which is most common in patients with membranous nephropathy, appears to be less common in the elderly. Four of the 31 (13%) elderly patients reported by Zech et al. (57) had renal vein thrombosis. Finally, in most of the reported series of adults with renal vein thrombosis, the majority were less than 60 years of age (250,252–254).

The diagnosis should be suspected when a patient with nephrotic syndrome presents with costo-vertebral angle pain associated with hematuria and/or an abrupt decline in kidney function. Symptoms and signs suggestive of pulmonary embolism may be the initial manifestation. The diagnosis of renal vein thrombosis depends on the demonstration of clots in the renal veins by venography. Noninvasive techniques, such as gray-scale ultrasonography, have been tried with variable success (255,256). Avasthi and associates (257) have suggested that the Doppler flowmetric method may be useful for the diagnosis and follow-up of patients with renal vein thrombosis.

There remains the question of whether to perform renal venography routinely in nephrotic patients. As we discussed, the incidence of renal vein thrombosis in elderly patients with primary glomerular disease (even those with membranous nephropathy) is sufficiently low that renal venography can be reserved for those patients in whom the clinical suspicion of thrombosis is increased by any of the symptoms or signs described above (258).

Once the diagnosis of renal vein thrombosis is made, anticoagulant therapy should be started. A 7- to 10-day course of heparin, followed by Warfarin, is the therapy of choice. This regimen has been found to result in significant improvement in creatinine clearance in patients presenting with rapid worsening in their GFR (250). There is not enough information as to how long anticoagulation should be continued in these patients. We have used 3 months as a guideline, keeping in mind the higher susceptibility of the elderly to bleeding. Longer-term therapy, using daily subcutaneous injection of low-molecular-weight heparin (251), should be considered in patients with recurrent pulmonary embolism. Success with fibrinolytic therapy (streptokinase) has been reported (259); however, further experience with a larger number of patients is needed before its routine use can be recommended.

E. Acute Renal Failure

Acute renal failure (ARF) as an initial presentation or a subsequent complication of nephrotic syndrome has been reported in over 80 adult patients. Although the true incidence is not clear, it is probably not a common phenomenon. Esparza et al. (260) found 4 patients with nephrotic syndrome out of 102 patients in whom a renal biopsy was performed for ARF. Whatever its true incidence, the condition seems to be more prevalent in the elderly. Of the reported patients where age has been documented, 52% were over the age of 60 (156,260–272).

In addition to edema and the other stigmata of nephrotic syndrome, which were generally severe, patients with ARF reported by Lowenstein et al. (264) were usually oliguric, tended to be hypertensive, and had a fractional excretion of sodium (FENa) which was less than 1%. Some patients require dialysis because of uremic complications. Kidney biopsy reveals minimal change nephropathy in over 87%, with focal glomerulosclerosis and membranous glomerulopathy in the remaining 13%. Since the histological findings were not severe enough to explain the change in renal function, several hypotheses have been proposed to explain the renal failure. In some cases, a temporal association has been found between the ARF and the use of analgesics and/or NSAIDs (269). Small-vessel thrombosis in the nephrotic kidney made ischemic by hypotension (260), acute tubular necrosis (271), and nephrosarca with subsequent increased intratubular pressure (264) are among the other mechanisms proposed. Contrary to previous suggestions, hypovolemia per se does not appear to play a role in the ARF associated with nephrotic syndrome, unless the patient has been aggressively diuresed without the support of a volume expander such as albumin.

Every patient with ARF and the nephrotic syndrome should receive a trial of albumin infusion with or without a diuretic to induce diuresis, which has been associated with prompt remission in some patients. In others, the course might be quite protracted. Since minimal change disease is by far the most commonly found histological diagnosis in these patients, steroid therapy should also be initiated. (See previous section, "Minimal Change Disease"). Seventy-nine percent of the patients reported recovered kidney function eventually. The remaining either expired (mainly those in whom the acute renal failure was the presenting manifestation of the nephrotic syndrome) or did not improve and had to be placed on maintenance dialysis or received a kidney transplant.

F. Superimposed Crescentic Glomerulonephritis

In some patients with known primary glomerular disease, a rapid decline in renal function may supervene, due to the development of crescentic glomerulonephritis. The incidence of this complication is not known, but it has been reported in patients with membranous glomerulopathy, mesangiocapillay glomerulonephritis, mesangial nephritis, and focal glomerulosclerosis (273–277). Anti-GBM antibodies have been found in some patients. It is postulated that preexisting immune complexes along the glomerular basement membrane may render the glomerulus more susceptible to additional injury. A repeat kidney biopsy is necessary to confirm the diagnosis. The prognosis, as expected, is usually poor. We suggest that plasmapheresis be tried for those with anti-GBM antibody and pulse steroid therapy for those without (277). However, there are no data to support this approach in the elderly.

G. Malignancy

A final consideration in patients with nephrotic syndrome is that of associated malignancy. Lee et al. (278) reported 11 patients with an underlying malignancy among 101 patients older than 40 years of age with de-novo onset of nephrotic syndrome. In a review of 48 patients with malignancy and nephrotic syndrome, 33 had membranous glomerulopathy, 4 had membranoproliferative glomerulonephritis, 3 had minimal change, 2 had amyloid, and in 6 various other glomerulopathies were present (279).

In five reports, including 103 elderly patients with membranous glomerulopathy, 12 patients (12%) had a malignancy (54,55,57,280,281). More than 50% of patients with lymphoma and nephrotic syndrome have minimal change disease on biopsy. Crescentic glomerulonephritis has been more commonly associated with solid tumors, usually of the lung and prostate (281–283). P or C ANCA may be present in some patients (284). Although tumor-associated antigen–antibody complex deposition (for patients with solid tumors) or production of a humoral substance (lymphokines in patients with lymphomas) have been suggested to play a pathogenetic role in the development of the glomerular injury associated with neoplasia, direct proof has been lacking in the vast majority of cases.

The nephrotic syndrome can develop concurrently or precede the diagnosis of malignancy by several months. If the neoplasm is diagnosed concurrently with the nephrotic syndrome, treatment of the former could result in remission of the latter. We do not think that an extensive search for malignancy should be undertaken in the elderly patient with either membranous nephropathy or minimal change disease. We believe in performing a detailed history and physical examination in these patients to alert us to the possibility of a malignancy. Since lung and bowel cancer are the most common associated with membranous nephropathy, a chest X-ray and serial stools for occult blood are recommended. In a long-term follow-up of a large number of patients in the U.S. Collaborative Study of Nephrotic syndrome (C. Coggins, personal communication), as well as in the study of Lund et al. (285), the development of malignancy was not been found to be a significant problem.

REFERENCES

1. Furci L, et al. Nephropathies in the elderly. In: Sessa A, Meroni M, Battini G, eds. Glomerulonephritis in the Elderly. Contrib Nephrol (Basel: Karger) 1993;105: 157–160.
2. Johnston PA, Coulshed SJ, Davison AM. Renal biopsy findings in patients older than 65 years of age presenting with the nephrotic syndrome. In: Sessa A, Meroni M, Battini G, eds. Glomerulonephritis in the Elderly. Contrib Nephrol (Basel: Karger) 1993; 105:127–132.
3. Feriozzi S, et al. Glomerulonephritis in elderly patients. In: Sessa A, Meroni M, Battini G, eds. Glomerulonephritis in the Elderly. Contrib Nephrol (Basel: Karger) 1993; 105:122–126.
4. Modesto-Segonds A, et al. Renal biopsy in the elderly. In: Sessa A, Maroni M, Battini G, eds. Glomerulonephritis in the Elderly. Contrib Nephrol (Basel: Karger) 1993; 105:107–116.
5. Colombo V, et al. Renal biopsies in the elderly. In: Sessa A, Meroni M, Battini G, eds. Glomerulonephritis in the Elderly. Contrib Nephrol (Basel: Karger) 1993;105: 102–106.
6. Falk RJ, Jennette JC. Glomerular disease in the elderly. In: Jacobson HR, Striker GE, Klahr S, eds. The Principles and Practice of Nephrology. 2d ed. St. Louis: Mosby, 1995:518–523.
7. Levison SP. Renal disease in the elderly: the role of the renal biopsy. Am J Kidney Dis 1990;16:300–306.
8. Diaz-Buxo JA, Donadio JV Jr. Complications of percutaneous renal biopsy: an analysis of 1,000 consecutive biopsies. Clin Nephrol 1975;4:223–227.
9. Davison AM, Johnson PA. Idiopathic glomerulonephritis in the elderly. In: Sessa A, Meroni M, Battini G, eds. Glomerulonephritis in the Elderly. Contrib Nephrol (Basel: Karger) 1993;105:38–48.
10. Cameron JS. The nephrotic syndrome and its complications. Am J Kidney Dis 1987;10:157–171.
11. Simon P, et al. Epidemiology of primary glomerular disease in the elderly. In: Sessa A, Meroni M, Battini G, eds. Glomerulonephritis in the Elderly. Contrib Nephrol (Basel: Karger) 1993;105:161–166.

12. Friedman SA, et al. Functional defects in the aging kidney. Ann Intern Med 1972;76:41–45.
13. Ginsberg JM, et al. Use of single voided urine samples to estimate quantitative proteinuria. N Engl J Med 1983;309:1543–1546.
14. Fliser D, et al. Proteinuria as a function of hypertension and age. In: Sessa A, Meroni M, Battini G, eds. Glomerulonephritis in the Elderly. Contrib Nephrol (Basel: Karger) 1993;105:25–32.
15. Rennke HG, Patel Y, Venkattachalam MA. Effect of molecular charge on glomerular permeability to proteins in the rat: clearance studies studies using neutral, anionic and cationic horseradish peroxidase. Kidney Int 1983;13:278.
16. Guasch A, Dean WM, Myers BD. Charge selectivity of the glomerular filtration barrier in healthy and nephrotic humans. J Clin Invest 1993;92:2274–2282.
17. Bohrer MP, et al. Mechanism of angiotensin II-induced proteinuria in the rat. Am J Physiol 1977;223:F13–F21.
18. Blau EB, Haas JE. Glomerular sialic acid and proteinuria in human renal disease. Lab Invest 1973;28:477–481.
19. Myers BD, et al. Mechanisms of proteinuria in human glomerulonephritis. J Clin Invest 1982;70:732–746.
20. Dean WM, et al. Heteroporous model of glomerular size selectivity: application to normal and nephrotic humans. Am J Physiol 1989;249:F374–F389.
20a. Blouch K, et al. Molecular configuration and glomerular size selectivity in healthy and nephrotic humans. Am J Physiol 1997;273:F430–F437.
21. Dorhout Mees EJ, et al. Observations on edema formation in the nephrotic syndrome in adults with minimal lesions. Am J Med 1979;67:378–384.
22. Krishna GG, Danovitch GM. Effects of water immersion on renal function in the nephrotic syndrome. Kidney Int 1982;21:395–401.
23. Dorhout Mees EJ, et al. Changes in plasma volume and renin activity during correction of edema in the nephrotic syndrome. Kidney Int 1984;25:163A.
24. Koomans HA, et al. Effects of plasma volume expansion on renal salt handling in patients with the nephrotic syndrome. Am J Nephrol 1984;4:227–234.
25. Berlyne GM, et al. Renal salt and water handling in water immersion in the nephrotic syndrome. Clin Sci 1981;61:605–610.
26. Berlyne GM, et al. Water immersion in nephrotic syndrome. Arch Intern Med 1981; 141:1275–1278.
27. Meltzer JI, et al. Nephrotic syndrome: vasoconstriction and hypovolemic types indicated by renin-sodium profiling. Ann Intern Med 1979;91:688–696.
28. Chonko AM, et al. The role of renin and aldosterone in the salt retention of edema. Am J Med 1977;63:881–889.
29. Brown EA, et al. Evidence that some mechanism other than the renin system causes sodium retention in nephrotic syndrome. Lancet 1982;2:1237–1239.
30. Dusing R, Vetter H, Kramer HJ. The renin-angiotensin-aldosterone system in patients with nephrotic syndrome. Effects of 1 sar-8-ala-angiotensin II. Nephron 1980;25: 187–192.
31. Kopp UC, DiBona GF. Neural control of volume homeostasis. In: Brenner BM, Stein JH, eds. Body Fluid homeostasis. Contrib Nephrol (New York: Churchill Livingstone) 1987;16:185–220.

32. Oliver WJ, Kelch RC, Chandler JP. Demonstration of increased catecholamine excretion in the nephrotic syndrome. Proc Soc Exp Biol Med 1967;125:1176–1180.
33. Geers AB, et al. Postural changes in the nephrotic syndrome (NS). Kidney Int 1984; 25:165A.
34. Hollister AS, et al. Clearance of atrial natriuretic factor by lung, liver and kidney in human subjects and the dog. J Clin Invest 1989;83:623–628.
35. Yamamoto Y, et al. Plasma concentration of human atrial natriuretic polypeptide in patients with impaired renal function. Clin Nephrol 1987;27:84–86.
36. Daniels H, Pederson EB. Atrial natriuretic peptide, angiotensin II and aldosterone in plasma in chronic glomerulonephritis during basal conditions and during excercise. Acta Med Scand 1988;224:61–67.
37. Zietse R, Schalekamp NA. Effect of synthetic human atrial natriuretic peptide (102–106) in nephrotic syndrome. Kidney Int 1988;34:717–724.
38. Perico N, Remuzzi G. Edema of the nephrotic syndrome: the role of the atrial peptide system. Am J Kidney Dis 1993;22:355–366.
39. Peterson C, et al. Atrial natriuretic peptide and the renal response to hypervolemia in nephrotic humans. Kidney Int 1988;34:828–831.
40. Pedersen EB, et al. Urinary prostaglandin E_2 and F_{2a} excretion in nephrotic syndrome during basal conditions, after water loading, and after remission of the syndrome. Acta Med Scand 1988;224:69–77.
41. Shapiro MD, et al. Role of glomerular filtration rate in the impaired sodium and water excretion in patients with the nephrotic syndrome. Am J Kidney Dis 1986;8:81–87.
42. Drumond MC, et al. Structural basis for reduced glomerular filtration capacity in nephrotic humans. J Clin Invest 1994;94:1187–1195.
43. Ichikawa I, et al. Role for intrarenal mechanisms in the impaired salt excretion of experimental nephrotic syndrome. J Clin Invest 1983;71:91–103.
44. Gransz H, Lieberman R, Earley LE. Effect of plasma albumin on sodium reabsorption in patients with nephrotic syndrome. Kidney Int 1972;1:47–54.
45. Koomans HA, et al. Sodium balance in renal failure. A comparison of patients with normal subjects under extreme sodium intake. Hypertension 1985;71:714–722.
46. Preston RA, Singer I, Epstein M. Renal parenchymal hypertension. Current concepts of pathogenesis and management. Arch Intern Med 1996;156:602–610.
46a. Messing EM, et al. The significance of asymptomatic microhematuria in men 50 or more years old. Findings of a home screening study using urinary dipsticks. J Urol 1987;137:919–922.
47. Rizzoni G, Braggion F, Zacchello G. Evaluation of glomerular and nonglomerular hematuria by phase-contrast microscopy. J Pediatr 1983;103:370–374.
48. Birch DF, et al. Urinary erythrocyte morphology in the diagnosis of glomerular hematuria. Clin Nephrol 1983;20:78–84.
49. Fassett RG, et al. Scanning electron microscopy of glomerular and nonglomerular red blood cells. Clin Nephrol 1983;20:11–16.
50. Haughstaine D, Bollens W, Wichielsen R. Detection of glomerular bleeding using a simple staining method for light microscopy. Lancet 1982;2:761.
51. Raman GV, et al. A blind controlled trial of phase-contrast microscopy by two observers for evaluating the source of hematuria. Nephron 1986;44:304–308.
52. Georgopoulos M, et al. Evaluation of asymptomatic microscopic hematuria, influ-

ence and clinical relevance of osmolality and PH on urinary erythrocyte morphology. Br J Urol 1996;78:192–196.
53. Pollack C, et al. Dysmorphism of urinary red blood cells. Value in diagnosis. Kidney Int 1989;36:1045–1049.
54. Moorthy AV, Zimmerman SW. Renal disease in the elderly: Clinico-pathologic analysis of renal disease in 115 elderly patients. Clin Nephrol 1980;14:223–229.
55. Kingswood JC, et al. Renal biopsy in the elderly: clinicopathological correlations in 143 patients. Clin Nephrol 1984;22:183–187.
56. Fawcett TW, et al. Nephrotic syndrome in the elderly. Br Med J 1971;2:387–388.
57. Zech P, et al. The nephrotic syndrome in adults aged over 60: Etiology, evolution and treatment of the cases. Clin Nephrol 1982;5:232–236.
58. Boner G, et al. Nephrotic syndrome in patients over 60 years of age. Abstr VII Int Cong of Nephrol, June 1978;18–26.
59. Noel LH, et al. Long-term prognosis of idiopathic membranous glomerulonephritis. Study of 116 untreated patients. Am J Med 1979;66:82–90.
60. Ehrenreich T, Churg J. Pathology of membranous nephropathy. Pathol Ann 1968;3: 145–186.
61. Gallo GR, Caulin-Glaser T, Lamm ME. Charge of circulating immune complexes as a factor in glomerular basement membrane localization in mice. J Clin Invest 1981; 67:1305–1313.
62. Couser WG, Salant DJ. Immunopathogenesis of glomereular capillary wall injury in nephrotic states. In Brenner BM, Stein JH, eds. Contemporary Issues in Nephrology. New York: Churchill Livingstone, 1982:47.
62a. Kon SP, et al. Urinary $C5_b$-9 excretion and clinical course in idiopathic human membranous nephropathy. Kidney Int 1995;48:1953–1958.
63. Bizzari D, et al. Idiopathic membranous glomerulonephritis in the elderly. In: Sessa A, Meroni M, Battini G, eds. Glomerulonephritis in the Elderly. Contrib Nephrol (Basel: Karger) 1993;105:65–70.
64. Rollino C, et al. Outcome of membranuous glomerulonephritis in the elderly. In: Sessa A, Meroni M, Battini G, eds. Glomerulonephritis in the Elderly. Contrib Nephrol (Basel: Karger) 1993;105:71–74.
65. Passerini P, et al. Idiopathic membranuous nephropathy in the elderly. Nephrol Dial Transplant 1993;8:1321–1325.
65a. Zent R, Nagai R, Cattran DC. Idiopathic membranous nephropathy in the elderly: a comparative study. Am J Kidney Dis 1997;29:200–206.
66. Wehrmann M, et al. Long-term prognosis of chronic idiopathic membranous glomerulonephritis. Clin Nephrol 1989;31:67–76.
67. Porush JG, Faubert PF. Treatment of idiopathic membranous glomerulopathy. In: Avram MM, ed. Proteinuria (New York: Plenum Medical) 1983;14:175–193.
68. Hogan SL, et al. A review of therapeutic studies of idiopathic membranuous glomerulopathy. Am J Kidney Dis 1995;25:862–875.
68a. Imperiale TF, Goldfarb S, Berns JS. Are cytotoxic agents beneficial in idiopathic membranous nephropathy? A meta-analysis of the controlled trials. J Am Soc Nephrol 1995;5:1553–1558.
69. Cattran DC, et al. A controlled trial of cyclosporine in patients with progressive membranuous nephropathy. Kidney Int 1995;47:1130–1135.

69a. Ambalavanan S, et al. Mechanism of the antiproteinuric effect of cyclosporine in membranous mephropathy. J Am Soc Nephrol 1996;7:290–298.
69b. Glassock RJ. Therapy of idiopathic nephrotic syndrome in adults. A conservative or aggressive therapeutic approach. Am J Nephrol 1993;13:422–428.
70. Warwick GL, Geddes CG, Boulton-Jones JM. Prednisolone and chlorambucil therapy for idiopathic membranous nephropathy with progressive renal failure. Quart J Med 1994;87:223–229.
70a. Pei Y, Cattran D, Greenwood C. Predicting chronic renal insufficiency in idiopathic membranous glomerulonephritis. Kidney Int 1992;42:960–955.
70b. Herbert LA: Therapy of membranous nephropathy: What to do after the after (meta) analyses. J Am Soc Nephrol 1995;5:1543–1545.
71. Cohen AH, Border WA. Mesangial proliferative glomerulonephritis. Sem Nephrol 1982;2:228.
72. Habib R, Churg J. Minimal change disease, mesangial proliferative glomerulonephritis and focal sclerosis: Individual entities or a spectrum of disease? In: Robinson RR, ed. Proceedings of the IXth International Congress of Nephrology. Nephrology 1984;1:634–644.
73. Nicholls KM, et al. The clinical course of mesangial IgA associated nephropathy in adults. Quart J Med 1984;210:227–250.
74. Clarkson AR, et al. IgA nephropathy: a syndrome of uniform morphology, diverse clinical features and uncertain prognosis. Clin Nephrol 1977;8:459–471.
75. Neela Kantappa K, Gallo GR, Baldwin DS. Proteinuria in IgA nephropathy. Kidney Int 1988;33:716–721.
76. Boyce NW, et al. Clinicopathological associations in mesangial IgA nephropathy. Am J Nephrol 1986;6:246–252.
77. Sinniah R. IgA mesangial nephropathy: Berger's disease. Am J Nephrol 1985;5:73–83.
78. Kobayashi Y, et al. IgA nephropathy: prognostic significance of proteinuria and histological alterations. Nephron 1983;34:146–153.
79. Yoskimura M, et al. Significance of IgA deposits on the glomerular capillary walls in IgA nephropathy. Am J Kidney Dis 1987;9:404–409.
80. Emancipator SN, Gallo GR, Lamm ME. IgA nephropathy: perspective on pathogenesis and classification. Clin Nephrol 1985;24:161–179.
81. Lai KN, et al. Increased binding of polymeric lamba-IgA to cultured human mesangial cells in IgA nephropathy. Kidney Int 1996;49:839–845.
82. Harper SJ, et al. Increased dimeric IgA producing B cells in the bone marrow of IgA nephropathy determined by in-situ hybridisation for J Chain mRNA. J Clin Pathol 1996;49:38–42.
83. Van Es LE: Pathogenesis of IgA nephropathy. Kidney Int 1992;41:1720–1729.
84. Monteiro RC, et al. Charge and size of mesangial IgA in IgA nephropathy. Kidney Int 1985;28:666–671.
85. Schena FP, Gesualdo L, Montinaro V. Immunopathological aspects of immunoglobulin A nephropathy and other mesangial proliferative glomerulonephritides. J Am Soc Nephrol 1992;2:S167–S172.
86. Praga M, et al. Acute worsening of renal function during episodes of macroscopic hematuria in IgA nephropathy. Kidney Int 1985;28:69–74.

87. Caillette A, et al. IgA mesangial nephropathy in over 75 year-old patients. In: Sessa A, Meroni M, Battini G, eds. Glomerulonephritis in the Elderly. Contrib Nephrol (Basel: Karger) 1993;105:152–156.
88. Ibels LS, Gyä ory AZ. IgA nephropathy: analysis of the natural history, important factors in the progression of renal disease, and a review of the literature. Medicine 1994;73:79–102.
89. Nomura S, et al. Gallium 67 scintigraphy as a predictor of renal prognosis in primary immunoglobulin A nephropathy. Am J Kidney Dis 1996;27:204–208.
90. Chida Y, Tomura S, Takeuchi. Renal Survival rate of IgA nephropathy. Nephron 1985;40:189–194.
91. Mustonen J, et al. Clincopathologic correlations in a series of 143 patients with IgA glomerulonephritis. Am J Nephrol 1985;5:150–157.
92. Lai KN, et al. Nephrotic range proteinuria—a good predictive index of disease in IgA nephropathy? Quart J Med 1985;222:677–688.
93. D'Amico G, et al. Prognostic indicators in idiopathic IgA mesangial nephropathy. Quart J Med. 1986;228:363–378.
94. Clarkson AR, et al. Controlled trial of phenytoin therapy in IgA nephropathy. Clin Nephrol 1980;13:215–218.
95. Egido J, et al. Phenytoin in IgA nephropathy: a long-term controlled trial. Nephron 1984;38:30–39.
96. Coppo R, et al. Ineffectiveness of phenytoin treatment on IgA-containing circulating immune complexes in IgA nephropathy. Nephron 1984;36:275–276.
97. Coppo R, et al. Immunological monitorization of plasma exchange in primary IgA nephropathy. Proc IX Int Cong Nephrol 1984:78A.
98. Genin C, et al. Efficiency of high dose steroids and plasma exchanges in severe mesangial IgA glomerulonephritis. Proc IX Int Cong Nephrol 1984:89A.
99. Glassock RJ, Kurokawa K. IgA nephropathy in Japan. Am J Nephrol 1985;5: 127–137.
100. Lai KN, et al. Cyclosporin treatment of IgA nephropathy: a short-term controlled trial. Br Med J 1987;295:1165–1168.
101. Hogg RJ, Waldo B. Advances in treatment: immunoglobulin A nephropathy. Sem Nephrol 1996;16:511–516.
102. Mustonen J, Pasternack A, Rantala I. The nephrotic syndrome in IgA glomerulonephritis: response to corticosteroid therapy. Clin Nephrol 1983;20:172–176.
103. Kobayashi Y, et al. Steroid therapy in IgA nephropathy: a prospective pilot study in moderate proteinuric cases. Quart J Med 1986;61:935–943.
104. Brown EA, et al. The clinical course of mesangial proliferative glomerulonephritis. Medicine 1979;58:295–303.
105. Yamamoto S, et al. Study on a predictive marker for evaluating the effectiveness of steroid therapy in IgA nephropathy. Significance of extracapillary changes. Nippon Jinzo Gakkai Shi 1996;38:74–83.
106. Donadio JV Jr, et al. A controlled trial of fish oil in IgA nephropathy. N Engl J Med 1994;331:1194–1198.
106a. Dillon JJ. Fish oil therapy for IgA nephropathy: efficacy and interstudy variability. J Am Soc Nephrol 1997;8:1739–1744.

107. Furci L, et al. Rapidly progressive glomerulonephritis in the elderly. Long-term results. In: Sessa A, Meroni M, Battini G, eds. Glomerulonephritis in the Elderly. Contrib Nephrol (Basel: Karger) 1993;105:98–101.
108. Velosa JA, Homburger HA, Holley KE. Prospective study of anti-neutrophil cytoplasmic auto antibody tests in the diagnosis of idiopathic necrotizing crescentic glomerulonephritis and renal vasculitis. Mayo Clin Proc 1993;68:561–565.
109. Bindi P, et al. Necrotizing crescentic glomerulonephritis without significant immune deposits: a clinical and serological study. Quart J Med 1993;86:55–68.
110. Pettersson EE, Sundelin B, Heigl Z. Incidence and outcome of pauci-immune necrotizing and crescentic glomerulonephritis in adults. Clin Nephrol 1995;43:141–149.
111. Franssem CFM, et al. Differences between anti-myeloperoxidase and anti-proteinase 3 associated renal disease. Kidney Int 1995;47:193–199.
112. Lewis EJ, Schwartz MM. Idiopathic crescentic glomerulonephritis. Sem Nephrol 1982;2:193–213.
113. Groggel GC, et al. Role of the terminal complement pathway in the heterologous phase of antiglomerular basement membrane nephritis in the rabbit. Kidney Int 1985;27:643–651.
114. Tucker BJ, et al. Effect of leucocyte depletion on glomerular dynamics during acute glomerular immune injury. Kidney Int 1985;28:28–35.
115. Bonsib SM. Glomerular basement membrane necrosis and crescent organization. Kidney Int 1988;33:966–974.
115a. Atkins RC, et al. Modulators of crescentic glomerulonephritis. J Am Soc Nephrol 1996;7:2271–2278.
116. Germuth FG Jr, et al. Fatal immune complex glomerulonephritis. Acta Path Microbiol Scand 1974;249(suppl):20–28.
117. Cohen AH, et al. Crescentic glomerulonephritis: immune vs. nonimmune mechanisms. Am J Nephrol 1981;1:78–83.
118. Olsen S, Peterson V, Hansen H. Immunofluorescence studies of extracapillary glomerulonephritis. Acta Path Microbiol Scand 1974;249(suppl):20–28.
119. Mrowka C, et al. Distribution of the granulocyte serine proteinases proteinase 3 and elastase in human glomerulonephritis. Am J Kidney Dis 1995;25:253–261.
120. Beirne GJ, et al. Idiopathic crescentic glomerulonephritis. Medicine 1977;56:349–381.
121. Wilson CB, Dixon FJ. Anti-glomerular basement membrane antibody-induced glomerulonephritis. Kidney Int 1973;3:74–89.
122. Morrin PAF, et al. Rapidly progressive glomerulonephritis. Am J Med 1978;65:446–460.
123. Simpson JJ, et al. Plasma exchange in Goodpasture's syndrome. Am J Nephrol 1982;2:301–311.
124. Flores JC, et al. Clinical and immunological evolution of oligoanuric anti GBM nephritis treated by hemodialysis. Lancet 1986;1:508.
125. Kelly PT, Haponik EF. Goodpasture syndrome: molecular and clinical advances. Medicine 1994;73:171–185.
126. Kline BW. Rapidly progressive glomerulonephritis. Sem Nephrol 1996;16:517–626.

127. Bosch X, et al. Antineutrophil cytoplasmic auto antibody-associated alveolar capillaritis in patients presenting with pulmonary hemorrhage. Arch Pathol Lab Med 1994;118:517–522.
128. Saxena R, et al. Circulating auto-antibodies as serological markers in the differential diagnosis of pulmonary renal syndrome. J Intern Med 1995;238:143–152.
129. Niles JL, et al. The syndrome of lung hemorrhage and nephritis is usually an ANCA-associated condition. Arch Intern Med 1996;156:440–445.
130. Sonsino E, et al. Extracapillary proliferative glomerulonephritis so-called malignant glomerulonephritis. Adv Nephrol 1972;2:121–163.
131. O'Neill WM Jr, Etheridge WB, Bloomer A. High dose corticosteroids. Their use in treating idiopathic rapidly progressive glomerulonephritis. Arch Intern Med 1979; 139:514–5128.
132. Kline Bolton W, Couser WG. Intravenous pulse methylprednisolone therapy of acute crescentic rapidly progressive glomerulonephritis. Am J Med 1979;66: 495–502.
133. Oredugba O, et al. Pulse methylprednisolone therapy in idiopathic, rapidly progressive glomerulonephritis. Ann Intern Med 1980;92:504–506.
134. Neild GH, et al. Rapidly progressive glomerulonephritis with extensive glomerular crescent formation. Quart J Med 1983;207:395–416.
135. Petterson EE, Sundelin B, Heigl Z. Incidence and outcome of pauci immune necrotizing and crescentic glomerulonephritis in adults. Clin Nephrol 1995;43:141–149.
136. Heilman RL, et al. Analysis of risk factors for patients and renal survival in crescentic glomerulonephritis. Kidney Int 1986;29:189A.
137. Johnson JP, et al. Therapy of anti-glomerular basement membrane antibody disease: analysis of prognostic significance of clinical, pathologic and treatment factors. Medicine 1985;64:219–227.
137a. Bosch X, et al. Prognostic implications of anti-neutrophil cytoplasmic antibodies with myeloperoxidase specificity in anti-glomerular basement membrane disease. Clin Nephrol 1991;36:107–113.
138. De'Oliviera J, et al. Relationship between disease activity and anti-neutrophil cytoplasmic antibody concentration in long term management of systemic vasculitis. Am J Kidney Dis 1995;25:380–389.
139. Gonzalo A, et al. Clinical significance of IgM mesangial deposits in the nephrotic syndrome. Nephron 1985;41:246–249.
140. Lawer W, et al. IgM associated primary diffuse mesangial proliferative glomerulonephritis. J Clin Pathol 1980;33:1029–1038.
141. Osakabe K, Matumoto K. Concavalin A-induced suppressor cell activity in lipoid nephrosis. Scand J Immunol 1981;14:161–166.
142. Schnaper HW, Aune TM. Identification of the lymphokine soluble immune response supressor in urine of nephrotic children. J Clin Invest 1985;76:341–349.
143. Levin M, et al. Steroid responsive nephrotic syndrome: a generalised disorder of membrane negative charge. Lancet 1985;2:239–242.
144. Kreisberg JE, et al. Rapid and focal loss of negative charge associated with mononuclear cell infiltration early in nephrotoxic serum nephritis. Kidney Int 1979;16: 290–300.
145. Lagrue G, Laurent J. Allergy and lipid nephrosis. Adv Nephrol 1983;12:151–175.

146. Bohrer MP, et al. Mechanisms of the puromycin-induced defects in the transglomerular passage of water and macromolecules. J Clin Invest. 1971;60:152–161.
147. Bohman SD, et al. Foot process fusion and glomerular filtration rate in minimal change nephrotic syndrome. Kidney Int 1984;25:696–700.
148. Bridges CR, et al. Glomerular charge alterations in human minimal change nephropathy. Kidney Int 1982;22:677–684.
149. Carrie BJ, Salyer WR, Myers BD. Minimal change nephropathy: an electrochemical disorder of the glomerular membrane. Am J Med 1981;70:262–268.
150. Hooper J Jr, et al. Lipoid nephrosis in 31 adult patients: renal biopsy study by light, electron and fluorescence microscopy with experience in treatment. Medicine 1970;49:321–341.
151. Hayslett JP, et al. Clinicopathological correlations in the nephrotic syndrome due to primary renal disease. Medicine 1973;52:93–120.
152. Cameron JS, et al. The nephrotic syndrome in adults with "minimal change" glomerular lesions. Quart J Med 1974;43:461–488.
153. Wang F, Looi LM, Chua CT. Minimal change glomerular disease in Maylasian adults and use of alternate day steroid therapy. Quart J Med 1982;203:312–328.
154. Palmieri PF, et al. In: Sessa A, Meroni M, Battini G, eds. Glomerulonephritis in the Elderly. Contrib Nephrol (Basel: Karger) 1993;105:58–64.
155. Sessa A, et al. Glomerulonephritis in the elderly aged over 65. In: Sessa A, Meroni M, Battini G, eds. Glomerulonephritis in the Elderly. Contrib Nephrol (Basel: Karger) 1993;105:85–92.
156. Nolasco F, Cameron JS, Heywood EF. Adult-onset minimal change nephrotic syndrome: a long term follow-up. Kidney Int 1986;29:1215–1223.
157. Korbet SM, Schwartz MM, Lewis EJ. Minimal-change glomerulopathy of adulthood. Am J Nephrol 1988;8:291–297.
158. Cameron JS. Nephrotic syndrome in the elderly. Sem Nephrol 1996;16:319–329.
159. Bourgoignie JJ, Meneses R, Pardo V. The nephropathy related to acquired immune deficiency syndrome. Adv Nephrol 1988;17:113–126.
160. D'Agati V. The many masks of focal segmental glomerulosclerosis. Kidney Int 1994;46:1223–1241.
161. Hoyer JR. Focal segmental glomerulosclerosis. Sem Nephrol 1982;2:253–263.
162. Savin VJ, et al. Circulating factor associated with increased glomerular permeability to albumin in recurrent focal segmental glomerulosclerosis. N Engl J Med 1996;334:878–883.
163. Matsumoto K, et al. Concavalin A-induced suppressor cell activity in focal glomerulosclerosis. Nephron 1978;20:307–315.
164. Nagai R, Cattran DC, Pei Y. Steroid therapy and prognosis of focal segmental glomerulosclerosis in the elderly. Clin Nephrol 1994;42:18–21.
165. Bolton WK, Westervelt FB, Sturgill BC. Nephrotic syndrome and focal glomerular sclerosis in aging man. Nephron 1978;20:307–315.
166. Winetz JA, et al. The nature of the glomerular injury in minimal change and focal sclerosing glomerulopathies. Am J Kidney Dis 1981;2:91–98.
167. Newman WJ, et al. Focal glomerulosclerosis: contrasting clinical patterns in children and adults. Medicine 1976;55:67–87.

168. Velosa JA, et al. Significance of proteinuria on the outcome of renal function in patients with focal segmental glomerulosclerosis. Mayo Clin Proc 1983;58:568–577.
169. Korbet SM, Schwartz MM, Lewis EJ. The prognosis of focal segmental glomerulosclerosis of adulthood. Medicine 1986;65:304–311.
170. Pei Y, et al. Evidence suggesting under-treatment in adults with idiopathic focal segmental glomerulosclerosis. Am J Med 1987;82:938–944.
171. Cameron JS, et al. The long-term prognosis of patients with focal segmental glomerulosclerosis. Clin Nephrol 1978;10:213–218.
172. Beaufils H, et al. Focal glomerulosclerosis: natural history and treatment. Nephron 1978;21:75–85.
173. Meyrier A, Simon P. Treatment of corticoresistant idiopathic nephrotic syndrome in the adult: minimal change disease and focal segmental glomerulosclerosis. Adv Nephrol 1988;17:127–150.
173a. Ponticelli C, et al. A randomized trial of cyclosporine in steroid-resistant idiopathic nephrotic syndrome. Kidney Int 1993;43:1377–1384.
174. Velosa JA, et al. Treatment of severe nephrotic syndrome with meclofenamate: an uncontrolled pilot study. Mayo Clin Proc 1985;60:586–592.
175. Anderson CF. Meclofenamate and the nephrotic syndrome: the use of the right drug in the right patient by the right physician. Mayo Clin Proc 1984;59:206–207.
176. Abreo K, Moorthy AV. Type 3 membranoproliferative glomerulonephritis. Clinicopathologic correlations and long term follow-up in nine patients. Arch Pathol Lab Med 1982;106:413–417.
177. Cameron JS, et al. Idiopathic mesangiocapillary glomerulonephritis. Comparison of types I and II in children and adults and long-term prognosis. Am J Med 1983;74: 175–192.
178. West CD. Pathogenesis and approaches to therapy of membrano-proliferative glomerulonephritis. Kidney Int 1976;9:1–7.
179. Davis CA, Marder H, West CD. Circulating immune complexes in membranoproliferative glomerulonephritis. Kidney Int 1981;20:728–732.
180. Ooi YM, Vallota EH, West CD. Classical complement pathway activation in membranoproliferative glomerulonephritis. Kidney Int 1976;9:46–53.
181. Whaley K, Ward D, Ruddy S. Modulation of the properdin amplification loop in membranoproliferative and other forms of glomerulonephritis. Clin Exp Immunol 1979;35:101–106.
182. Nuñez NJ, et al. Glomerular nephropathy in persons older than 50 years. Kidney Int 1985;28:587A.
183. Zimmerman SW, et al. Prospective trial of Warfarin and dipyridamole in patients with membranoproliferative glomerulonephritis. Am J Med 1983;75:920–927.
184. Zäuner I, for the Collaborative Glomerulonephritis Therapy Study Group. Effect of aspirin and dipyridamole on proteinuria in idiopathic membrane proliferative glomerulonephritis: a multicentre prospective clinical trial. Nephrol Dial Transplant 1994;9:619–622.
185. Donadio JV Jr, et al. Membranoproliferative glomerulonephritis. A prospective clinical trial of platelet-inhibitor therapy. N Engl J Med 1984;310:1421–1426.

186. Mowry JA, McCarthy ET. Cyclosporine in glomerular disease. Sem Nephrol 1996; 16:548–554.
187. Montoliu J, et al. Acute and rapidly progressive forms of glomerulonephritis in the elderly. J Am Geriatr Soc 1981;29:108–116.
188. Volpi A, et al. Postinfectious glomerulonephritis in the elderly. Am J Nephrol 1988; 8:431–432.
189. Rodriguez-Iturbe B, et al. Circulating immune complexes and serum immunoglobulins in acute poststreptococcal glomerulonephritis: evidence for circulating immune complex pathogenesis. Clin Nephrol 1980;13:1–5.
190. Van De Rijn I, Fillet H, Brandeis WE. Serial studies on circulating immune complexes in poststreptococcal sequelae. Clin Exp Immunol 1978;34:318–325.
191. Oite T, et al. Quantitative studies of in-situ immune complex glomerulonephritis in the rat induced by planted, cationized antigen. J Exp Med 1982;155:4360–474.
192. Batsford SR, Talamiya H, Vogt A. A model of in-situ immune complex glomerulonephritis in the rat employing cationized ferritin. Clin Nephrol 1980;14: 211–216.
193. Mclntosh RM, et al. Evidence of autologous immune complex pathogenic mechanism in acute poststreptoccal glomerulonephritis. Kidney Int 1978;14:501–510.
194. Abrams CK. Glomerulonephritis in the elderly. Am J Nephrol 1985;5:409–418.
195. Zhao-Long W, et al. The presentation, treatment and outcome of acute glomerulonephritis in the elderly. Clin Nephrol 1996;45:277–279.
196. Samiy AH, Field RA, Merrill JP. Acute glomerulonephritis in elderly patients. Report of seven cases over sixty years of age. Ann Intern Med 1961;54:603–609.
197. Nesson R, Robbins SL. Glomerulonephritis in older age groups. Arch Intern Med 1960;105:47–56.
198. Lee HA, Stirling G, Sharpstone P. Acute glomerulonephritis in middle-aged and elderly patients. Br Med J 1966;2:1361–1363.
199. Arieff A, Anderson RJ, Massry SG. Acute glomerulonephritis in the elderly. Geriatrics 1971;26:74–84.
200. Lien JWK, Matthew TH, Meadows R. Acute post-streptococcal glomerulonephritis in adults: a long-term study. Quart J Med 1979;189:99–111.
201. Kaplan EL, Wanamaker LW. Suppression of the antistreptococcal response by cholesterol and by lipid extracts of rabbit skin. J Exp Med 1976;144:754–767.
202. Montoliu J, et al. Primary acute glomerular disorders in the elderly. Arch Intern Med 1980;140:755–756.
203. Sapir DG, Yardley JH, Walker WG. Acute glomerulonephritis in older patients. Johns Hopkins Med J 1968;132:145–152.
204. Vogel W, et al. Long-term prognosis for endocapillary glomerulonephritis of poststreptococcal type in children and adults. Nephron 1986;44:58–65.
205. Coggins CH. Management of nephrotic syndrome. In: Brenner BM, Stein J, eds. Contemporary Issues in Nephtology. Vol 9. New York: Churchill Livingston, 1982; 283–296.
206. Kirchner KA, Voelker JR, Brater DC. Tubular resistance to furosemide contributes to the attenuated diuretic response in nephrotic rats. J Am Soc Nephrol 1992;2: 1201–1207.

207. Kaysen GA, et al. Effect of dietary protein intake on albumin hemostatis in nephrotic patients. Kidney Int 1986;29:572–577.
208. Rosenberg ME, et al. Glomerular and hormonal responses to dietary protein intake in human renal disease. Am J Physiol 1987;253:F1083–F1090.
209. de Jong PE, Anderson S, de Zeeuur D. Glomerular preload and after-load reduction as a tool to lower urinary protein leakage: will such treatments also help to improve renal function outcome? J Am Soc Nephrol 1993;3:1333–1341.
210. Ruilope LM, et al. Additive antiproteinuric effect of converting enzyme inhibition and a low protein intake. J Am Soc Nephrol 1992;3:1307–1311.
211. Golbetz H, et al. Mechanism of the antiproteinuric effect of indomethacin in nephrotic humans. Am J Physiol 1989;256:F44–F51.
212. Velosa JA, Torres VE. Benefits and risks of nonsteroidal antiinflammatory drugs in steroid resistant nephrotic syndrome. Am J Kidney Dis 1986;8:345–350.
213. Chopra JS, Mallick NP, Stone MC. Hyperlipoproteinaemia in nephrotic syndrome. Lancet 1971;1:317–320.
214. Appel GB, et al. The hyperlipidemia of the nephrotic syndrome. Relation to plasma albumin concentration, oncotic pressure and viscosity. N Engl J Med 1985;312: 1544–1548.
215. Newmark SR, Anderson CF, Donadio JV Jr. Lipoprotein profiles in adult nephrotics. Mayo Clin Proc 1975;50:359–364.
216. Short CP, et al. Serum and urinary high density lipoproteins in glomerular diseases with proteinuria. Kidney Int 1986;29:1224–1228.
217. Warwick GL, et al. Low-density lipoprotein metabolism in the nephrotic syndrome. Metabolism 1990;39:187–192.
218. Vega GL, Toto RD, Grundy SM. Metabolism of low density lipoproteins in nephrotic dyslipidemia: comparison of hypercholesterolemia alone and combined hyperlipidemia. Kidney Int 1995;47:579–586.
219. Staprans J, Felts JM. The effect of alpha-acid glycoprotein (orosomucoid) on triglyceride metabolism in the nephrotic syndrome. Biochem Biophys Res Commun 1977;79:1272–1278.
220. Felts JM, Mayerle JA. Urinary loss of plasma high density lipoprotein. A possible cause of the hyperlipidemia of the nephrotic syndrome. Circulation 1974;49–50(suppl 3):263A.
221. Saku K, et al. High-density lipoprotein apolipoprotein AI and AII turnover in moderate and severe proteinuria. Nephron 1988;50:112–115.
222. Mallick NP, Short CD. The nephrotic syndrome and ischemic heart disease. Nephron 1981;27:54–57.
223. Wass V, Cameron JS. Cardiovascular disease and the nephrotic syndrome: the other side of the coin. Nephron 1981;27:58–61.
224. Ordonez, et al. The risk of coronary artery disease among patients with nephrotic syndrome. Kidney Int 1990;37:243A.
225. Grone EF, et al. The role of lipids in nephrosclerosis and glomerulosclerosis. Atherosclerosis 1994;107:1–13.
226. Grundy SM, et al. The place of HDL in cholesterol management. Arch Intern Med 1989;149:505–510.

227. Grundy SM. Managemenmt of hyperlipidemia of kidney disease. Kidney Int 1990; 37:847–853.
228. Golper TA, et al. Lovastatin in the treatment of multifactorial hyperlipidemia associated with proteinuria. Am J Kidney Dis 1989;13:312–329.
229. Vega GL, Grundy SM. Lovastatin therapy in nephrotic hyperlipidemia: effects on lipoprotein metabolism. Kidney Int 1988;33:1160–1168.
230. Rabelink AJ, et al. Effects of simvastatin and cholestyramine on lipoprotein profile in hyperlipidemia of nephrotic syndrome. Lancet 1988;2:1335–1338.
231. Kasiske BL, et al. The effects of lovastatin in hyperlipidemic patients with the nephrotic syndrome. Am J Kidney Dis 1990;15:8–15.
232. Goldstein DA, et al. Vitamin D metabolites and calcium metabolism in patients with nephrotic syndrome and normal renal function. J Clin Endocrinol Metab 1981;52:116–121.
233. Goldstein DA, et al. Blood levels of 25- hydroxyvitamin D in nephrotic syndrome: studies in 26 patients. Ann Intern Med 1977;87:664–668.
234. Sato KA, Gray RW, Lemann J Jr. Urinary excretion of 25- hydroxyvitamin D in health and the nephrotic syndrome. J Lab Clin Med 1982;99:325–330.
235. Malluche HH, Goldstein DA, Massry SG. Osteomalacia and hyperparathyroid bone disease in patients with nephrotic syndrome. J Clin Invest 1979;63:494–500.
236. Malluche HH, et al. Bone histology in incipient and advanced renal failure. Kidney Int 1976;9:355–362.
237. Klein RG, et al. Intestinal calcium absorption in exogenous hypercortisonism. Role of 25-hydroxyvitamin D and corticosteroid dose. J Clin Invest 1977;60:253–259.
238. Canalis E. Mechanisms of glucocorticoid action in bone: implications to glucocorticoid-induced osteoporosis. J Clin Endocr 1996;81:3441–3447.
238a. Reid IR: Glucocorticord osteoporosis. Mechanisms and management. Eur J Endocrinol 1997;137:209–217.
239. Lips P, et al. The effect of vitamin D supplementation on vitamin D status and parathyroid function in elderly subjects. J Clin Endocrinol Metab 1988;67:644–650.
240. Dykman TR, et al. Effect of oral 1,25-dihydroxyvitamin D and calcium on glucocorticoid-induced osteopenia in patients with rheumatic diseases. Arthr Rheum 1984;27:1336–1343.
241. Cosio FG, et al. Plasma concentrations of the natural anticoagulants protein C and protein S in patients with proteinuria. J Lab Clin Med 1985;106:218–222.
242. Manucci PM, et al. High plasma levels of protein C activity and antigen in the nephrotic syndrome. Thromb Haemost 1986;55:31–33.
243. Allon M, et al. Protein S and C antigen levels in proteinuric patients, dependency on type of glomerular pathology. Am J Hematol 1989;31:96–101.
244. Vigano-D'Angelo S, et al. Protein S deficiency occurs in the nephrotic syndrome. Ann Intern Med 1987;107:42–47.
245. Du XH, et al. Nephrotic syndrome with renal vein thrombosis: pathogenetic importance of a plasmin inhibitor ($\propto_2$-antiplasmin). Clin Nephrol 1985;24:186–191.
246. Remuzzi G, et al. Platelet hyperaggregability and the nephrotic syndrome. Thromb Res 1979;16:345–354.

247. Machleidt C, et al. Multifactorial genesis of enhanced platelet aggregability in patients with nephrotic syndrome. Kidney Int 1989;36:1119–1124.
248. Llach F. Hypercoagulability, renal vein thrombosis and other thrombotic complications of nephrotic syndrome. Kidney Int 1985;28:429–439.
249. Andrassy K, Ritze E, Bommer J. Hypercoagulability in the nephrotic syndrome. Klin Wochenschr 1980;58:1029–1036.
250. Llach F, Papper S, Massry SG. The clinical spectrum of renal vein thrombosis, acute and chronic. Am J Med 1980;69:819–827.
251. Rostoker G, et al. Prevention of thrombotic complications of the nephrotic syndrome by the low molecular-weight heparin enoxaparin. Nephron 1995;69:20–28.
252. Wagoner RD, et al. Renal vein thrombosis in idiopathic membranous glomerulopathy and nephrotic syndrome: incidence and significance. Kidney Int 1983;23: 368–374.
253. Trew PA, et al. Renal vein thrombosis in membranous glomerulopathy: incidence and association. Medicine 1978;57:69–82.
254. Llach F, Arieff Al, Massry SG. Renal vein thrombosis and nephrotic syndrome. A prospective study of 36 adult patients. Ann Intern Med 1975;83:8–14.
255. Rosenfield AT, et al. Ultrasound in experimental and clinical renal vein thrombosis. Radiology 1980;137:735–741.
256. Braun B, Weilemann LS, Weigand W. Ultrasonographic demonstration of renal vein thrombosis. Radiology 1981;138:157–158.
257. Avasthi PS, et al. Noninvasive diagnosis of renal vein thrombosis by ultrasonic echo-Doppler flowmetry. Kidney Int 1983;23:882–887.
258. Harrington JT, Kassirer JP. Renal vein thrombosis. Annu Rev Med 1982;33:255–262.
259. Crowley JP, et al. Fibrinolytic therapy for bilateral renal vein thrombosis. Arch Intern Med 1984;144:159–160.
260. Esparza AR, et al. Spectrum of acute renal failure in nephrotic syndrome with minimal (or minor) glomerular lesions. Lab Invest 1981;45:510–521.
261. Chamberlain MJ, Pringle A, Wrong OM. Oliguric renal failure in the nephrotic syndrome. Quart J Med 1966;138:215–235.
262. Conally ME, Wrong OM, Jones NF. Reversible renal failure in idiopathic nephrotic syndrome with minimal glomerular changes. Lancet 1968;1:665–668.
263. Raij L, et al. Irreversible acute renal failure in idiopathic nephrotic syndrome. Am J Med 1976;61:207–214.
264. Lowenstein J, Schacht RG, Baldwin DS. Renal failure in minimal change nephrotic syndrome. Am J Med 1981;70:227–233.
265. Case records of the Massachusetts General Hospital. N Engl J Med 1978;299:136–145.
266. Hulter HN, Bonner EL Jr. Lipoid nephrosis appearing as acute oliguric renal failure. Arch Intern Med 1980;140:403–405.
267. Imbasciati E, et al. Acute renal failure in idiopathic nephrotic syndrome. Nephron 1981;28:186–191.
268. Sjoberg RJ, et al. Renal failure with minimal change nephrotic syndrome: reversal with hemodialysis. Clin Nephrol 1983;20:98–100.

269. Searle M, et al. Reversibility of acute renal failure in elderly patients with the nephotic syndrome. Postgrad Med 1985;61:741–744.
270. Thompson H, Odell M. Reversible uraemia in normotensive nephrotic syndrome. Br Med J 1979;274:705–706.
271. Jennette JC, Falk RJ. Adult minimal change glomerulopathy with acute renal failure. Am J Kidney Dis 1990;16:432–437.
272. Furuga R, et al. Reversible acute renal failure in idiopatic nephrotic syndrome. Intern Med 1993;32:31–35.
273. Moorthy AV, et al. Association of crescentic glomerulonephritis with membranous glomerulopathy: a report of three cases. Clin Nephrol 1976;6:319–325.
274. Hill GS, et al. An unusual variant of membranous nephropathy with abundant crescent formation and recurrence in the transplanted kidney. Clin Nephrol 1978;10: 114–120.
275. Bennett WM, Kincaid-Smith P. Macroscopic hematuria in mesangial IgA nephropathy: correlation with glomerular crescents and renal dysfunction. Kidney Int 1983; 23:393–400.
276. Abrielo GJ, et al. Crescentic IgA nephropathy. Medicine 1984;63:396–406.
277. Koethe JD, et al. Progression of membranous nephropathy to acute crescentic rapidly progressive glomerulonephritis and response to pulse methylprednisolone. Am J Nephrol 1986;6:224–228.
278. Lee JC, Yamauchi H, Hooper J Jr. The association of cancer and the nephrotic syndrome. Ann Intern Med 1966;64:41–51.
279. Eagen JW, Lewis EJ. Glomerulopathies of neoplasia. Kidney Int 1977;11:297–306.
280. Hooper J Jr, Trew PA, Biava CG. Membranous nephropathy: its relative benignity in women. Nephron 1981;29:18–24.
281. Faubert PF, Porush JG. Unpublished observations, 1990.
282. Biava CG, et al. Crescentic glomerulonephritis associated with nonrenal malignancies. Am J Nephrol 1984;4:208–214.
283. Haskell LP, et al. Crescentic glomerulonephritis associated with prostatic carcinoma: evidence of immune-mediated glomerular injury. Am J Med 1990;88: 189–192.
284. Edgar JDM, et al. An association between ANCA positive renal disease and malignancy. Clin Nephrol 1993;40:22–25.
285. Lund L, Jacobsen BA, Schmidt EB. The occurrence of malignant disease in adult nephrotic syndrome. J Intern Med 1989;226:201–203.

7

Renal Involvement in Systemic Diseases

I. DIABETIC NEPHROPATHY

A. Incidence and Prevalence

Diabetic nephropathy is the most common form of secondary glomerular disease, as well as one of the most common causes of end-stage renal disease (ESRD) in the elderly. Thirty-one percent of individuals 65 years and older enrolled in the United States ESRD program from 1989 to 1993 had type II diabetic nephropathy (1). It is estimated that in the United States, 10–40% of patients with type II diabetes mellitus will develop diabetic nephropathy (2,3). The incidence of nephropathy in type II diabetes varies among countries and even among groups within a given country. For instance, in the United States, diabetic nephropathy occurs with a higher frequency among Blacks, Mexican Americans, and Native Americans (more so among Pima Indians) than among Whites with diabetes mellitus, suggesting that genetic factors play a role. Besides genetics, the duration of diabetes, family history of hypertension, cigarette smoking, and degree of glycemic control are important contributory factors (4–7).

B. Pathology

The early changes on light microscopy consist of widening of the glomerular mesangium and Bowman's capsule. As the disease progresses, the capillary basement membrane thickens, the capillaries undergo aneurysmal dilatation, and the mesangial matrix continues to expand. The latter takes two morphological forms, a diffuse one and a nodular one (Kimmelsteil-Wilson nodules). Hyaline deposits are seen in Bowman's capsule, the mesangium, or in the lumen of dilated capillaries. Ultimately, the glomerulus ends up completely sclerosed. With electron microscopy, one sees thickening of the glomerular basement membrane (GBM), and thick strands of mesangial matrix aggregating into nodules. A loose network of pores, about 8 nm in diameter, develops along the GBM. The density of negatively charged molecules such as heparin sulfate proteoglycans is decreased (8). With immunofluorescence microscopy, linear deposits of immunoglobulins (IgG), albumin, or fibrinogen may be found along the glomerular and tubular basement membranes.

C. Pathogenesis

The mechanisms by which patients with diabetes mellitus develop nephropathy are not clear. As noted, it is quite likely that this form of kidney disease results from the interplay of various environmental and genetic factors. Variations in extracellular levels of glucose have been found to stimulate collagen production by mesangial cells (9). Also, in mice, prolonged exposure of protein to glucose results in the formation of advanced glycation end products, which increases extracellular matrix gene expression, similar to that seen in patients with diabetic nephropathy (10). Furthermore, hyperglycemia, perhaps through deactivation of the tubuloglomerular feedback, can induce glomerular hyperfiltration. Indeed, the glomerular filtration rate (GFR) is elevated in most patients with type II diabetes mellitus when compared to controls (4,4a) (Fig. 1). Also contributing to the hyperfiltration is an increase in glomerular capillary flow due, in part, to a decrease in glomerular contractile responsiveness to angiotensin II (AII), as suggested by the reduced All receptor density seen in rats with streptozotocin-induced diabetes mellitus (11). The resulting glomerular capillary hypertension has been shown to play a role in the glomerular injury associated with experimental diabetes mellitus (12).

Intensive, tight control of the blood glucose level could retard the progression of the microvascular complications of diabetes (13). However, factors other than hyperglycemia are involved, since nephropathy develops in only 10–40% of type II diabetics, and the disease may become manifest in patients with mild, previously undiagnosed diabetes mellitus. Proteinuria is more common in smokers with type II diabetes mellitus than in former smokers and nonsmokers (14). A hypertensive diabetic is more likely to develop proteinuria than is a nonhypertensive (4), which may be environmental or genetic.

As for the genetic factors, the risk of nephropathy increases significantly for a diabetic who has a parent or a sibling with diabetic nephropathy. As noted, nephropathy develop more frequently in Blacks and Mexican or Native Ameri-

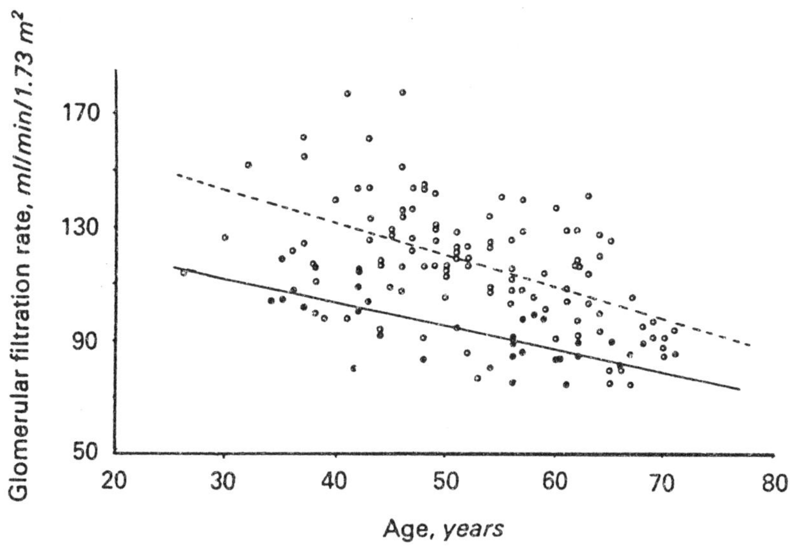

Figure 1 Relationship between glomerular filtration rate and age in non-insulin-dependent diabetics (open circles) (N = 110) and normal subjects (N = 32). (From Vora JP, et al. Renal hemodynamics in newly presenting non-insulin dependent diabetes mellitus. Kidney Int 1992; 41:829–835.

cans with diabetes mellitus (4). Finally, the angiotensin-converting enzyme (ACE) *DD* genotype carries a high prognostic value for the development of microalbuminuria and for rapid deterioration of kidney function in patients with diabetic nephropathy (15,15a).

D. Clinical Manifestations

1. Proteinuria

Microalbuminuria, defined as an albumin excretion rate of 20–200 µg/min, is considered the earliest manifestation of diabetic renal disease and is present in a significant number of elderly at the time of diagnosis of diabetes mellitus. Males are affected more often than females (16). The average duration of clinical type II diabetes in patients with microalbuminuria is 9.4 years, compared to 7.9 years for those with a normal albumin excretion (17). Retinopathy is present in 62% (17) of those patients with microalbuminuria. Hypertension is twice as common as in the general population (16). Even in normotensive patients, there may be a loss in diurnal blood pressure variation, which is known to be related to an increased occurrence of target organ damage in essential hypertension (18). In general, the smaller the night-time systolic dip in the blood pressure, the higher is the albumin excretion rate in these patients.

GFR is either higher or similar to that of age-matched nondiabetics (16,16a). It has been postulated that the proteinuria seen in these patients may be the result of impaired proximal tubular reabsorption of albumin. However, recent studies in microalbuminuric patients with type I diabetes mellitus demonstrated that the infusion of ANP results in a significant increase in the excretion of albumin and IgG in these patients compared to controls, suggesting the presence of a dysfunction of the glomerular barrier (19).

Macroalbuminuria (albumin excretion > 200 μg/min) ensues in 22% of elderly patients with microalbuminuria (16). Experience with Pima Indians has shown that the higher the albumin excretion during the microalbuminuric stage, the greater is the risk of developing macroalbuminuria, compatible with the hypothesis that enhanced protein flux across the glomerular capillary wall contributes to progressive glomerular damage (16a). Patients with macroalbuminuria have a history of clinical diabetes mellitus for approximately 11 years (17). Retinopathy is usually present in 75% and hypertension in more than 90% of these patients.

GFR will vary according to the stage at which the diagnosis is made; however, some degree of renal insufficiency is present in the majority of patients with macroalbuminuria. As noted, the proteinuria develops as a function of impairment in the GBM size selectivity, due to an increase in the number of large pores (shunt pathway) (20). The renal insufficiency is the result of a loss of ultrafiltration capacity of the glomerular capillaries (21,22) due to the mesangial expansion (23).

2. *Hematuria*

In a prospective study of 30 patients of varying ages with a diagnosis of diabetic nephropathy, microscopic hematuria was found in 30% and red cell casts in 13% (24). The incidence of hematuria in the elderly has been somewhat lower in our experience, closer to the 14%, as reported by Lopes de Faria et al. (25). In these patients the decision to undertake extensive urological evaluation depends on the characteristics of the hematuria, which appears to be of glomerular origin in the majority of patients (see Chapter 6). For those with apparent nonglomerular bleeding, the incidence of a superimposed urological disorder, other than benign prostatic hypertrophy in the male, has been low in our experience.

3. *Hypertension*

As noted earlier, hypertension is more common in diabetics compared to the general population and tends to occur early, even prior to the microalbuminuric phase (4). The prevalence of hypertension in older diabetics is 58% in males and 72% in females aged 65–74 years, 55% in males and 71% in females aged 75–84 years, and 42% in males and 73% in females 85 years and older (26). In a randomly selected group of 155 type II patients attending a diabetic clinic, 39% were found to have hypertension, compared to 16% in controls (27). A positive correlation has been found between systolic BP and 24-hr urinary albumin excretion in these patients (27). This positive correlation has not been universally present, however, since either it has not been found at all (28, 29) or has been present only in those hypertensives who failed to have a night-time reduction in mean arterial pressure of 5–10% (30,31). Since the blood pressure rises progressively with decreasing renal function, the hypertension in patients with established diabetic glomerulosclerosis is probably largely a consequence of the kidney disease (32).

According to De Chatel and associates (33), at an early stage of diabetic nephropathy there is a significant increase in exchangeable sodium (Na), even in nonhypertensive subjects, despite the presence of plasma and blood volumes which were similar to normal controls. As hypertension sets in, however, both plasma and blood volume increase significantly. Even though basal levels of plasma renin, aldosterone, and catecholamines are identical in diabetics and normals, the pressor responsiveness of diabetes to norepinephrine (NE) and AII is exaggerated (34). This increased sensitivity to AII must be selective and limited to the hypertensive diabetics, since AII receptor density is reduced in platelets (35) and in the glomerular capillary (7) of insulin-dependent diabetics. The mechanism responsible for the Na retention is not clear (36), but may be due, in part, to the endogenous hyperinsulinemia that is generally present in type II diabetics, as insulin has been shown to increase renal tubular Na reabsorption (37,38). Intracellular Na metabolism (estimated by Na/lithium countertransport and Na/potassium cotransport) is similar in type II hypertensive diabetics and type II normotensive diabetics (39). Treatment with a thiazide diuretic often improves blood pressure and restores total body sodium to control levels and improves the cardiovascular responsiveness to NE and AII as well (40).

Based on an increased ratio of urinary kallikrein activity to supine plasma renin activity (a ratio which apparently correlates with renal blood flow), it has been suggested that abnormalities in the metabolism of these vasodilatory renal enzyme systems may play a pathogenetic role in the hypertension of type II diabetics (41). The possible therapeutic implications of these findings remain to be determined. A marked defect in calcium ATPase activity has been found in the erythrocytes of hypertensive type II diabetics (42). This defect is associated with an increase in intracellular calcium and appears to result partly from diabetes-induced alterations in calmodulin rather than from an intrinsic defect in pump function (43). Hyperglycemia also has been shown to increase the intracellular calcium and to stimulate proliferation of vascular smooth muscle cells, with the end result being an increase in muscle tone and vascular resistance (44).

E. Natural History and Therapy

Microalbuminuria is a good predictor for subsequent development of macroalbuminuria and renal impairment in type II diabetes, as it is in type I diabetics (6,16,45,45a). The prevalence of microalbuminuria in the former varies between 12% and 50% (4a,16). As noted, macroalbuminuria develops in 22% of elderly patients with microalbuminuria, compared to 5% of those with an albumin excretion rate of less than 30 μg/min (16). The mechanisms responsible for the transition from micro- to macroalbuminuria are not clear, and the time course of the transition differs markedly among patients (45).

The presence of macroalbuminemia in a diabetic patient usually translates into progressive renal impairment with subsequent end-stage renal disease. The course of 16 such patients is illustrated in Fig. 2.

Although it is not entirely clear that tight glycemic control slows or avoids the progression from micro- to macroalbuminemia in type II diabetics (45–47), we recommend that every effort be made to maintain blood glucose levels as close to normal as possible, since the overall rate of microvascular complications is decreased with better glycemic control (48–49a). Whether the patient has micro- or macroalbuminuria, we suggest keeping the Hgb A_{1c} level between 8% and 9%, keeping in mind that the Hgb A_{1c} increases with age in normals (50,51). Whether a Hgb A_{1c} level, less than 8%, has added benefit is a matter of controversy (52). Given the fact that the risk of hypoglycemia increases with more intensive therapy, we suggest that levels below 8% are not advisable and, in fact, may not always be achievable, particularly in the frail disabled elderly who have to rely on others for their care.

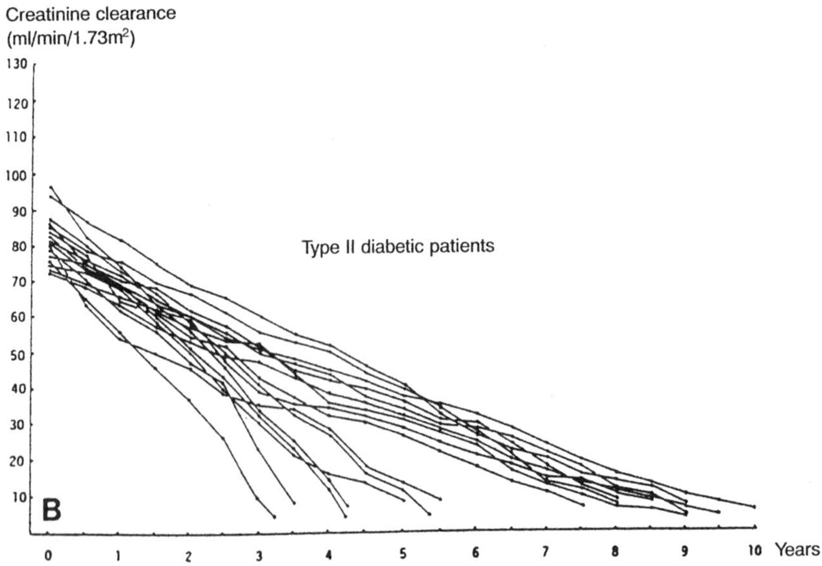

Figure 2 Change in creatinine clearance in 16 patients with type II diabetes mellitus. (From Ritz E, Stefanski A. Diabetic nephropathy in type II diabetes. Am J Kidney Dis 1996; 27:167–194.)

In virtually every study published so far, an ACE inhibitor has been found to slow the rate or prevent the conversion from micro- to macroalbuminuria in normotensive type I and type II diabetics (53–58a). Captopril, 25–50 mg every 12 hr, enalapril, 5–20 mg daily, lisinopril, 20 mg daily, or benazepril, 10 mg daily, have all been used successfully.

In general, hypertension should be rigorously controlled in the elderly diabetic, no matter what the albumin excretion rate is. Blood pressure control in the normoalbuminuric patient has been shown to delay the development of microalbuminuria, using either conventional antihypertensive drugs or ACE inhibitors (59–61).

In hypertensive patients with micro- or macroalbuminemia, there is some controversy whether ACE inhibitors or calcium channel blockers (CCB) confer additional renospecific benefit, independent of their blood pressure-lowering effect (61a). Kasiske et al. (62), in a meta-analysis of 100 studies published up to 1993, concluded that ACE inhibitors decrease proteinuria and slow the loss of GFR in patients with either type I or type II diabetes, independent of the systemic blood pressure (62). A similar conclusion has been reached more recently by Gansevoort et al. (63). Based on these findings and the possible direct effect of ACE inhibitors on the cellular mechanisms leading to the development of diabetic nephropathy (64), we recommend that an ACE inhibitor be started first and the dose titrated upward until the blood pressure is controlled or the maximum dose is reached (our goal is to keep the BP as close as 120/80 mmHg). In patients who are not adequately controlled with an ACE inhibitor, a calcium channel blocker, preferably a nondihydropyridine such as verapamil or diltiazem should be used (65). If a dihydropyridine CCB is necessary to control the blood pressure, a second generation (felodipine, nifedipine GITS, etc.) should be used. If one can extrapolate to the elderly with type II diabetes, the results from the long-term study in type I diabetes suggest that rigorous BP control and the use of an ACE inhibitor is associated with improved survival as well as a slowing of the decline in kidney function in patients with nephropathy (66).

Patients with superimposed renal insufficiency very often require a low-sodium diet (2–3 g) (67) and/or furosemide, at a dose tailored to the patient's GFR and diuretic response. Caloric reduction is necessary in the obese patient because weight loss, per se, may facilitate blood pressure control (68). In addition to improving glycemic control, protein restriction (0.6–0.8 gm/kg/day) should be initiated (69). Attempts also should be made to keep the serum cholesterol within the normal range (70,70a). Smokers are encouraged to stop.

Occasionally, a hypertensive elderly diabetic has supine hypertension and symptomatic orthostatic hypotension. These patients can be managed with a combination of antihypertensives and 9-alpha-fluorohydrocortisone, 0.05–0.3 mg/day. Volume status must be carefully monitored to prevent fluid overload (71).

F. Differential Diagnosis

The diagnosis of diabetic nephropathy is most often made on clinical grounds when the triad of retinopathy, proteinuria, and hypertension exists in a patient with long-standing diabetes mellitus; however, the development of proteinuria and or the nephrotic syndrome in a long-standing diabetic does not necessarily imply diabetic glomerulopathy, particularly in type II diabetes, given the uncertainty with respect to time of onset of the disease and a lower prevalence of retinopathy than in type I patients (72).

In 47 patients with long-standing type II diabetes mellitus biopsied by Hatch et al. (73), six (13%) showed histological findings other than diabetic glomerulosclerosis. Two had chronic glomerulonephritis, two had nephrosclerosis, one had membranous glomerulopathy, and one had acute endoproliferative glomerulonephritis. Chihara and associates (74) found a glomerular disease other than diabetic glomerulosclerosis in 36 (22%) of 164 diabetic patients. The reason these 164 diabetic patients were biopsied is not stated by the authors. They noted that those diabetics with glomerular disease were older, had their diabetes mellitus for a shorter period of time, and 70% of them had hematuria (compared to 28% of those with diabetic glomerulosclerosis). Retinopathy was detected in 82% of patients with diabetic glomerulosclerosis and in only 41% of those with superimposed glomerular disease. Similar observations were made by Parving et al. (75), Suzuki et al. (76), and Schwartz et al. (76a), who noted that 23%, 16%, and 9%, respectively, of their type II diabetic patients had a glomerulopathy other than diabetic glomerulosclerosis.

The glomerular diseases commonly found in 83 diabetics reported in the literature were mesangial proliferative (45%), membranous nephropathy (23%), acute endoproliferative glomerulonephritis (14%), and lipoid nephrosis (5%) (73–83). In some of these patients, several factors raised the suspicion of a diagnosis other than diabetic nephropathy, including rapid onset of proteinuria and microscopic hematuria in a patient without retinopathy (confirmed by fluorescein angiography), normal blood pressure, rapid deterioration of kidney function in an otherwise stable patient, gross hematuria, and difficulty in controlling the blood pressure in a patient previously controlled, or the absence of neuropathy (84). In others, however, no significant clinical difference could be detected between the patients with a primary glomerulopathy and those with diabetic nephropathy (76). The presence of diabetes mellitus does not seem to alter the natural history of the glomerulopathy, so the management should be the same as for nondiabetics (Chapter 6). It should be noted, however, that the relatively high prevalence of nondiabetic glomerular disease in patients with diabetes mellitus has not been found by others (76b).

Immune complex glomerular disease superimposed on preexisting diabetic glomerulosclerosis has also been reported (85,86), occurring in one-third of biopsied elderly patients with diabetes mellitus in one study (87). No significant difference was noted in age, mean duration of diabetes, kidney function, protein excretion, or mean arterial pressure between those with diabetic nephropathy alone and those with diabetic nephropathy and an immune complex glomerular disease. As expected, immunofluorescence and electron microscopic examination were essential for a final diagnosis. Acute endocapillary glomerulonephritis was the most common disease found. There is no information concerning the long-term renal outcome in such patients, but our inclination is not to treat the superimposed glomerular disease specifically.

As discussed in Chapter 13, ischemic nephropathy is more prevalent among diabetics. The approach to these patients should be individualized, keeping in mind that the mortality rate after surgical repair is higher in diabetics and that age per se, the preexisting history of heart disease, and renal insufficiency are independent predictors to time to death or to dialysis (88). The only time we pursue the diagnosis of ischemic nephropathy in an elderly diabetic is when there is severe hypertension, not controlled with multiple-drug therapy, and evidence of vascular disease elsewhere (Chapter 13).

II. KIDNEY DISEASES ASSOCIATED WITH DYSPROTEINEMIA AND PARAPROTEINEMIA

As seen in Table 1, which represents the combined experience of eight studies (89–91; Refs. 3–6 and 9 in Chapter 6) and our own and includes only patients in whom biopsies were performed, after diabetes, dysglobulinemias account for the majority of renal diseases due to a systemic disease in the elderly. This group includes amyloidosis, multiple myeloma associated with cast nephropathy or light chain nephropathy, essential mixed cryoglobulinemia, macroglobulinemia, and fibrillary glomerulonephritis.

A. Amyloidosis

Amyloidosis encompasses a group of diseases characterized by the extracellular deposition of a proteinaceous material in a variety of tissues, with the classification based on the biochemical composition of the protein subunit deposited (92,93) (Table 2), which accounts for 85% of the deposited amyloid. The remaining 15% of the deposited material consists of other proteins and glycoproteins common to all types of amyloidosis. Since renal amyloidosis in the elderly is almost entirely limited to AL and AA protein, this discussion will involve these two entities only.

1. Incidence

Primary amyloidosis (AL, amyloid light chain protein) is relatively common in the elderly and should be considered in the differential diagnosis of any elderly

Table 1 Incidence of Renal Involvement in Systemic Disease in the Elderly[a]

Disease	Number of patients (%)
Dysproteinemia and paraproteinemia	239 (59)
Amyloidosis	
Multiple myeloma	
Cast nephropathy	
Light chain nephropathy	
Glomerular disease with fibrillary deposits	
Cryoglobulinemia	
Waldenstrom's macroglobulinemia	
Vasculitis	99 (24)
Periarteritis nodosa	
Wegener's granulomatosis	
Microscopic polyarteritis	
Giant cell arteritis	
Henoch-Schonlein purpura	
Collagen vascular diseases	39 (10)
Systemic lupus erythematosus	
Scleroderma	
Others	28 (7)
Hemolytic uremic syndrome	
Thrombotic thrombocytopenic purpura	
Rheumatoid arthritis	
Sjögren's syndrome	
Infections and glomerular diseases	
Sarcoidosis	

[a]Diabetes mellitus not included; includes only biopsy-proven cases.

patient presenting with the nephrotic syndrome. In a large series of patients with amyloidosis reported by Kyle and Gertz (94), 66% were over the age of 60. The elderly made up 60–63% of the patients with renal involvement (95).

The reported incidence of secondary amyloidosis (AA, amyloid A protein) in the elderly has been quite variable. In 32 patients reported by Triger and Joekes (96), three (10%) were over 60 years, whereas in the series reported by Browning et al. (97), 36 of 75 patients (48%) were over 60 years of age. The most common diseases associated with AA amyloidosis in the elderly are rheumatoid arthritis, bronchiectasis, chronic osteomyelitis, tuberculosis, Hodgkin's disease, carcinoma of the kidney, and inflammatory bowel diseases.

2. *Pathology*

The diagnosis of renal amyloidosis depends on the demonstration of amyloid deposits, using appropriate staining procedures, such as Congo red, crystal violet

Table 2 Classification of Amyloidosis

Type of amyloidosis	Associated diseases	Designation
Primary (light chain kappa, lambda)	Myeloma, macroglobulinemia, related plasma cell neoplasms	AL
Secondary (amyloid A protein)	Chronic infections, inflammatory diseases, malignancies	AA
Familial (prealbumin)	Many familial types	AF
Senile cardiac (prealbumin)	—	SSA
Dialysis amyloid (beta-$_2$ microglobulin)	—	Aβ_2M
Localized (calcitonin)	Medullary carcinoma of thyroid	AE
Cerebral (alpha-4 or beta)	Senile dementia, Down's syndrome	CAA

Source: Adapted from Franklin EC. Immunopathology of the amyloid diseases. Hosp Pract 1980; 15:70–77, and Gertz MA, Kyle RA. Primary systemic amyloidosis-A diagnostic primer. Mayo Clin Proc 1989; 64:1505–1519.

or thioflavin T. With light microscopy, deposits of amyloid are found in the mesangium and in the capillary walls. In the former, nodules of various sizes or diffuse infiltrates are seen which expand the intercapillary space and compress the lumina. In the latter, the deposits are present in the basement membrane and appear in a pattern of perpendicular projections on the epithelial side, referred to as spicules. These spicules are of prognostic significance, since they are associated morphologically with accelerated amyloid deposition and clinically with a fulminant clinical course (98). The severity of the proteinuria has also been found to correlate with the presence of spicules (98). Under electron microscopy, the deposits take the form of fine, nonbranching fibrils arranged in bundles. With immunofluorescence microscopy, kappa or lambda light chain deposits are found in AL amyloidosis, whereas A protein deposits are present in AA amyloidosis.

3. Pathogenesis

In AL amyloidosis, a clone of plasma cells secrete an excessive amount of light chains, some of which are incompletely digested by phagocytes while others escape degradation. The amyloid fibrils result from incorporation of light chain fragments alone or with whole light chains that have bypassed degradation. Fibrils, singly and in aggregates, may then deposit in the kidneys (92).

The A protein in AA amyloidosis results from cleavage by monocytes of serum AA (SAA), a substance secreted by hepatocytes. The A protein in turn aggregates into fibrils and is deposited between renal cells. The concentration of AA protein in the serum has been found to be markedly increased in some patients with rheumatoid arthritis and Crohn's disease. The level appears to correspond to the incidence of systemic amyloidosis in these patients (99). Besides the increased serum level of AA protein, decreased activity of a serum factor capable of degrading AA fibrils has also been described (100). It thus appears that both primary and secondary amyloidosis occur in situations in which the immune system becomes overwhelmed by an antigenic load or has undergone neoplastic transformation. The specific immunological defect remains to be unraveled.

4. *Clinical Manifestations*

Since amyloid proteins can deposit in several organs, the initial manifestations associated with the syndrome are quite variable (101). Proteinuria is the most common renal manifestation associated with both AL and AA amyloidosis. In AL amyloidosis, proteinuria was found in 29–86% of reported cases (89–91,94,95,97). Nephrotic syndrome was present in 35% of these patients. Sixty-six percent of patients without myeloma-associated AL have monoclonal light chains in their urine, whereas the incidence is 93% for those with myeloma. The proteinuria is usually nonselective. The urine sediment is usually benign, although macroscopic or microscopic hematuria has occasionally been described (94,95). Renal insufficiency (serum creatinine > 2 mg/dl) was found in 25–43% of patients at initial diagnosis. Hypertension was found in 42% of patients, whereas orthostatic hypotension was present in 10–20%. As might be expected, 11% of patients with myeloma had associated hypercalcemia (Ca > 11 mg/dl), compared to only 2% in those without myeloma. The kidney size varies considerably among patients at the time of diagnosis.

In AA amyloidosis, proteinuria occurred in 57% of the patients, half of whom had the nephrotic syndrome (96,97).

5. *Natural History and Treatment*

Renal disease due to amyloidosis is usually progressive, with virtually all patients reaching end stage or dying from other complications within a relatively short period of time (1–3 years). The prognosis appears to be better in those with AA amyloidosis, where survival up to 11 years has been reported (97). We have observed a precipitous and irreversible decrease in renal function in some of our patients with AL amyloidosis without a morphological or hemodynamic explanation, which has been reported by others (98). Specifically, renal vein thrombosis was ruled out in our patients.

Several forms of therapy have been tried in patients with amyloidosis, with little success, in general. There are a few case reports describing disappearance of the amyloid deposits (in patients with the AA form) after treatment of the chronic infection or removal of a renal cell carcinoma (102–105). Based on these reports, every attempt should be made either to treat or to correct the underlying condition judged responsible for the amyloidosis. D-Penicillamine, alone or in combination with chlorambucil, has been tried in patients with rheumatoid arthritis and AA amyloidosis with varied success (106,107). Colchicine has been shown to prevent amyloidosis in high-risk patients with familial Mediterranean fever and also prevent deterioration of renal function in those with amyloidosis and proteinuria, but not the nephrotic syndrome (108). Whether this drug will benefit other patients with AA amyloidosis is worth investigating.

In a recent prospective randomized study, the combination of prednisone and melphalan with or without colchicine was found to be superior to colchicine alone in prolonging survival in patients with AL amyloidosis (109). Proteinuria decreased more than 50% in 12 of 68 patients with nephrotic syndrome managed with this regimen and in 2 of the 35 patients managed with colchicine alone ($p = 0.23$). Forty-three percent of the patients given colchicine alone and 38% of the patients treated with melphalan-prednisone with or without colchicine developed end-stage renal failure. No difference was noted between treatment groups from the time of randomization to the time of dialysis initiation. Five percent of the treated patients developed acute nonlymphocytic leukemia or myelodysplasia. The dose of melphalan was 0.15 mg/kg given in two divided doses and prednisone 0.8 mg/kg given in four divided doses daily. The treatment schedule in the study was 7 days of treatment repeated every 6 weeks and continued for a minimum of 1 year. Colchicine was used at the dose of 0.6 mg twice daily. The 5-year survival rate was 78% for those patients who responded to this regimen, compared to a 5-year survival rate of 7% for those who did not respond (110).

It should be noted that in patients who do not tolerate this regimen, colchicine alone is still associated with a better outcome than no therapy at all, even in patients with AL protein (111). Dimethyl sulfoxide (DMSO), an agent which theoretically can accelerate the destruction of the amyloid fibril, has also been tried with some success (112,113).

Besides the amyloid fibrils, which consist of nonglycosylated polypeptide chains, amyloid deposits may also contain a nonfibrillar glycoprotein called amyloid P component (AP). It has been postulated that AP forms a protective coating over the amyloid fibrils; if so, methyl 4,6-O-(1-carboxyethylident)-B-D-galactopyranoside (MOBDG), a substance capable of dissociating AP from amyloid fibrils, might open a new therapeutic avenue in patients with amyloidosis (114).

Patients with orthostatic hypotension (commonly seen with amyloidosis) may be treated with midodrine, an alpha-agonist, 5–10 mg every 8 hr (110,110a).

B. Multiple Myeloma

The renal lesions associated with multiple myeloma can be divided into two broad categories, as discussed by Hill et al. (115): (a) cast nephropathy (also called myeloma kidney), and (b) tissue deposition of paraproteins, either amyloid (discussed above) or light chains (rarely, heavy chains). The latter condition is also referred to as light chain nephropathy. Cast and light chain nephropathy tend to be mutually exclusive, since few or no myeloma casts are seen in patients with diffuse tissue deposition of light chains and, in patients with cast nephropathy, mesangial, interstitial, or vascular deposits of amyloid or light chains are seen only occasionally. The reason a given patient develops one form or the other is not clear. The nature and characteristics of the monoclonal protein (or M component) produced undoubtedly plays an important role, however (116).

1. Cast Nephropathy (Myeloma Kidney)

a. Incidence. The elderly account for 62% of reported cases of multiple myeloma (117). The incidence of renal failure in patients of all age groups with multiple myeloma is 40–50%. The incidence in the elderly is 58%, suggesting that age per se is only a minor risk factor for developing renal insufficiency (117). The elderly male:female ratio is 3:2. Cast nephropathy is responsible for 63–78% of the cases of renal involvement associated with myeloma in the elderly (89–91).

b. Pathology. The pathological hallmark of the myeloma kidney is the presence of intratubular protein casts seen with light microscopy. These casts have a granular appearance, with a characteristic "fracture line." Multinucleated giant cells can be seen engulfing the casts. Marked tubular atrophy and degeneration are found in advanced cases with renal insufficiency and are associated with a poor outcome (118). In general, the amount of interstitial fibrosis present parallels the amount of tubular atrophy. Flecks of calcium in tubular cast or the interstitium have occasionally been reported (119). With immunofluorescent studies, the casts may contain all classes of immunoglobulins, and kappa and lambda light chains. Albumin, Tamm-Horsfall protein, and complement components are also found occasionally. With electron microscopy, the casts are composed of homogeneous, finely granular material. Tears in the tubular basement membrane and intracytoplasmic inclusions may be seen. Rarely, finely granular, electron-dense amorphous deposits may be seen in the mesangium, subendothelial, or intramembranous (120).

c. Pathogenesis. A strong association exists between the presence of light chain proteinuria and the development of renal insufficiency in the myeloma patient (121). Light chains, because of their molecular weight, are easily filtered and reabsorbed by the tubular cells through a saturable process (122). In multiple myeloma, the amount of light chains produced frequently exceeds the reabsorptive capacity of the tubular cells. As a consequence, these unreabsorbed free proteins may precipitate in the lumen, particularly in the presence of volume contraction, ischemia produced by hypercalcemia, sepsis, or exposure to iodinated contrast agents. Also, light chains may be directly toxic to tubule cells, as evidenced by the presence of varying degrees of proximal tubule damage, such as cell desquamation, vacuolation, and coagulation necrosis (123). In studies by DeFronzo et al. (124), creatinine clearance and PAH clearance (effective renal plasma flow) were statistically lower in myeloma patients with Bence Jones proteinuria compared to those without. Urinary pH, after ammonium chloride loading, was higher, and urinary osmolality, after overnight fast and ADH administration, was lower in the patients with Bence Jones proteinuria. It should be emphasized that the typical myeloma cast is not a universal finding in the myeloma patient with renal insufficiency; thus, factors other than the presence of light chains are involved in the pathogenesis of the renal disease. Patients with abundant light chain proteinuria have been followed for years without any renal functional abnormality (125), and, in patients with renal insufficiency, GFR can improve despite the persistence of light chain proteinuria (126).

Besides the intrinsic structure of monoclonal proteins, their glycosylation pattern (126a) or their isoelectric point (pi) may also be a determinant of pathogenicity. A negative correlation between the pi and creatinine clearance has been found in patients studied by Coward et al. (127). Acute reversible renal failure has been associated with light chains of low pi and the chronic irreversible renal failure with light chains of high pi (128); however, this has not been a consistent finding (118,129). Further studies are obviously needed to clarify the exact role of pi in the pathogenesis of cast nephropathy.

d. Clinical Manifestations. In the majority of patients with renal involvement (90–93%), the process is insidious and usually progresses over a period of several months to years. In the remaining 7–10%, the disease presents abruptly with acute renal failure. In as many as 40–50% of these patients, the diagnosis of both myeloma and acute renal failure are made simultaneously, making it mandatory that multiple myeloma be considered in the elderly with unexplained acute renal failure (130,131). In some of these patients, nonsteroidal antiinflammatory drugs, dehydration, sepsis, hypercalcemia, or contrast agents have been the precipitating factor (118,132). Fifty percent of patients with acute renal failure are oliguric. Bence Jones proteinuria, 850 to 2000 mg/24 hr, is found in patients with either the chronic or the acute form of the disease. The presence of a low anion gap in a patient with renal failure and proteinuria should raise the suspicion of multiple myeloma (133,134). The low gap is due to the presence of cationic paraproteins.

Fanconi syndrome (glycosuria, aminoaciduria, phosphaturia, renal tubular acidosis) and hyporeninemic hypoaldosteronism have been reported in association with multiple myeloma. Their incidence in the elderly is not known (135).

The presence of a monoclonal protein (M protein) in the serum of an elderly subject in association with renal insufficiency does not necessarily confirm the diagnosis of cast nephropathy, as other entities, such as plasmacytoma, macroglobulinemia, lymphoma, chronic lymphocytic leukemia, and AL amyloidosis can also present in this manner. It should be noted that 3% of subjects over the age of 70 years (Blacks more than Whites) have a monoclonal gammopathy of undetermined significance (136). This entity is characterized by a relatively low serum M-protein concentration, fewer than 10% plasma cells in the bone marrow, and the absence of hypercalcemia and/or lytic bone lesions. The M-protein level tends to remain stable (<3 g/dl) over time. In these patients, a different etiology for the renal disease should be suspected. No therapy is necessary for the patient with monoclonal gammopathy of undetermined significance.

e. Natural History and Treatment. An attempt should be made to uncover the presence of a precipitating factor leading to acute renal failure in patients with myeloma. Aggressive treatment of hypercalcemia has been found to reverse the renal failure in 67% of the patients reported by Bernstein and Humes (137). Volume should be replaced in the dehydrated patient and sepsis treated with the appropriate antibiotics. Alkalinization of the urine, without any attempt at characterizing the pi of the light chain, has been found to have a marginal benefit (126).

The primary therapy for the renal disease is that recommended for the multiple myeloma, and these patients should be followed in concert with an oncologist. A discussion of the currently used cytotoxic agents is beyond the scope of this chapter, and the reader is referred to a recent review (138). The addition of plasma exchange to cytotoxic agents has been found to be more effective than chemotherapy alone in reversing renal failure in patients with rapidly deteriorating kidney function (139). Five recent reports have added additional evidence for the possible benefits of plasma exchange added to chemotherapy (140–144). In the Italian Collaborative Study, patients who received plasma exchange in addition to chemotherapy recovered renal function more frequently (61%) than those treated with chemotherapy alone (27%) (140). Thirty-seven of the 50 reported patients were 60 years or older. Twenty-five received chemotherapy and plasma exchange (group I), whereas 12 received chemotherapy alone (group II). The average time of follow-up was 11.0 ± 3.9 months for group II and 13.0 ± 2.7 months for group I. Forty-two percent of the patients in group II and 32% in group I were alive at the end of the follow-up period. Despite the beneficial effect on recovery of kidney function, it appears that plasma exchange did not prolong survival of myeloma patients. Zucchelli et al. (141), however, noted a 1-year survival rate of 66% in patients treated with plasmapheresis, compared to 28% of untreated patients. Further studies are needed before this approach can be routinely recommended. We suggest that a kidney biopsy be performed before considering plasma exchange, since the presence of large numbers of tubular casts and chronic tubulointerstitial changes is associated with a rather poor response (140).

The use of plasmapheresis in patients with cast nephropathy has not been standardized. We use the approach outlined by Zucchelli et al. (141). Initially, therapy consists of intravenous pulse steroids (the equivalent of 20/mg/kg/day of methylprednisolone) given on 3 consecutive days, followed by oral prednisone (20–30 mg/m^2/day) for 7 days. Cyclophosphamide (200 mg/m^2/day) is simultaneously administered parenterally for 5 days. Daily plasma exchange (3–4 L) is performed for 5 consecutive days. Maintenance therapy consists of prednisone (60 mg/m^2/day) and cyclophosphamide (100 mg/m^2/day) orally for 4 days at 4- to 6-week intervals. In general, patients who will respond do so within the first month after therapy is initiated. We usually discontinue therapy in patients who do not respond after a 6-month trial. Sixty-two percent of the patients who improved did so within 1 month of treatment, and only 15% of the patients who did not improve within 1 month eventually did (145).

Dialysis should not be withheld from the patient with multiple myeloma and associated end-stage renal failure (144,145a,146). The 1-year survival rate for this group is similar to that of the general myeloma population (147). Cytotoxic therapy for the myeloma should be continued or initiated in these patients, since patients occasionally may recover enough kidney function to survive without dialysis (148,149). The response of the tumor to chemotherapy is independent of recovery of renal function and clearly remains the critical feature in all patients.

2. *Light Chain Nephropathy*

a. Incidence. The true incidence of light chain nephropathy is not known. Of a total of 46 patients, including those reported in the literature where age is given, and our personal experience, 16 (35%) were over the age of 60. In the elderly, the ratio of males to females was 3:2 (150–160). Sixty to seventy percent of patients with light chain nephropathy have multiple myeloma. The remaining 30–40% either have other myelomatosis monoclonal gammopathies or do not have any associated condition (161). Twenty-two to twenty-seven percent of patients with renal involvement due to myeloma have light chain nephropathy (145).

b. Pathology. The pathology of light chain nephropathy, like that of amyloidosis, is mainly glomerular, rather than tubulointerstitial as in cast nephropathy. With light microscopy, the most common finding is the nodular accumulation in the mesangium of PAS-positive material, which may be indistinguishable from the intercapillary nodule of diabetic glomerulosclerosis (153,155). The tubular basement membranes have a thickened refractile appearance and are outlined on their external aspect by ribbonlike continuous deposits, mainly along the distal tubules and loops of Henle. Occasional tubular casts are found. With immunofluorescence microscopy, either kappa or lambda light chains are found in a linear pattern along glomerular and tubular basement membranes or as granular to nodular deposits in the mesangium. In some patients, immunofluorescence microscopy is entirely negative. With electron microscopy, continuous granular deposits may be found in the subendothelial space and the lamina rara interna of the GBM. In others, the electron-dense material tends to accumulate in the area between the lamina densa and the lamina rara interna. Mesangial and paramesangial nodules of granular electron-dense material continuous with those in the subendothelial space may also be noted. Aneurysmal dilatation of the capillaries secondary to loss of endothelial cell lining and disruption of mesangial anchoring points of the basement membrane is frequently found (162).

c. Pathogenesis. The deposits in light chain nephropathy, as in amyloidosis, are extracellular and present in multiple organs. The precise mechanism of tissue precipitation is not known. In 5 of 6 patients studied by Ganeval et al. (160), abnormal immunoglobulin chains were produced. The authors postulated that these structural immunoglobulin abnormalities could possibly trigger their visceral deposition.

d. Clinical Manifestations. Clinical features of chronic renal disease are the initial manifestations in the majority of the patients (150–161). In others the disease is found during the course of established multiple myeloma. Renal insufficiency of varying severity and a nonselective proteinuria are found in all patients. Nephrotic syndrome is present in 20–30% of patients, and hypertension in 63%. The extrarenal manifestations of the disease may be present during the initial investigation of the renal disease or can appear later; these include involvement of the liver and heart, with hepatic or cardiac failure a consequence.

e. Natural History and Treatment. Renal disease associated with light chain nephropathy is usually rapidly progressive; therefore, chemotherapy with prednisone and melphalan is recommended for all patients and should be initiated early. In general, patients who started therapy with a serum creatinine less than 4 mg/dl do better, with either improvement or stabilization in their kidney function (163,164). The dosage, regimen, and length of therapy are the same as those for patients with amyloidosis.

C. Glomerular Diseases with Fibrillary Deposits

This group of glomerular disease is characterized by fibrillary deposits in various parts of the glomerulus. These fibrils are distinct from amyloid in that they are not only larger but they do not stain with congo red or thioflavin T and are divided into microfibrillar collagen, fibrillary, and immunotactoid fibrils.

Microfibrillar collagen glomerulopathies have a familial tendency and become manifest earlier in life than the others with proteinuria, sometimes in the nephrotic range. Kidney function is generally well maintained. In the collagen type III form, the deposits have a 60-nm periodicity and are seen in the subendothelial region and mesangium. In the fibronectin form, fibrillary and amorphous deposits are present in the subendothelial and mesangial areas (165).

Both fibrillary and immunotactoid glomerulonephritis have been reported in the elderly. The fibrillary form is five times more common than the immunotactoid form in the adult population; the latter, however, is more common in the elderly. Both entities share common renal manifestations, with proteinuria (usually in the nephrotic range) a universal finding. Renal insufficiency is present in 80% of the elderly, hematuria in 70%, and hypertension in 80%. In fibrillary glomerulonephritis, the disease is limited to the kidneys, whereas a large percentage of patients with immunotactoid glomerulonephritis have an associated lympho-proliferative disorder. The ultrastructural patterns for either entity are shown in Table 3.

Both diseases tend to progress, with the fibrillary form having a more aggressive course. There is no specific therapy available for either form of the disease (166–169).

D. Cryoglobulinemia

Cryoglobulinemias can occur in association with a variety of disorders (170,171). The presence of the cryoglobulins per se does not significantly alter the clinical course of the underlying disease, and renal involvement is rare. By contrast, in patients with so-called mixed essential cryoglobulinemia, a syndrome characterized by the presence of arthralgia, purpura, liver involvement, and Raynaud's phenomenon, renal disease often dominates the clinical picture and plays a major role in the prognosis (172). It should be emphasized that cryo-immunoglobulins are commonly found in low concentrations (less than 20 mg/dl) in patients with various forms of primary glomerular diseases and appear to have neither diagnostic nor prognostic significance (173).

Table 3 Morphological Features of Fibrillary and Immunotactoid Glomerulonephritis

	Fibrillary glomerulonephritis	Immunotactoid glomerulonephritis
Light microscopy	Diffuse or focal segmental proliferative Lobular Crescents may be present	Diffuse or focal segmental proliferative Membranous Crescents usually absent
Immunofluorescence microscopy	Mainly IgG and C_3, in mesangium and occasionally in glomerular basement membrane (granular)	IgG and C_3, granular along the glomerular basement membrane
Electron microscopy	Fibrils randomly oriented in mesangium, endothelium, epithelium, and/or vascular walls; average diameter 20 nm	Large microtubules arrayed in parallel in mesangium and glomerular capillary wall; diameter >30 nm

Antibodies to hepatitis C or viral RNA are detected in over 80% of patients and may be of etiological significance (174,175). Hepatitis B virus is present in a very small number of patients.

1. *Incidence*

In 231 patients with essential mixed cryoglobulinemia reported in the literature, 52 (23%) were 60 years and older (176–184). The overall incidence of kidney involvement varied between 50% and 60%, and 20% of patients were 60 years and older, suggesting that age per se is not a risk factor for developing renal disease in essential mixed cryoglobulinemia. The female:male ratio was 3:1.

2. *Pathology*

The light microscopic appearance is that of mesangiocapillary glomerulonephritis. The glomeruli have a lobular appearance, with increased mesangial matrix and cellularity. Endothelial cell swelling and focal areas of necrosis with extensive "splitting" of the GBM are usually seen. In 18% of patients, an acute necrotizing vasculitis, involving medium-sized arteries and small arterioles with polymorphonuclear white blood cell infiltration, is found. A pattern of diffuse or focal mesangial proliferative glomerulonephritis can be seen. Crescents may be present in some glomeruli. With immunofluorescence microscopy, granular IgM, IgG, and C_3 deposits are found along the glomerular capillary wall and in the mesangium. Less common are IgA, C_{1q}, and C_4 deposits. With electron microscopy, the capillary lumen is obliterated by swollen endothelial cells, by cells with the characteristics of macrophages, and by intraluminal thrombi. Large crystalloid deposits are seen in the subendothelial areas (185).

3. *Pathogenesis*

Circulating immune complexes are frequently detected in the serum of patients with mixed cryoglobulinemia (186). In those infected with hepatitis C or B virus, these immune complexes probably represent an interaction between a viral antigen and a polyclonal IgG. The reaction of an IgM monoclonal rheumatoid factor with the Fc portion of the IgG results in the formation of the cryoimmunoglobulins. The deposition of these cryoglobulins in the glomeruli subsequently initiates glomerular inflammation and damage (183,187). Indeed, patients with more severe histological changes and greater renal functional impairment have been shown to display antiglobulin activity (181). Neither the mechanism involved in the glomerular deposition of these immune complexes nor the basis for the glomerular injury are well understood. A decrease has been found in the clearance of immune complexes by the mononuclear phagocytic system of patients with essential mixed cryoglobulinemia. In this situation, more of the complexes could theoretically reach the kidneys, thereby increasing their likelihood of being entrapped and causing injury (188). It is also possible that the mononuclear macrophages found on histological examination in these patients are responsible, in part, for the glomerular injury and proteinuria, as is postulated for other glomerulonephritides (189). Finally, the complement system probably plays a role in the pathogenesis of the renal disease.

4. *Clinical Manifestations*

The diagnosis of essential mixed cryoglobulinemia should be suspected in any elderly patient presenting with weakness, purpura, arthralgia, and renal disease. An analysis of 38 elderly patients with these symptoms revealed that proteinuria (present in 71%) and renal insufficiency (present in 68%) were the most common manifestations (176–184). Nephrotic syndrome was found in 24%. Microscopic hematuria is a universal finding, and red blood cell casts are frequently present. At the time of diagnosis, 80% of patients are hypertensive. Serum C_3 and/or C_4 is depressed in 84% of patients. Acute renal failure as the initial manifestation of kidney involvement has been reported (185).

5. *Natural History and Treatment*

The development of kidney disease in patients with essential mixed cryoglobulinemia is associated with a poor prognosis. Of 20 patients followed by Gorevic et al. (172) for an average of 5.6 years, 70% with renal failure died, versus 31% with normal kidney function. Generally, the prognosis is worse in the elderly compared to younger patients (190). The causes of death were extrarenal complications, such as systemic vasculitis and cardiovascular and cerebrovascular accidents, and lymphoproliferative diseases. Patients with mixed cryglobulinemias and hepatitis C should be treated with alpha-interferon (191). The recommended regimen consists of 4.5–6 million units subcutaneously thrice weekly for 6 months. If a response (as assessed by serum anti-hepatitis C virus antibody activity) is noted, then therapy is continued with 3 million units thrice weekly for another 6 months. The drug is then tapered over the next 6 months. Dosage adjustment can be made according to tolerance of the treatment. Follow-up evaluation of hepatitis C RNA in the serum is carried out twice yearly. In a recent study of relatively younger patients with mixed cryoglobulinemia and renal disease, interferon therapy was associated with a significant reduction in proteinuria, but no improvement in renal function (192). Relapse of proteinuria and renal disease was common following discontinuation of therapy.

Other therapeutic modalities have had some success (182,193–196). The major problem with these studies, however, is that none was controlled, and the number of patients involved has been rather small. Nevertheless, for the patient with rapid deterioration in kidney function or rapidly increasing proteinuria, we recommend a 3-day course of 1 g of intravenous "pulse" methylprednisolone (or its equivalent), followed by a maintenance dose of 0.4–0.6 mg/kg/day of prednisone together with 1–2 mg/kg/day of cyclophosphamide (or chlorambucil, 0.1 mg/kg/day). In addition, plasmapheresis is used simultaneously 10 to 15 times, depending on changes in cryocrit, serum creatinine, and proteinuria.

In patients with less progressive renal disease, the long-term course is quite variable, with spontaneous remissions, either partial or complete, occurring in as many as 33%. End-stage renal disease develops in 10% (190,197). Since the natural history of the renal disease in these patients is so unpredictable, therapy, as outlined above, should probably be reserved only for control of the extrarenal manifestations of the disease. The optimal length of therapy is not known. Some authors have stopped once a response occurs, while others have continued for a total of 12 months (181,193–196).

E. Waldenström's Macroglobulinemia

Waldenström's macroglobulinemia most likely represents a spectrum of malignant disorders identified as separate from other malignant diseases by the presence of an increase in the IgM protein in plasma (198). Even though diffuse interstitial infiltrate with lymphoid cells similar to those found in the bone marrow commonly has been seen in the kidney on autopsy, overt renal disease does not usually accompany the syndrome (199). The majority of reported patients with renal disease were 60 years and older. The most specific histological lesion found in Waldenstrom's macroglobulinemia is large eosinophilic hyaline thrombi within the capillary loops. On immunofluorescence, the thrombi stain strongly with IgM. The latter has a fibrillar structure when viewed by electron microscopy (200).

The renal disease can manifest itself either as acute or chronic renal failure, with moderate to severe renal insufficiency and/or proteinuria, hematuria, and hypertension. In 15 elderly patients with proteinuria and/or chronic renal disease, 5 had the characteristic large glomerular thrombi described above; no detectable glomerular lesion was found in 4, whereas 3 had amyloidosis and there was 1 case each of mesangiocapillary glomerulonephritis, intercapillary glomerulosclerosis (light chain nephropathy), and crescentic glomerulonephritis (200–202). It should be noted that crescentic glomerulonephritis can be seen as the initial manifestation of other plasma cell dyscrasias. Several such elderly patients have been reported (202,203). In 2 patients reported with acute renal failure, 1 had mesangiocapillary glomerulonephritis and the other the characteristic thrombi (204).

There is not enough information concerning the response of the kidneys to specific forms of therapy for the disease. Since the physical characteristics of the IgM protein are frequently responsible for a great majority of the patient's clinical manifestations (hyperviscosity syndrome), therapy should be directed at reducing the serum concentration of IgM by plasmapheresis. Drugs such as busulfan or cyclophosphamide can be added to plasmapheresis. Whereas this regimen might benefit the patient with the characteristic lesion, other forms of therapy (e.g, melphalan and prednisone for those with amyloidosis, pulse steroids for those with crescentic disease) may be needed as well. The presence of amyloidosis in patients with Waldenstrom's macroglobulinemia is associated with a poor prognosis (205a).

F. Glomerular Disease in the Elderly with Neoplasia

In the previous chapter we discussed the probable association between membranous nephropathy and extracapillary glomerulonephritis and solid tumors, as well as between minimal change disease (lipoid nephrosis) and lymphomas. Recently, an increasing number of patients with glomerular disease associated with chronic lymphocytic leukemia (CLL) has been reported (205). In most of these patients the CLL was diagnosed simultaneously with or prior to the kidney disease. Ten of the reported patients were over 60 years. Kidney biopsy revealed mesangiocapillary glomerulonephritis in five, membranous nephropathy in two, focal glomerulosclerosis in one, minimal change disease in one, and focal nephritis in one (206–213). The preponderance of mesangiocapillary glomerulonephritis has also been noted in younger patients with CLL (212). The reason for this association is not clear; however, because of the putative role of immune complexes in the generation of the idiopathic form of mesangiocapillary glomerulonephritis, immune complexes should be considered the prime pathogenetic candidate in patients with CLL-associated glomerulonephritis (212,213). Remission of the renal disease has been reported following chemotherapy-induced remission of the CLL (213).

An association has also been reported between positive ANCA renal involvement and solid tumors (213a). The renal histology in these cases has been one of vasculitis related glomerulopathy (see below).

III. VASCULITIS

The term *vasculitis* refers to a heterogeneous group of disorders that have in common inflammatory destruction of blood vessel walls occurring de novo (in contrast to the vasculitis which occurs as a secondary feature of diseases, for example, systemic lupus erythematosus and rheumatoid arthritis) (214). Several forms of classification have been proposed. A list of these vasculitides based on the size of the blood vessels involved is shown in Table 4. Even though sufficient clinical and laboratory information is usually available to classify a given patient into one disease group or the other (e.g., periarteritis nodosa versus Wegener's granulomatosis),

Table 4 Classification of Vasculitis According to Size of the Involved Artery

Large artery	Medium artery	Small artery
Giant cell	Periarteritis nodosa	Wegener's granulomatosis
Takayasu's disease	Churg-Strauss syndrome	Microscopic polyangitis
		Necrotizing glomerulonephritis (see Chapter 6)
		Hypersensitivity angiitis

overlap is common (215–218). Since the renal histological lesions associated with this group of disorders, known as systemic necrotizing arteritis, are rather strikingly homogeneous, we will discuss them as a group, emphasizing the specific points which might help in the differential diagnosis (214).

A. Incidence

The incidence of renal involvement in the elderly with systemic vasculitis is not known; however, in most series of patients with vasculitis and renal disease for which information concerning age group is given, 30–63% were elderly (219–221). It appears that the elderly with vasculitis are more prone to renal involvement.

B. Pathology

As noted by Serra et al. (219), it is difficult on histological examination of the renal tissue alone to categorize a given patient into a specific classification of vasculitis, since the histological changes in the kidney may be similar among the various vasculitic diseases.

Both vascular and glomerular structures can be involved, either alone or in combination. The vascular involvement is characterized by fibrinoid necrosis of the vessel wall, with polymorphonuclear, eosinophilic, and mononuclear cell infiltration. In Wegener's granulomatosis the infiltrating cells are mainly lymphocytes and monocytes (222), and one sees segmental necrotizing glomerulitis with crescent formation. In periarteritis, there is nonspecific ischemic shrinkage of the capillary tuft. When there are numerous crescents, pathological differentiation from idiopathic, rapidly progressive crescentic glomerulonephritis may be difficult. With immunofluorescent microscopy, various patterns of immunoglobulins, albumin, complement, and/or fibrinogen in the vessel wall have been reported. In cases of necrotizing glomerulitis, immunofluorescence studies are usually negative. The presence of IgA and C_3 should raise the suspicion of Henoch-Schonlein, and IgG, IgA, IgM, C_3, and C_4 suggests systemic lupus erythematosus (see appropriate section).

With electron microscopy, fibrin and poorly defined electron-dense deposits may be seen, and in patients with segmental necrotizing glomerulitis, degeneration, swelling and hypertrophy of endothelial and mesangial cells are common. Localized subepithelial or subendothelial deposits have also been described (219). It should be noted that bacterial endocarditis, rheumatoid vasculitis, and Goodpasture's syndrome may also show necrotizing glomerulitis on kidney biopsy (223,224).

C. Pathogenesis

The pathogenesis of the tissue inflammation and resulting damage to the vessel wall in the various forms of vasculitis is not known. Immune complexes probably play an important role, since these complexes have been found to be present in a large number of patients using different methods of measurement (225). Moreover, a close association between active disease and circulating immune complexes has been reported in patients with Wegener's granulomatosis and kidney disease (226). The nature of the antigenic challenge could be chemical (allopurinol, phenytoin, etc.), bacterial, viral, or tumor related, with the individual immune response of the host the ultimate determinant of the type and/or extent of the vasculitic process (227). The absence of detectable vascular electron-dense deposits (with the exception of patients with Henoch-Schönlein purpura) (228), however, raises important questions concerning this hypothesis. This discrepancy has been explained by two hypotheses: (a) rapid removal of these deposits by phagocytosis or other means, or (b) the binding of complement or activation of coagulation mechanisms by circulating immune complexes at the level of vascular lumen, causing endothelial injury without intramural deposits (229). This process includes chemotaxis and attraction of polymorphonuclear leukocytes, which release lysosomal enzymes with generation of H_2O_2. The latter is converted into hydroxyl radicals (230). The end point is vascular injury and necrosis. Platelets, monocytes, and basophils may also release vasoactive amines that increase the permeability of vessel wall, thereby contributing to the inflammatory response (231,232). Another pathogenic alternative is direct cytopathic effects on the arterial endothelium by certain infectious agents resulting in injury, independent of circulating immune complexes (233).

As noted in Chapter 6, the primary necrotizing vasculitides are frequently associated with auto-antibodies directed against lysosomal enzymes (proteinase-3 and myeloperoxidase) of neutrophils and monocytes (217,221,234). At the present time it is not clear whether those antibodies are directly responsible for the vascular lesions, or represent only a secondary phenomenom. Recent observations tend to suggest that these circulating antibodies may reflect the severity of the inflammatory process rather than being involved directly in the pathogenesis of the vasculitis (235).

Glomerulonephritis associated with antimyeloperoxidase (MPO) antibodies is more common in the elderly than antiproteinase-3 (PR3) antibodies.

D. Clinical Manifestations, Natural History, and Treatment

The diagnosis of vasculitis should be suspected in any elderly patient with a multisystem disease presenting with microscopic hematuria and proteinuria. Kidney function is normal in about half of these patients, with the remaining presenting with varying degrees of renal failure. Age has been found by some (236,237) but not by others (234,238) to be associated with a worse prognosis. In some patients, complete loss of kidney function can develop in a relatively short period of time.

E. Wegener's Granulomatosis

Renal involvement occurs in 70–85% of patients with Wegener's granulomatosis (239). In an analysis of 55 elderly patients, the lung was involved in 96%, the upper airway in 78%, both in 75%, which preceded clinical manifestations of renal disease by weeks or months. In some patients, rapidly progressive glomerulonephritis may antedate the extrarenal manifestations by months or even years (240). Hematuria was a universal finding, as well as red blood cell casts (found in 14 of 14 cases where mentioned). Proteinuria, 500–1800 mg/24 hr, was present in 65% of patients and nephrotic syndrome in an additional 6%. Renal insufficiency was initially present in 70% of the patients. In some of the patients the progression to end-stage kidney disease was rather rapid, with crescentic disease found on histological examination. ANCA (anti-PR_3 in over two-thirds) was positive in 95% of patients with Wegener's granulomatosis (217,241–254).

All the patients were treated with cyclophosphamide, with or without the addition of steroids. Plasmapheresis was attempted in some. Among the 28 patients with renal insufficiency, follow-up in 15 showed that 11 responded with improved kidney function, whereas the remaining 4 either died while still in renal failure or were started on dialysis. In general, patients who are treated prior to the onset of severe renal damage do better (255). The regimen we have adopted consists of cyclophosphamide, 2 mg/kg/day, and prednisone, 1 mg/kg, administered daily for 2–4 weeks, with gradual conversion to an alternate-day regimen over a 1- to 2-month period. Cyclophosphamide is usually continued for a full year and then decreased by 25 mg/day every 2–3 months.

Azathiophrine, 1.5–2.0 mg/kg/day, can be substituted during the maintenance phase in those elderly who do not tolerate cyclophosphamide (238). ANCA levels should be monitored, since the risk of relapse is high when the level increases or remains persistently elevated (256). In patients with fulminant and rapidly progressive disease, a higher dose of cyclophosphamide, 3–4 mg/kg (using the WBC count to guide dosage adjustment), together with oral or parenteral steroids, 2 mg/kg/day, is recommended (239). As noted earlier, plasmapheresis has also been used and should be limited to patients who present with renal insufficiency severe enough to require dialysis (257,258). Trimethoprim 160 mg/sulfamethoxazole 800 mg, 2 times a day, should not be used alone in treating the elderly with Wegener's associated glomerulonephritis. The drug, however, might reduce the incidence of relapse and is worth trying in patients who achieved a remission following conventional therapy (259,260). Therapy of Wegener's granulomatosis is relatively well tolerated in the elderly (221, 253,254), with 1-year survival of 63–79%, similar to younger patients (238, 261).

Acute renal failure due to obstructive uropathy has also been reported in patients with Wegener's granulomatosis (261a).

F. Periarteritis Nodosa

The elderly patient with periarteritis nodosa usually presents with fever, weight loss, fatigue, and involvement of the musculoskeletal and neurological (peripheral neuropathy) systems. The kidneys are involved in 60–70% of patients and always in association with other system involvement. Hematuria is present in 40–80% of patients, with red cell casts in 40%. Seventy-five to ninety percent of the patients have proteinuria; nephrotic syndrome, however, is rare. Renal insufficiency is present in approximately 50% of patients, and hypertension in 30–70%. ANCA (anti-MPO) is positive in only 30% of patients (217). Crescentic disease, angiitis, and ischemic glomerular lesions are usually found on histological examination (220,262). In one study, patients with periarteritis nodosa and renal involvement treated with steroids and cytotoxic agents had a better outcome than patients treated with steroids alone (263). Others have not found any difference in the outcome between patients treated with corticosteroids alone and those treated with a combination of corticosteroids and a cytotoxic agent (either azathioprine or cyclophosphamide) (264). The current recommendations is to use steroids and cyclophosphamide, as outlined above for patients with Wegener's granulomatosis (265). If azathioprine is used, the dose is 1.5–2 mg/kg/day. The efficacy of intermittent pulse therapy with methylprednisolone or plasma exchange cannot yet be assessed. There are virtually no data available to recommend how long therapy should be continued or its effect on the natural history of the kidney disease in the elderly. ANCA levels should be followed in those patients who are positive, to evaluate the response to therapy.

G. Giant Cell Arteritis

The incidence of renal involvement in patients with giant cell arteritis is not known. Klein et al. (266) found red cell casts in 10 of 86 patients (12%). Of 8 patients reported with renal disease, hematuria was present in 7 (4 had red cell casts) and proteinuria in 6 (2 had nephrotic syndrome) (246,265–271). Four had normal kidney function, and 4 had renal failure (3 chronic, 1 acute). Histology varied from interstitial mononuclear cell infiltration with increased cellularity in the glomerular tuft to necrotizing glomerulonephritis. One patient had membranous nephropathy, which might have been coincidental. Therapy with glucocorticoids is usually effective, even in patients with advanced renal failure.

Whether a kidney biopsy should be performed in all elderly patients with proven giant cell arteritis and kidney involvement is not clear. A legitimate approach might be to treat with steroids and monitor kidney function and/or the urinary sediment. If the patient fails to respond, a biopsy is necessary to rule out other renal diseases such as amyloidosis, which can occur with giant cell arteritis (272). Also ANCA should be determined in such patients, since the temporal artery may rarely be involved with Wegener's granulomatosis or periarteritis nodosa (273). The recommended treatment for giant cell arteritis is prednisone, 40–60 mg/day, since the alternate-day regimen is ineffective in controlling symptoms (274). When control of the disease has been achieved, as indicated by a decrease in the erythrocyte sedimentation rate (ESR), prednisone is tapered to a maintenance dose, generally 7.5–10 mg/day. Therapy should be continued for a period of 1–2 years (275).

H. Henoch-Schonlein Nephritis

Henoch-Schonlein nephritis is not rare in the elderly, who comprise 20–30% of the patients reported in the adult population (276). In a total of 37 elderly patients with renal involvement reported in the literature (246,277–282), including some seen by us, cutaneous vasculitis (purpura) was found in the lower extremities in 31, joint pains in 4, and abdominal complaints in 9. Seven were taking medication at the time of diagnosis; 2 antibiotics, 2 analgesics, 2 diuretics, 1 an antiarrhythmic drug. In some patients a malignancy or chronic ethanol abuse were considered potential triggering factors (282). All patients had hematuria (red cell casts in 5), with mild to moderate proteinuria in 13 (5 had nephrotic range proteinuria). Kidney function was abnormal at the time of diagnosis in 19 patients. Hypertension was present in 20. The disease was transient and self-limiting, with complete recovery in all the patients with normal kidney function. In general, the kidney biopsy revealed only focal proliferative glomerulonephritis with IgA and C_3 deposits. The patients with renal insufficiency had diffuse proliferative glomerulonephritis with crescents. Three of the 19 had partial recovery of kidney function; not enough follow-up information is available on the other 16. Cyclophosphamide and plasmapheresis have been used in patients in whom the disease persists or progresses (281); however, this treatment should be considered experimental at this time.

I. Other Vasculitides

Patients with microscopic polyangiitis usually present with arthralgia, purpura, and pulmonary hemorrhage (283). Renal involvement is common. Hematuria and renal insufficiency are seen universally. Proteinuria is present in 91% of the patients, with 41% in the nephrotic range. ANCA is positive in 75% of the patients (with anti-MPO present in 45%). Extracapillary glomerulonephritis (see Chapter 6) is considered a form of microscopic polyangiitis with minimal extrarenal manifestation.

Churg-Strauss syndrome should be considered in any elderly with asthma, eosinophilia, and renal disease (284). The presence of proteinuria and/or renal insufficiency is associated with a higher mortality rate (285). ANCA (anti-MPO) is positive in 70%. Renal histology in both types of vasculitis is that of a necrotizing glomerulonephritis with crescents.

Some patients have clinical and pathological features characteristic of two different vasculitides, such as periarteritis nodosa and allergic granulomatous angiitis or periarteritis nodosa and Wegener's granulomatosis, but do not fit precisely into either category. This situation has been labeled the "overlap syndrome." Therapy for all the vasculitides described above should consist of cyclophosphamide and steroids. Relapses, which occur in a significant percentage of patients, generally respond to retreatment (285a,285b).

Hypocomplementemic urticarial vasculitis is a syndrome manifested by urticarial vasculitis, arthralgia or arthritis, and lung disease (obstructive) (286). ANCA is usually negative, ANA can be positive, but anti-DNA is always negative. C_3 and/or C_4 may be decreased in some, and C1q is decreased in every patient (287). This syndrome is more common in younger patients, and the incidence in the elderly is not known. Renal involvement, manifested as mild proteinuria, occurs in 50% of the patients. Nephrotic syndrome may be seen. Renal histology is that of an immune complex disease with mesangial proliferative glomerulonephritis, deposits (IgG, IgM, C_3, C_4) by immunofluorescence and electron microscopy (intramembranous). Therapy, consisting of prednisone and azathioprine in the dose mentioned above, should be limited to those patients with heavy proteinuria and/or worsening of kidney function.

IV. SYSTEMIC LUPUS ERYTHEMATOSUS

A. Incidence

Systemic lupus erythematosus (SLE) is not uncommon in the elderly, with a reported incidence of 7–17% in large series of patients (288,289). Most authors agree that, in general, the disease tends to follow a more benign course in the elderly (290). Although some authors have found a significant positive correlation between age and the prevalence of nephritis (291), renal involvement is less common in the elderly compared with younger patients (12% versus 29%) (292). The diagnosis of lupus nephritis is made in 7–8% of all renal biopsies from subjects younger than 65 years, compared to 1–3% from subjects older than 65 years (Ref. 2–5, Chapter 6). In a 10 year period (1978–1987) we saw 80 patients with SLE with evidence of kidney disease (defined as the presence of RBC casts, proteinuria > 1 g/24 hr, serum creatinine > 1.5 mg/dl, or biopsy-proven disease), 10 (13%) of whom were 55 years or older (8 females and 2 males) with biopsy-proven lupus nephritis.

B. Pathology

The glomerulonephritis of lupus has been classified into six different types (WHO classification) (293):

Type I: Normal or minimal changes.

Type II: Pure mesangial alteration with mild to moderate mesangial widening and/or proliferation. With immunofluorescent microscopy, the deposits are usually limited to the mesangium.

Type III: Focal segmental glomerulonephritis with one or multiple segmental necrotizing lesions in a given glomerulus. Deposits are localized to the affected areas.

Type IV: Diffuse proliferative glomerulonephritis with at least 80% of the glomeruli involved with mesangial and endothelial cell proliferation. Areas of necrosis may be found as well as epithelial cell proliferation (crescents). Deposits are usually diffuse.

Type V: Membranous glomerulonephritis (see description of pathology in Chapter 4) is the most common histological form found in our elderly patients (60%). Mesangial cellularity with deposits or focal segmental or diffuse proliferative changes may be seen in addition. These latter changes should help differentiate membranous lupus from idiopathic membranous nephropathy.

Type VI: Mixed patterns—an interstitial nephritis, characterized by plasma cells, histiocytes, lymphocytes, and polymorphonuclear cells, may be seen with or without glomerular changes. Deposits are seen along the tubular basement membrane (294).

Acute necrotizing arteritis, consisting of focal areas of necrosis and infiltration of the vessel wall by inflammatory cells, may be seen in lupus and may affect the kidney.

C. Pathogenesis

The renal disease in SLE is the consequence of glomerular (or tubular basement membrane) deposits of immune complexes with subsequent inflammation and tissue damage. These complexes are composed mainly of DNA (either double or single stranded) and anti-DNA or, to a lesser extent, ribonucleoprotein and immunoglobulins (IgG, IgM) and their respective antibodies. The factors responsible for the deposition of these immune complexes in the glomerulus and for the various histological patterns are not completely understood. The two major proposals are that the complexes are derived from the circulation or formed in situ as a result of the combination of circulating antibodies with glomerular antigens (either structural components of the glomerulus or "planted" antigens). It is also possible that an immunological mechanism other than immune complex formation, such as delayed hypersensitivity, contributes to glomerular injury (295).

D. Clinical Manifestations

The nonrenal clinical features in the elderly with lupus nephritis are similar to those in younger patients (296,297). Females outnumber males by 4:1. Renal insufficiency is present in 75% of patients, hematuria in 80%, and proteinuria in 82%. Nephrotic syndrome is less common in the elderly than in younger patients (Refs. 2–5, Chapter 6). Complement (C_3, C_4) is decreased in 70% of patients. Antiphospholipid antibody is uncommon in the elderly. Hypertension is a universal finding. In our 10 patients, membranous histology (type V) was found in 6, diffuse proliferative (type IV) in 3, and vasculitis in 1. The decrease in GFR in this disease is probably secondary to a curtailment of the filtration surface area due to glomerular obliteration by either mesangial matrix expansion or glomerular cell swelling, proliferation, or infiltration (298). The proteinuria results from the presence of a subpopulation of large protein-permeable pores that are not present in normals (298). These changes may be reversed by immunosuppressive therapy.

As noted earlier, interstitial nephritis may be seen in patients with lupus glomerulonephritis, but may also occur in the absence of glomerular disease (299–301). This histological variation also seems to be immunologically mediated, since granular deposits may be found along the tubular basement membrane with immunofluorescence microscopy. In the patients reported, acute or chronic renal insufficiency was present. Proteinuria was usually < 1 g/24 hr, and the urinary sediment was generally benign (300). Tubular abnormalities, as evidenced by the increased excretion of β_2 microglobulin, are common in these patients (302), and hyperkalemia due to a defect in the distal nephron's ability to maximally secrete potassium or due to hyporenin-hypoaldosteronism has also been reported (303,304). The incidence and course of lupus interstitial nephritis in the elderly is not known.

E. Natural History and Treatment

Our approach to the treatment of lupus nephritis in the elderly is similar to that in younger patients, since in our experience the natural history of a given histological form is similar in all age groups. In patients with rapidly worsening kidney function, "pulse therapy," consisting of 1 g of methylprednisolone (or its equivalent) given intravenously over 30 min for 3 successive days, followed by maintenance oral therapy (60–80 mg/day of prednisone) is recommended (305). If kidney function in stable, we start the patient on oral prednisone, 60–80 mg/day. If the patient responds, we switch to alternate-day therapy after a period of 6–12 weeks and then gradually titer down the dose. If these is no response to steroids, cyclophosphamide, 2 mg/kg/day, or azathioprine, 1.5–2.0 mg/kg/day, is added. Monthly and/or quarterly intravenous cyclophosphamide, as outlined below, may be used as an alternative to oral therapy. In general, the patient is maintained on a dose of prednisone necessary for control of extrarenal manifestation of the lupus.

Some investigators believe that patients with diffuse proliferative glomerulonephritis should be treated with monthly infusions of cyclophosphamide (0.5–1.0 g/m^2) for the first 6 months, followed by quarterly infusion for 2 more years (306), with prednisone used to control the extrarenal manifestations of the disease. Plasma exchange added to immunosuppressive therapy does not have any role in the management of lupus nephritis (307,308).

Patients with lupus nephritis should be biopsied and treated early, as delay in the diagnosis and treatment affects the long-term prognosis (308a). The patient's response to therapy is usually a good indicator of long-term outcome (308b). Hypertension should be managed aggressively (308c). The presence of renal insufficiency at the time of diagnosis is considered a negative prognostic factor (308d).

Patients with interstitial nephritis should receive a course of steroids as outlined above. When present, hyperkalemia may also respond to steroids or can be treated as described in Chapter 3.

V. SCLERODERMA

A. Incidence

Scleroderma (progressive systemic sclerosis) is a syndrome characterized by excessive collagen deposition and vascular changes in multiple organ systems, with skin (Raynaud's phenomenon), gastrointestinal tract, lungs, heart, and kidneys most frequently involved. The incidence of renal involvement in scleroderma (15–58%) does not vary much among various age groups (309–312).

B. Pathology

Light microscopy of the kidney reveals mild to moderate nonspecific increase in the mesangial matrix. Areas of patchy interstitial fibrosis with associated tubular atrophy can be seen. As is the case of malignant hypertension, the major changes involve the vessel wall, with intimal fibrosis in the arcuate and interlobular arteries. Fibrinoid degeneration or thrombi are seen in arterioles. Fibrinoid necrosis of afferent arterioles and capillary loops have been reported. Immunofluorescence microscopy may show immune deposits of C_3 and immunoglobulins (usually IgM) in the intima of arcuate and intralobular arteries. With electron microscopy, the most common finding is wrinkling of the glomerular basement membrane. Electron-dense deposits are not usually found.

C. Pathogenesis

The mechanisms underlying the vascular changes seen in the kidneys (and elsewhere) in scleroderma are not known. Studies by Kahaleh and colleagues (313) have provided evidence for the presence of a serum factor that is specifically toxic to endothelial cells. The response to this substance is either periadventitial fibrosis with subsequent obliteration of capillaries and lymphatics or endothelial cell migration into the media. Once there, these cells proliferate and produce excessive amounts of connective tissue components. The source of this serum factor is not clear but seems to result from activation of both T and B cells, by an immunological, infectious, endocrine, or other insult in a susceptible host (314).

Whatever the pathogenesis, the end point is repeated vascular insults with a proliferative vascular response, luminal narrowing, reduced blood flow, and local ischemia.

D. Clinical Manifestations

Involvement of the kidneys in scleroderma can take the form of chronic renal insufficiency or scleroderma renal crisis. The incidence of either and possible interrelationships in the elderly are not known.

In general, older age is associated with reduced survival (315). In elderly patients with scleroderma and chronic renal insufficiency, the serum creatinine varied from 1.7 to 11.0 mg/dl at the time of diagnosis (316–318). Proteinuria, usually less than 2 g/24 hr, was present in over 80% of patients. Hypertension of varying severity was present in all the patients with renal insufficiency and in 20% of those with normal kidney function. The relationship between the histological findings in the kidney and the presence of renal insufficiency and/or hypertension are not clear, since these changes can be present in patients with normal kidney function and normotension (319). Furthermore, improvement in kidney function may take place despite persistence of the same histological findings (318).

Scleroderma renal crisis is characterized by a sudden rise in blood pressure, hypertensive retinopathy, and rapid deterioration of renal function. This complication occurs in 8–10% of patients with scleroderma and, in general, tends to occur relatively early in the course of the disease and is more common in older patients (320–321). The rise in blood pressure can be modest. The cause of this complication is not clear. It seems to occur more commonly during the winter months and is associated with a marked elevation of plasma renin activity, suggesting the following scenario. Most patients with scleroderma have compromised renal cortical blood flow, as demonstrated by Cannon et al. (309). Given an appropriate stimulus (e.g., cold weather) the renal vasculature undergoes further vasoconstriction (equivalent of a Raynaud's phenomenon), the juxtaglomerular apparatus is stimulated, causing an excessive release of renin and leading to further vasoconstriction, worsening kidney function, and uncontrolled hypertension.

It has not been possible on clinical or laboratory grounds to predict which patients will develop this complication. Several markers have been found; however, their application to the individual patient is not clear. Nevertheless, it is important to note that an unexplained increase in PRA in an otherwise stable patient (322), a greater than 2.0 ng/ml/hr rise in PRA in response to the cold pressor test (319), or rapidly progressive skin thickening (275) associated with the development of anemia, pericardial effusion, or congestive heart failure (323,324) all point to the possible supervening of scleroderma renal crisis. The use of corticosteroid is also associated with an increase risk of developing scleroderma renal crisis (321).

E. Natural History and Treatment

In a study of 358 hospitalized male veterans with scleroderma, the 17 patients with renal insufficiency died within 10 months (325).

Up to a decade ago, scleroderma renal crisis was invariably fatal, with the hypertension usually refractory to therapy and the majority of patients succumbing in 2–3 months after onset of the crisis. In some instances it was necessary to do bilateral nephrectomy to bring the blood pressure down. Over the last decade, several reports have appeared showing a beneficial effect of the ACE inhibitor captopril on the natural history of both the chronic renal insufficiency and acute renal crisis in patients with scleroderma (317,318,320,326). Since recovery of renal function with ACE inhibitor may take place in the latter group even after months of dialysis, nephrectomy should not be performed in these patients (327). ACE inhibitors should be considered the drugs of choice in the therapy of the scleroderma in patients with hypertension, with or without renal insufficiency (318); however, the renal insufficiency may not improve or may even progress despite control of the blood pressure (328). If the GFR is above 30 ml/min, either captopril or enalapril can be used at maximum recommended dose. For enalapril, a starting dose of 2.5 mg is recommended for a GFR less than 30 ml/min, with upward titration. For captopril, Beckett and associates (318) have recommended a maximum dose of 100 mg if the GFR is 20–30 ml/min, 75 mg for a GFR of 10–20 ml/min and 50 mg for a GFR less than 10 ml/min. In some patients, despite a maximum dose of an ACE inhibitor, the blood pressure may not be adequately controlled. In these instances a calcium channel blocker should be used, since the effect of All on the renal vasculature is critically dependent on transmembrane calcium ion transport (329,330).

The patient with scleroderma and renal disease should also be followed by a rheumatologist, as other therapeutic modalities aimed at controlling disease activity in other organ systems commonly involved in such patients are under active investigation (331).

VI. HEMOLYTIC UREMIC SYNDROME/THROMBOTIC THROMBOCYTOPENIC PURPURA

Hemolytic uremic syndrome (HUS) and thrombotic thrombocytopenic purpura (TTP) most likely represent the spectrum of a single syndrome, HUS occurring mainly in children and involving predominantly the kidneys, and TTP occurring in adults and involving other organ systems as well. The diagnosis of HUS should be considered in any elderly patient presenting with hemolytic anemia, thrombocytopenia, and acute renal failure, while TTP should be considered if there is also fever and neurological disease. In general, the syndrome is rare in the elderly, comprising approximately 6% of the reported cases; however, renal involvement is seen in 77% of elderly with HUS/TTP (332,333).

Damage to the kidney and other organ vasculature results from several abnormalities of the coagulation system (334). The production and activity of tissue plasminogen activator, as well as circulating levels of prostacyclin, are decreased in these patients. There is an increase in the plasma concentration of platelet-activating factors. A deficiency of the protease enzyme responsible for converting the large von Willebrand factor multimers into smaller-molecular-weight forms and endothelial cell damage also contribute to the pathogenesis of the disease (335,336). The triggering factors for these various abnormalities have not been characterized but may be facilitated by bacterial endotoxins, vasoactive amines, anticancer drug therapy, cyclosporine, or metastatic disease (337,338).

Moderate to marked thickening of the glomerular capillary wall with luminal obliteration is usually seen on biopsy. Arteries and arterioles with intimal thickening of varying severity might be of prognostic significance, since patients with less intimal thickening have a better chance of recovering kidney function (339). Interstitial fibrosis and tubular atrophy may be seen. Immunofluorescence studies reveal the presence of fibrinogen in vessels and glomerular capillary loops, sometimes accompanied by C3. Immunoglobulins are usually not seen. With electron microscopy, the intima of the arterial wall shows cellular proliferation, granular material containing red cells, red cell fragments, and degenerative thrombotic material. The glomerular capillary walls reveal wrinkling and irregular thickening of the basement membrane.

The most common renal manifestation is hematuria with or without RBC casts. Proteinuria is seen in 70–80% of patients, occasionally in the nephrotic range. Elevated BUN and serum creatinine is seen in over 80% of patients. The renal disease may progress rapidly to end stage, but may follow a more variable course or even reverse (340). In some patients, factors such as volume depletion superimposed on hemolysis might contribute to the genesis of the renal failure.

Several forms of therapy have been tried on patients with HUS/TTP, including platelet function inhibitors (340), high doses of prednisone, and splenectomy, with varying degrees of success (333). Recently, vincristine has been advocated for the form of the disease caused by mitomycin (337). At present, plasmapheresis with replacement by fresh-frozen plasma seems to be the therapy of choice and is associated with a survival rate similar to that of younger patients. Approximately one plasma volume (40 ml/kg) is exchanged during each session. It is not clear whether prednisone and/or antiplatelet agents (aspirin and dipyridamole) can potentiate the therapeutic benefits of plasmapheresis (332,333,336,341–343). High-dose intravenous gamma-immunoglobulin infusion may be tried in patients who fail to respond to plasmapheresis (334).

VII. RHEUMATOID ARTHRITIS

The percentage of elderly patients with rheumatoid arthritis who develop kidney disease (manifested by either proteinuria, hematuria, or an elevated serum creatinine) is not known. Of those who ultimately undergo renal biopsy, a variety of histological pictures may be seen.

Amyloidosis or mesangial nephritis is present in 73% of the patients biopsied, while interstitial nephritis and various other glomerulopathies contribute to the remaining 27% (91,344–346). Nephrotic-range proteinuria and renal insufficiency are more commonly found in those patients with amyloidosis. In patients with membranous nephropathy, kidney function is generally well preserved, with the disease occurring earlier in the history of rheumatoid arthritis compared with amyloidosis (346). History of treatment with D-penicillamine and gold is common in patients with membranous nephropathy. In patients with mesangial nephritis, glomerular immunofluorescence is dominated by IgM and/or C_3. Management of these varied lesions is similar to that in patients without rheumatoid arthritis.

Systemic vasculitis complicates the course of long-standing rheumatoid arthritis in a small percentage of patients. The lesion can involve blood vessels of all sizes, with a predilection for the small digital arteries. Renal involvement is present in 24–40% of these patients (347,348). Glomerular changes are usually minimal, since the lesion is localized primarily to the arcuate arteries and includes both acute necrotizing injury and intimal scarring with organized thrombi (349,350). Focal segmental necrotizing glomerulonephritis has also been reported (350a). ANCA (MPO) is positive in most of these patients. A kidney biopsy is needed to differentiate between those patients with vasculitis and those with the histological findings described earlier. For instance, of the 12 patients with evidence of systemic vasculitis reported by Scott et al. (348), 4 had amyloidosis and 2 had chronic nonspecific changes on renal biopsy. The mortality rate is higher in patients with renal involvement, particularly in older patients (348). A regimen consisting of intravenous methylprednisolone (500 mg) and cyclophosphamide (500 mg), administered on days 1, 8, 29, and 50, followed by an oral maintenance dose of cyclophosphamide (1.5 mg/kg/day) or azathioprine (2 mg/kg/day), appears to be the best form of therapy presently available, and has been associated with long-lasting remissions in a significant number of patients (348,350,350a).

VIII. RELAPSING POLYCHONDRITIS

Relapsing polychondritis is diagnosed when three or more of the following clinical features are present: (a) bilateral auricular chondritis; (b) nonerosive seronegative inflammatory polyarthritis; (c) nasal chondritis; (d) ocular inflammation; (e) respiratory tract chondritis; and (f) audio-vestibular damage. Thirteen percent of reported patients were 60 years and older when the diagnosis was made (351).

Renal involvement is quite rare, but has been reported with a higher frequency in the elderly (352). When present, it takes the form of acute renal failure with hematuria and proteinuria. Histological examination of the kidney reveals the presence of glomerulonephritis with segmental fibrinoid necrosis and abundant crescents or segmental glomerulosclerosis (352–354). Interstitial cellular infiltrates and fibrosis are also commonly seen. With immunofluorescence microscopy, immunoglobulins (IgG, IgM) and complement (C_3) are frequently found, predominantly in the mesangium. Electron-dense deposits have been noted in the basement membrane and mesangium. Prednisone (60–100 mg/day) is the treatment of choice. Cyclophosphamide may also be tried if prednisone fails or the patient is intolerant of steroids. 4,4'-Diaminodiphenylsulfone (Dapsone) and prednisone in combination have also been tried (354). The prognosis is, in general, worse in patients with renal involvement.

IX. SJÖGREN'S SYNDROME

Sjögren's syndrome is a chronic inflammatory disorder which may occur as a primary disease (sicca syndrome) or in association with other autoimmune diseases, particularly rheumatoid arthritis, systemic lupus erythematosus, primary biliary cirrhosis, or scleroderma. The disease primarily affects postmenopausal women. In those series where age is given, 21% of the patients were over the age of 60 (355–356). Renal involvement can take the forms of tubulo-interstitial disease or a glomerulonephritis.

Tubulo-interstitial disease may present as a urinary concentrating defect, most likely due to impaired water permeability of the cortical collecting tubule (357). A distal renal tubular acidosis (type I) may also be seen in 67% of patients (358–359a). Kidney function is usually normal in these patients and proteinuria uncommon. Hypocitraturia and a decrease in tubular reabsorption of phosphate are also quite common (359a). On kidney biopsy, diffuse interstitial inflammatory cell infiltration, composed predominantly of plasma cells and lymphocytes, with relatively well preserved glomerular morphology has been found. The contribution of the infiltrates to the pathogenesis of the tubular dysfunction is not clear. It is interesting to note, however, that in a repeat kidney biopsy in one such patient after treatment with steroids and remission of the renal tubular acidosis, the interstitial inflammation was also gone (360). Moderate renal insufficiency with mild proteinuria (<1 g/24 hr) is occasionally found in patients with chronic interstitial nephritis (361). Both cyclophosphamide and low-dose prednisone (30 mg daily) have been used with some success in these patients.

Glomerulonephritis as a complication of Sjögren's syndrome is rare. Its presence should suggest the possibility of cryoglobulinemia, which occurs in up to one-third of patients. Clinical manifestations associated with glomerulonephritis include hematuria, renal insufficiency of varying severity, and proteinuria, occasionally in the nephrotic range. Circulating immune complexes have been found in some of the patients. Their presence seems to be of pathogenetic significance, since their level decreases concomitantly with drug-induced improvement in kidney function (362).

A picture of mesangiocapillary glomerulonephritis (with low C3), membranous nephropathy with endocapillary hypercellularity, or even necrotizing arteriolitis may be found on histological examination of kidney tissue. The response to moderate doses of prednisone (20–30 mg/day) in two of our elderly patients with Sjögren's syndrome and mesangiocapillary glomerulonephritis has not been as good as described by Motsopoulos et al. (362). In one patient, kidney function acutely worsened, and death was due to septic shock. The other died from GI bleeding with renal insufficiency (serum creatinine 4 mg/dl). She had been previously treated with cyclophosphamide and prednisone.

X. DRUG-INDUCED GLOMERULAR DISEASE

A. Nonsteroidal Antiinflammatory Drugs (NSAIDs)

The adverse effects of NSAIDs in the kidney are multiple and will be dealt with under separate headings according to the specific complication. In this section we discuss the problem of nephrotic syndrome which can occur with or without renal insufficiency. Kidney biopsy will show either minimal changes in the glomeruli with prominent interstitial infiltrates or membranous nephropathy.

1. Incidence

Nephrotic syndrome is seen mainly in the elderly, with the ratio of females to males at 2:1 in those patients with the acute interstitial nephritis form (363–367). In the membranous form, males are involved as frequently as females (368). The reason for the high incidence in the elderly is not clear. It is not simply because the use of those agents increases with age, since the incidence of all side effects of NSAIDs increases disproportionately with age (369). The drugs most commonly associated with the nephrotic syndrome are fenoprofen, diclofenamate, sulindac, tolmetin, ibuprofen, and naproxen. Zomepirac, phenylbutazone, and indomethacin have also been implicated.

2. Pathology

a. Interstitial Nephritis. With light microscopy, the glomeruli are normal. Most of the abnormalities are located in the interstitium, with edema and cellular infiltrates made up mainly of lymphocytes, histiocytes, and eosinophils. Granulomatous interstitial changes have also been reported (370). Tubular degeneration and atrophy have been described on occasion. Immunofluorescent studies are normal in most patients. Variable staining for IgG, IgA, IgM, and C3 may be seen in the interstitium or in the tubular basement membrane. With electron microscopy, fusion of foot processes is the major finding, similar to idiopathic minimal-change disease. In general, it is not possible to separate patients with renal failure from those without by histological findings alone.

b. Membranous Nephropathy. The histological picture is indistinguishable from that of idiopathic membranous nephropathy. Most patients had stage I disease (Chapter 6).

3. Pathogenesis

The pathogenesis of the renal injury associated with interstitial nephritis is not clear and is most likely multifactorial, including direct glomerular and tubular toxicity, delayed hypersensitivity reaction, and specific facilitation of lymphocytic interstitial infiltration through augmentation of polyenoic acid synthesis from arachidonic acid (363,367).

In the membranous form, the deposition of IgG and C3 in the glomerulus suggests the involvement of an immune mechanism. At present, it is not clear whether the drug itself acts as an antigen or facilitates the immune response to another antigen.

4. Clinical Manifestations

In those patients with an acute interstitial nephritis, duration of exposure to the drug before the apparent onset of the nephropathy can vary from days to years. The hypersensitivity response of fever, skin rash, eosinophilia, and/or eosinophiluria, so commonly associated with allergic interstitial nephritis, is unusual with NSAIDs, occurring in only 20% of patients. Renal insufficiency is present in 87% of patients, with approximately one-third requiring dialysis. Edema is the most common presenting complaint, followed by oliguria or anuria and general malaise. Besides proteinuria, microscopic hematuria and granular casts are present in half of the patients (363–367,371).

Patients with the membranous form usually present with the nephrotic syndrome and relatively well preserved kidney function. Eosinophilia may be present in some patients. Clinical manifestations suggestive of an allergic reaction are generally absent (368).

5. Natural History

Following discontinuation of the offending agent, almost all patients with the interstitial form eventually recover, although a varying degree of renal insufficiency may occasionally persist. The period of time required for complete recovery has been quite variable, so the therapeutic benefit from steroids has been difficult to assess. It is recommended that steroid therapy be reserved for patients with severe disease (e.g., those requiring dialysis) or who fail to improve in 1–2 weeks after the offending agent has been removed (363–367,371).

A clinical picture identical to that associated with NSAIDs has been reported in an elderly man during therapy with rifampin (372).

In those patients with membranous nephropathy, protein excretion usually decreases to below 1 g in an average of 25 weeks after discontinuation of the drug. Management should be supportive only (368).

B. Penicillamine

Proteinuria occurs in 16% of elderly patients with rheumatoid arthritis who are treated with penicillamine (373). This complication seems to be related, in part, to the rate at which the dose is increased and can appear at any time during therapy. It should be remembered that oral iron inhibits penicillamine absorption by chelation in the gut. If the iron is stopped, a larger amount of the maintenance dose of penicillamine will be reabsorbed, making drug toxicity more likely. Such was the case in 4 of 16 patients reported by Harkness and Blake (374). The proteinuria is usually in the nephrotic range. Kidney function is generally well preserved. On biopsy the findings are those of membranous nephropathy, making an immune pathogenesis quite likely. Minimal-change disease and mesangial proliferation with electron-dense deposits have also been reported (375). The proteinuria and histological changes remit after discontinuing the drug; however, it may take up to 16 months. Other modalities of therapy for the rheumatoid arthritis should then be considered, since a recrudescence of proteinuria has been observed upon restarting penicillamine (376). Rapidly progressive glomerulonephritis with a renal histological picture identical to Goodpasture's syndrome has also been reported with penicillamine. ANCA (MPO) may be positive (377). Treatment with plasmapheresis and immunosuppressives is worth trying (378–381).

C. Gold

Nephropathy occurs in 5–25% of patients treated with the parenteral form of gold and in 3% of those who receive the oral form (382). The majority of patients (42%) present with moderate proteinuria (1–3.5 g/day). Mild proteinuria (<1 g/day) develops in 37%, and the remaining 21% have nephrotic syndrome. As with penicillamine use, kidney function is, in general, well preserved, and the renal histology is predominantly that of membranous nephropathy. Other histological forms, such as minimal-change disease and mesangial nephritis, have also been reported (383,384). The development of renal disease does not appear to be dose related. The pathogenesis is not clear but very likely is immune related. Patients with rheumatoid arthritis with beta-lymphocyte alloantigens HLA-DRW3 or B8 are at increased risk of developing proteinuria with parenteral gold therapy (385,386). The level of circulating metallothioneine may also be involved in the relationship between chrysotherapy and nephrotoxicity (387). The proteinuria usually disappears upon discontinuing the gold. It is recommended that these patients not be rechallenged with the drug.

D. Captopril

The use of captopril has been associated with membranous nephropathy and proteinuria in the elderly. This rather rare complication has been reported in patients taking large doses (400–600 mg/day) or patients with underlying renal disease (388,389). Generally, the proteinuria disappears (or decreases to predrug levels in those with underlying disease) after discontinuation of the drug; however, persistent proteinuria has been reported (390).

E. Other Drugs

Besides the two patterns of glomerular injury discussed earlier (minimal-change disease and membranous glomerulopathy), proliferative glomerulonephritis associated with systemic vasculitis has been reported in association with a variety of drugs (391). No data are available, however, as to how often these occur in the elderly.

XI. INFECTIONS AND GLOMERULAR DISEASE

Glomerulonephritis can occur as a complication of infections. This complication appears to be rare in the elderly, although the true incidence is not known.

A. Bacterial Endocarditis

Approximately 10% of elderly patients with either acute or subacute bacterial endocarditis develop a renal complication (392), usually manifested by acute renal failure, proteinuria, and hematuria. The renal failure can be progressive, with some patients requiring dialysis. Serum complement (C3, C4) is decreased in most patients. In patients with subacute bacterial endocarditis, kidney biopsy reveals the presence of diffuse mesangial proliferation, which may be accompanied by epithelial crescents. Mesangial and subendothelial electron-dense deposits may be found on electron microscopy; with immunofluorescent microscopy, diffuse granular deposits of IgG (less commonly IgM or IgA) and C3 in subendothelial and mesangial areas may be found. In patients with acute bacterial endocarditis, the renal lesion resembles that of acute poststreptococcal glomerulonephritis (see Chapter 6). The association of severe renal failure and diffuse glomerulonephritis heralds a poor prognosis as far as recovery of kidney function is concerned (393). Also, patients with diffuse glomerulonephritis may have persistent hematuria or proteinuria, despite bacteriological cure of the endocarditis, although clinical recovery from the primary disease is usually associated with complete resolution of the glomerulonephritis (394). The treatment is that of the underlying infection. In general, older age increases the risk of death (395).

B. Visceral Suppuration

Glomerulonephritis can complicate other organ infection, particularly the lungs or retroperitoneal space (arterial graft) in the elderly. The clinical manifestations and laboratory data are identical to that of bacterial endocarditis. The serum complement (C3, C4), however, is usually normal. The prognosis is closely related to the course of the infection. In 3 patients reported by Forrest et al. (395), capsular antigen for the organism was localized in the glomeruli of all the patients. Other investigators have reported a high intraglomerular monocytic infiltration (396), a finding that may provide a clue to the diagnosis of visceral infection in cases where the diagnosis is not apparent (397,398).

Glomerulonephritis can complicate the course of methicillin-resistant staphylococcal infection and associated abscess or sepsis (399). Clinical manifestations become manifest between the second and tenth weeks of infection. Hematuria and proteinuria are seen in every patient. In 75% of patients the proteinuria is in the nephrotic range and in 88% renal insufficiency is seen, severe enough to require dialytic therapy in some. With light microscopy, endocapillary and/or mesangio-proliferative glomerulonephritis, with or without crescents, is seen. With immunofluorescence microscopy, IgG, IgA, IgM, and/or C3 are found. It has been postulated that the glomerular lesions result from the action of circulating immune complexes, following cytokine-induced polyclonal activation of IgG and IgA (399). Methicillin-resistant staphylococcus produces enterotoxins C and A and toxic shock syndrome produces toxin-1, known to act as superantigens. These superantigens are probably responsible for the release of the cytokines. Half of the patients had either improvement in kidney function or a decrease in proteinuria with cure of infection. Mortality rate is high (25%).

C. Viral Infections

A clinical picture identical to that seen with periarteritis nodosa and mixed cryoglobulinemia may be seen with hepatitis B virus. The renal manifestations are similar to the non-hepatitis-induced forms of either disease entity.

ANCA (MPO) is positive in 4% of the patients with vasculitis. Suggested treatment includes a 3-week course of vidarabine, plasma exchange, and a 2-week course of prednisone. Interferon-2b may be substituted for the vidarabine (400). The long-term efficacy of this regimen remains to be shown.

Hepatitis C virus, as discussed earlier, is the major cause of mixed cryoglobulinemia (401,402). The renal histology is that of mesangiocapillary glomerulonephritis (vide supra). However, a significant number of patients with glomerulonephritis and hepatitis C do not have cryoglobulinemia. Besides mesangiocapillary glomerulonephritis, other glomerulopathies such as acute exudative and proliferative glomerulonephritis and membranous nephropathy have been reported (403). These patients should also be treated with alpha-interferon as discussed earlier.

Focal segmental glomerulosclerosis and various other immune-mediated glomerulonephritides, such as acute endocapillary glomerulonephritis, mesangiocapillary glomerulonephritis, or membranous nephropathy, as well as tubulointerstitial disease, have been reported in HIV-positive patients (404). These entities are rarely seen in a geriatric practice, as most patients with HIV disease are either diagnosed or die at a younger age.

Several mechanisms have been proposed by which infections induce glomerular damage: (a) circulating immune complexes of microorganism antigen-antibody may become trapped in the glomerular capillary with subsequent inflammatory reaction; (b) there may be direct glomerular toxicity of microorganism products; (c) other pathogenic mechanisms may be triggered by the infectious process.

XII. SARCOIDOSIS

Glomerulonephritis (membranous, focal glomerulosclerosis, and mesangiocapillary glomerulonephritis) has been reported in association with sarcoidosis. The frequency of the problem in the elderly is not known. Also, it is not clear whether therapy should be directed to the sarcoidosis alone (steroids) or also to the specific glomerulopathy, where appropriate.

Although interstitial granulomas in the kidney are not uncommon in patients with sarcoidosis, only rarely have they been associated with renal impairment in the absence of nephrocalcinosis and hypercalcemia. Most of the well-documented patients with granulomatous interstitial nephritis as the only cause of renal insufficiency have been elderly (405,406). Steroids (prednisone 60 mg/day) should be tried in these patients.

REFERENCES

1. United States Renal Data System. 1996 annual data report II. Incidence and prevalence of ESRD. Am J Kidney Dis 1996;28(suppl 2):S34–S47.
2. Rodby RA, Firth LM, Lewis EJ. An economic analysis of captopril in the treatment of diabetic nephropathy. Diabetes Care 1996;19:1051–1061.
3. Savage S, et al. Urinary albumin excretion as a predictor of diabetic retinopathy, neuropathy and cardiovascular disease. Diabetes Care 1996;19:1243–1248.
4. Ritz E, Stefanski A. Diabetic nephropathy in type II diabetes. Am J Kidney Dis 1996;27:167–194.

4a. Keller CK, et al. Renal findings in patients with short-term type 2 diabetes. J Am Soc Nephrol 1996;7:2627–2635.

5. Greene DA. Acute and chronic complications of diabetes mellitus in older patients. Am J Med 1986;80(suppl 5A):39–53.
6. Schmitz A, Vaeth M. Microalbuminemia: a major risk factor in non-insulin-dependant diabetes. A 10-year follow-up study of 503 patients. Diabetic Med 1988;5:126–134.

7. Keinzelman CL, et al. Incidence of proteinuria in type 2 diabetes mellitus in the Pima Indians. Kidney Int 1989;35:681–687.
8. Makino H, et al. Ultrastructural changes of extracellular matrices in diabetic nephropathy revealed by high resolution scanning and immunoelectron microscopy. Lab Invest 1993;68:45–55.
9. Takenci A, et al. Periodic high extracellular glucose enhances production of collagens III and IV by mesangial cells. Am J Physiol 1995;268:13F–19F.
10. Yang C-W, et al. Advanced glycation end products up-regulate gene expression found in diabetic glomerular disease. Proc Natl Acad Sci USA 1994;91:9436–9440.
11. Ballerman BJ, Skorecki KL, Brenner BM. Reduced glomerular angiotensin II receptor density in early untreated diabetes mellitus in the rat. Am J Physiol 1984;247: F110–F116.
12. Zatz R, et al. Prevention of diabetic glomerulopathy by pharmacological amelioration of glomerular capillary hypertension. J Clin Invest 1986;77:1925–1930.
13. Reichard P, Nilsson B-Y, Rosengvist U. The effect of long-term intensified insulin treatment on the development of microvascular complications of diabetes mellitus. N Engl J Med 1993;329:304–309.
14. Olivarius NF, et al. Epidemiology of renal involvement in newly-diagnosed middle-aged and elderly diabetic patients. Diabetologia 1993;36:1007–1016.
15. Yoshida H, et al. Angiotensin I converting enzyne gene polymorphism in non-insulin-dependant diabetes mellitus. Kidney Int 1996;50:657–664.
15a. Dudley CRK, et al. UK prospective diabetes study XV: relationship of renin-angiotensin gene polymorphisms with microalbuminuria in non-insulin dependant diabetes mellitus. Kidney Int 1995;48:1907–1911.
16. Damsgaard EM, Mogensen CE. Microalbuminuria in elderly hyperglycaemic patients and controls. Diabetes Med 1986;3:340–345.
16a. Nelson RG, et al. Development and progression of renal disease in Pima Indians with non-insulin dependant diabetes mellitus. N Engl J Med 1996;335:1636–1642.
17. Savage S, et al. Urinary albumin excretion as a predictor of diabetic retinopathy, neuropathy, and cardiovascular disease in NIDDM. Diabetes Care 1996;19:1243–1248.
18. Lindsay RS, et al. Reduced diurnal variation of blood pressure in non-insulin dependant diabetic patients with microalbuminuria. J Hum Hypertens 1995;9:223–227.
19. Zietse R, et al. Effect of atrial natriuretic peptide on renal and vascular permeability in diabetes mellitus. J Am Soc Nephrol 1995;5:2057–2066.
20. Gall MA, et al. Glomerular size and charge selectivity in type 2 (non-insulin-dependant) diabetic patients with diabetic nephropathy. Diabetologia 1994;37:195–201.
21. Tomlanovich S, et al. Functional nature of glomerular injury in progressive diabetic glomerulopathy. Diabetes 1987;36:556–565.
22. Osterby R, et al. A strong correlation between glomerular filtration rate and filtration surface in diabetic nephropathy. Diabetologia 1988;31:265–270.
23. Mauer SM, et al. Structural-functional relationships in diabetic nephropathy. J Clin Invest 1984;74:1143–1155.
24. O'Neill WM Jr, Wallin JD, Walker PD. Hematuria and red cell casts in typical diabetic nephropathy. Am J Med 1983;74:389–395.
25. Lopes de Faria JB, et al. Glomerular hematuria in diabetics. Clin Nephrol 1988;30: 117–121.

26. Klein R, et al. Blood pressure and hypertension in diabetes. Am J Epidemiol 1985;122:75–89.
27. Ferriss JB, et al. Blood pressure in diabetic patients: relationships with exchangeable sodium and renin activity. Diabetic Nephropathy 1986;5:27–30.
28. Jerumus G, et al. Spectrum of proteinuria in type I and type II diabetes. Diabetes Care 1987;10:419–427.
29. Jarrett RJ, et al. Microalbuminemia predicts mortality in non-insulin dependant diabetes. Diabetic Med 1984;1:17–19.
30. Fogari R, et al. Urinary albumin excretion and nocturnal blood pressure in hypertensive patients with type II diabetes mellitus. Am J Hypertens 1994;7:808–813.
31. Equiluz-Bruck S, et al. Nondipping of nocturnal blood pressure is related to urinary albumin excretion rate in patients with type II diabetes mellitus. Am J Hypertens 1996;9:1139–1143.
32. Reubi FC, Franz KA, Horber F. Hypertension as related to renal function in diabetes mellitus. Hypertension 1985;7(suppl II):1121–1128.
33. De Chatel, et al. Sodium, renin, aldosterone, catecholamines and blood pressure in diabetes mellitus. Kidney Int 1977;12:412–421.
34. Weidmann P, Beretta-Piccoli C, Trost BN. Pressor factors and responsiveness in hypertension accompanying diabetes mellitus. Hypertension 1985;7(suppl II):1133–1142.
35. Connell JMC, et al. Reduced number of angiotensin II receptors on platelets in insulin-dependant diabetes. Clin Sci 1986;71:217–220.
36. Trujillo A, et al. Renin regulation in type II diabetes mellitus: influence of dietary sodium. Hypertension 1989;13:200–205.
37. DeFronzo RA, et al. The effect of insulin on renal handling of sodium, potassium, calcium and phosphate in man. J Clin Invest 1975;55:845–855.
38. DeFronzo RA, Goldberg M, Agus Z. The effects of glucose and insulin on renal electrolyte transport. J Clin Invest 1976;58:83–90.
39. Trevison M, et al. Hypertension, non-insulin dependant diabetes and intracellular sodium metabolism. Hypertension 1988;11:264–268.
40. Weidmann P, et al. Sodium-volume factor, cardiovascular reactivity and hypotensive mechanisms of diuretic therapy in hypertension associated with diabetes mellitus. Am J Med 1979;67:779–784.
41. Oshan AR, et al. Hypertension in adult onset diabetes mellitus: abnormal renal hemodynamics and endogenous vasoregulatory factors. Am J Kidney Dis 1982;2: 271–279.
42. Zemel MB, et al. Altered cation transport in diabetic hypertension. Clin Res 1987;35:853A.
43. Zemel MB, et al. Role of impaired calcium (Ca^{++}) transport in obesity-associated hypertension. FASEB J 1988;2:A502.
44. Sowers JR, et al. Hyperinsulinemia, insulin resistance, and hyperglycemia: contributing factors in the pathogenesis of hypertension and atherosclerosis. Am J Hypertens 1993;6:260S–270S.
45. Gilbert RE, et al. Long-term glycemic control and the rate of progression of early diabetic kidney disease. Kidney Int 1993;44:855–859.

45a. Berrut G, et al: Microalbuminuria as a predictor of a drop in glomerular filtration rate

in subjects with non-insulin dependant diabetes mellitus and hypertension. Clin Nephrol 1997;48:92–97.
46. Ravid M, et al. Proteinuria, renal impairment, metabolic control, and blood pressure in type 2 diabetes mellitus. Arch Intern Med 1992;152:1225–1229.
47. Microalbuminuria Collaborative Study Group, UK. Intensive therapy and progression to clinical albuminuria in patients with insulin dependant diabetes mellitus and microalbuminuria. Br Med J 1995;311:973–977.
48. Diabetes Control and Complications Trial Research Group. The effect of intensive treatment of diabetes on the developemnt and progression of long-term complications in insulin-dependent diabetes mellitus. N Engl J Med 1993;329:977–986.
49. Richard P, Nilsson B-Y, Rosenguist U. The effect of long term intensified insulin treatment on the development of microvascular complications of diabetes mellitus. N Engl J Med 1993;329:304–309.
49a. Ohkubo Y, et al. Intensive insulin therapy prevents the progression of diabetic microvascular complications in Japanese patients with non-insulin-dependent diabetes mellitus: a randomized prospective 6-year study. Diabetes Res Clin Pract 1995;28: 103–107.
50. Krolewski AS, et al. Glycosylated hemoglobin and the risk of micro albuminuria in patients with insulin-dependant diabetes mellitus. N Engl J Med 1995;332:1251–1255.
51. Kilpatrick ES, Dominiczak MH, Small M. The effects of aging on glycation and the interpretation of glycaemic control in type 2 diabetes Q J Med 1996;89:307–312.
52. Diabetes Control and Complications Trial Research Group. The absence of a glycemic treshold for the development of long term complications: the perspective of the diabetes control and complications trial. Diabetes 1996;45:1289–1298.
53. Viberti G. Effect of captopril on progression to clinical proteinuria in patients with insulin-dependant diabetes mellitus and microalbuminuria. JAMA 1994;271: 275–279.
54. Microalbuminuria Captopril Study Group. Captopril reduces the risk of nephropathy in IDDM patients with microalbuminuria. Diabetologia 1996;39:587–593.
55. Sano T, et al. Effects of long-term enalapril treatment on persistent microalbuminuria in normotensive type 2 diabetic patients: results of a 4-year prospective, randomized study. Diabetic Med 1996;13:120–124.
56. Ravid M, et al. Long-term renoprotective effect of angiotensin-converting enzyme inhibition in non-insulin-dependant diabetes mellitus. A 7-year follow-up study. Arch Intern Med 1996;156:286–289.
57. Laffel LM, McGill JB, Gans DJ. The beneficial effect of angiotensin converting enzyme inhibition with captopril on diabetic nephropathy in normotensive IDDM patients with microabluminuria. Am J Med 1995;99:497–504.
58. O'Donnell MJ, et al. Placebo-controlled trial of lisinopril in normotensive diabetic patients with incipient nephropathy. J Hum Hypertens 1993;7:327–332.
58a. DeCesaris R, et al. Effects of benazepril and nicardipine on microalbuminuria in normotensive and hypertensive patients with diabetes. Clin Pharmacol Ther 1996;60: 472–478.
59. Melbourne Diabetic Nephropathy Study Group. Comparison between perindopril and nifedipine in treating non-insulin-dependant diabetes mellitus associated with hypertension. Br Med J 1991;302:210–216.

60. Lacourciere Y, et al. Captopril or conventional therapy in hypertensive type II diabetics. Three-year analysis. Hypertension 1993;21:786–794.
61. Velussi M, et al. Effects of cilazapril and amlodipine on kidney function in hypertensive NIDDM patients. Diabetes 1996;45:216–222.
61a. Parving H-H, Tarnow L, Rossing P. Renal protection in diabetes: an emerging role for calcium antagonists. J Hypertens 1996;14(suppl 4):S21–S25.
62. Kasiske BL, et al. Effects of antihypertensive therapy on the kidney in patients with diabetes: a meta-regression analysis. Ann Intern Med 1993;118:129–138.
63. Gansevoort RT, et al. Antiproteinuric effect of blood pressure-lowering agents: a meta analysis of comparative trials. Nephrol Dial Transplant 1995;10:1963–1974.
64. Nakamura T, et al. Enalapril attenuates increased gene expression of extracellular matrix components in diabetic rats. J Am Soc Nephrol 1995;5:1492–1497.
65. Bakris GL, et al. Calcium channel blockers versus other anti-hypertensive therapies on progression of NIDDM associated nephropathy. Kidney Int 1996;50:1641–1650.
66. Parving H-H, et al. Angiotensin-converting enzyme inhibition in diabetic nephropathy: ten year's experience. Am J Kidney Dis 1995;26:99–107.
67. Dodson PM, et al. Sodium restriction and blood pressure in hypertensive type II diabetics: randomized blind controlled and crossover studies of moderate sodium restriction and sodium supplementation. Br Med J 1989;298:227–230.
68. Tuck ML, et al. Reductions in plasma catecholamines and blood pressure during weight loss in obese subjects. Acta Endocrinol 1983;102:252–257.
69. Zeller K, et al. Effect of restricting dietary protein on the progression of renal failure in patients with insulin-dependent diabetes mellitus. N Engl J Med 1991;324:78–84.
70. Mulec H, et al. Cholesterol: a renal risk factor in diabetic nephropathy? Am J Kidney Dis 1993;22:196–201.
70a. Ravid M, et al. Plasma lipids and the progression of nephropathy in diabetes mellitus type II: effect of ACE inhibitors. Kidney Int 1995;47:907–910.
71. Working Group on Hypertension in Diabetes. Statement on hypertension in diabetes mellitus. Arch Intern Med 1987;147:830–842.
72. Richards NT, et al. Increased prevalence of renal biopsy findings other than diabetic glomerulopathy in type II diabetes mellitus. Nephrol Dial Transplant 1992;7:397–399.
73. Hatch FE, et al. Diabetic glomerulosclerosis. A long term follow-up study based on renal biopsies. Am J Med 1961;31:216–230.
74. Chihara J, et al. Glomerulonephritis in diabetic patients and its effects on the prognosis. Nephron 1986;43:45–49.
75. Parving H-H, et al. Prevalence and causes of albuminuria in non-insulin dependant diabetic patients. Kidney Int 1992;41:758–762.
76. Suzuki Y, et al. A light microscopic study of glomerulosclerosis in Japanese patients with non-insulin dependant diabetes mellitus;the relationship between clinical and histological features. Clin Nephrol 1994;42:155–162.
76a. Schwartz MM, Lewis EJ, Leonard-Martin TC. Renal clinicopathology of type II diabetes mellitus. J Am Soc Nephrol 1996;7:1364:A0596.
76b. Waldherr R, Ilkenhans C, Ritz E. How frequent is glomerulonephritis in diabetes mellitus type II? Clin Nephrol 1992;37:271–273.

77. Gellman DD, et al. Diabetic nephropathy: a clinical and pathologic study based on renal biopsies. Medicine 1959;38:321–367.
78. Murphy WM, et al. Immunopathologic studies in glomerular diseases with membranous lesions. Am J Clin Pathol 1959;60:364–376.
79. Warms PC, et al. Idiopathic membranous glomerulonephritis occurring with diabetes mellitus. Arch Intern Med 1973;132:735–738.
80. Sharma HM, Yum MN, Kleit S. Acute glomerulonephritis with diabetes mellitus. Report of a case. Arch Pathol 1974;97:152–154.
81. Olivero J, Suki WN. Acute glomerulonephritis complicating diabetic nephropathy. Arch Intern Med 1977;137:732–734.
82. Wass JAH, et al. Renal failure, glomerular disease and diabetes mellitus. Nephron 1978;21:289–296.
83. Rao KV, Crosson JT. Idiopathic membranous glomerulonephritis in diabetic patients. Report of three cases and review of the literature. Arch Intern Med 1980;140: 624–627.
84. Amoaah E, et al. Clinical identification of non-diabetic renal disease in diabetic patients with type I and type II disease presenting with renal dysfunction. Am J Nephrol 1988;8:204–211.
85. Cavallo T, Pinto JA, Rajaraman S. Immune complex disease complicating diabetic glomerulosclerosis. Am J Nephrol 1984;4:347–354.
86. Bertani T, et al. Superimposed nephritis: a separate entity among glomerular diseases? Am J Kidney Dis 1986;7:205–212.
87. Gambara V, et al. Heterogenous nature of renal lesions in type II diabetes. J Am Soc Nephrol 1993;3:1458–1466.
88. Hansen KJ, et al. Is renal revascularization in diabetic patients worthwhile? J Vasc Surg 1996;24:383–393.
89. Moorthy AV, Zimmerman SW. Renal disease in the elderly: clinicopathologic analysis of renal disease in 115 elderly patients. Clin Nephrol 1980;14:223–229.
90. Zech P, et al. The nephrotic syndrome in adults aged over 60: etiology, evolution and treatment of 76 cases. Clin Nephrol 1982;18:232–236.
91. Kingswood JC, et al. Renal biopsy in the elderly: clinicopathological correlations in 143 patients. Clin Nephrol 1984;22:183–187.
92. Franklin EC. Immunopathology of the amyloid diseases. Hosp Pract 1980;15:70–77.
93. Gertz MA, Kyle RA. Primary systemic amyloidosis—a diagnostic primer. Mayo Clin Proc 1989;64:1505–1519.
94. Kyle RA, Gertz MA. Primary systemic amyloidosis: clinical and laboratory features in 474 cases. Sem Hematol 1995;32:45–59.
95. Ogg CS, et al. Presentation and course of primary amyloidosis of the kidney. Clin Nephrol 1981;15:9–13.
96. Triger DR, Joekes AM. Renal amyloidosis. A fourteen-year follow-up. Q J Med 1973;165:15–40.
97. Browning MJ, et al. Ten years' experience of an amyloid clinic—a clinicopathological survey. Q J Med 1985;215:213–227.
98. Dikman SH, Chur J, Kahn T. Morphologic and clinical correlates in renal amyloidosis. Hum Pathol 1981;12:160–169.

99. DeBeer FC, et al. Serum amyloid-A protein concentrations in inflammatory diseases and its relationship to the incidence of reactive systemic amyloidosis. Lancet 1982;2:231–234.
100. Maury CPJ, Teppo AM. Mechanism of reduced amyloid A degrading activity in serum of patients with secondary amyloidosis. Lancet 1982;2:234–237.
101. Kyle RA, Bayrd ED. Amyloidosis: review of 236 cases. Medicine 1975;54:271–299.
102. Parkins RA, Bywaters EGL. Regression of amyloidosis secondary to rheumatoid arthritis. Br Med J 1959;50:536–540.
103. Lowenstein J, Gallo G. Remission of the nephrotic syndrome in renal amyloidosis. N Engl J Med 1970;282:128–131.
104. Dikman SH, et al. Resolution of renal amyloidosis. Am J Med 1977;63:430–433.
105. Karenty G, et al. Clinical and histological resolution of systemic amyloidosis after renal cell carcinoma removal. Nephron 1985;40:232–234.
106. Bacon PA, et al. Rheumatoid disease, amyloidosis and its treatment with penicillamine. Eur J Rheumatol Inflamm 1979;3:70–74.
107. Berglund K, Thysell H, Keller C. Results, principles and pitfalls in the management of renal AA-amyloidosis, a 10–21 year follow-up of 16 patients with rheumatic disease treated with alkylating cytostatics. J Rheumatol 1993;20:2051–2057.
108. Zemer D, et al. Colchicine in the prevention and treatment of the amyloidosis of familial mediterranean fever. N Engl J Med 1986;314:1001–1005.
109. Kyle RA, et al: A trial of three regimens for primary amyloidosis: colchicine alone, melphalan and prednisone, and melphalan, prednisone and colchicine. N Engl J Med 1997;336:1202–1207.
110. Merlini G. Treatment of primary amyloidosis. Sem Hematol 1995;32:60–7.
110a. Low PA, et al. Efficacy of midodrine vs. placebo in neurogenic orthostatic hypotension. A randomized, double-blind multicenter study. JAMA 1997;277:1046–1051.
111. Cohen AS, et al. Survival of patients with primary (AL) amyloidosis colchicine-treated cases from 1976–1983 compared with cases seen in previous years (1961–1973). Am J Med 1987;82:1182–1190.
112. Scheinberg MA, Pernambuco JC, Benson MD. DMSO and colchicine therapy in amyloid disease. Ann Rheum Dis 1984;43:421–423.
113. Glenner GG. Amyloid deposits and amyloidosis. N Engl J Med 1980;302:1283–1292.
114. Hind CRK, et al. Specific chemical dissociation of fibrillar and non-fibrillar components of amyloid deposits. Lancet 1984;2:376–379.
115. Hill GS, et al. Renal lesions in multiple myeloma: their relationship to associated protein abnormalities. Am J Kidney Dis 1983;2:423–438.
116. Ganeval D, et al. Visceral deposition of monoclonal light chains and immunoglobulins: a study of renal and immunopathologic abnormalities. Adv Nephrol 1982;11:25–63.
117. Kyle RA. Multiple myeloma. Review of 869 cases. Mayo Clin Proc 1975;50:29–40.
118. Rofa S, et al. Multiple myeloma and severe renal failure: a clinicopathologic study of outcome and prognosis in 34 patients. Medicine 1987;66:126–137.

119. Hill GS, et al. Renal lesions in multiple myeloma: their relationship to associated protein abnormalities. Am J Kidney Dis 1983;2:423–438.
120. Pirani CL, et al. Renal lesions in plasma cell dyscrasias, ultrastructural observations. Am J Kidney Dis 1987;10:208–211.
121. Coward RA, Mallick NP, Delamore IW. Tubular function in multiple myeloma. Clin Nephrol 1985;24:180–185.
122. Beaufils M, Morel-Maroger L. Pathogenesis of renal disease in monoclonal gammopathies: current concept. Nephron 1978;20:125–131.
123. Sanders PW, et al. Morphologic alterations of the proximal tubules in light chain related disease. Kidney Int 1988;33:881–889.
124. DeFronzo RA, et al. Renal function in patients with multiple myeloma. Medicine 1978;57:151–166.
125. Perry MC, Kyle RA. The clinical significance of Bence Jones proteinuria. Mayo Clin Proc 1975;50:234–238.
126. MRC working party on leukemia in adults: analysis and management of renal failure in fourth MRC myelomatosis trial. Br Med J 1984;288:1411–1415.
126a. Kagimoto T, et al. Differential glycosylation of Bence Jones protein and kidney impairment in patients with plasma cell dyscrasia. J Lab Clin Med 1997;129:217–223.
127. Coward RA, et al. The importance of urinary immunoglobulin light chain isoelectric point (pl) in nephrotoxicity in multiple myeloma. Clin Sci 1984;66:229–232.
128. Melcion C, et al. Renal failure in myeloma: relationship with isoelectric point of immunoglobulin light chains. Clin Nephrol 1984;22:138–143.
129. Norden AGW, et al. Renal impairment in myeloma: negative association with isoelectric point of excreted Bence-Jones protein. J Clin Pathol 1989;42:59–62.
130. DeFronzo RA, et al. Acute renal failure in multiple myeloma. Medicine 1975;54:209–223.
131. Cohen DJ, et al. Acute renal failure in patients with multiple myeloma. Am J Med 1984;76:247–256.
132. Olmer M, Berland Y, Schutz G. Acute renal failure (ARF) and multiple myeloma. Miner Electrol Metab 1986;12:268A.
133. Murray T, Long W, Narins RG. Multiple myeloma and the anion gap. N Engl J Med 1975;292:574–575.
134. Flanagan NG, Ridway JC, Irving AG. The anion gap as a screening procedure for occult myeloma in the elderly. J Roy Soc Med 1988;81:27–28.
135. Mehta BR, et al. Hyporeninemic hypoaldosteronism in a patient with multiple myeloma. Am J Kidney Dis 1984;4:175–178.
136. Kyle RA. Monoclonal gammopathy of undetermined significance (MGUS). Baillieres Clin Haematol 1995;8:761–781.
137. Bernstein SP, Humes HD. Reversible renal insufficiency in multiple myeloma. Arch Intern Med 1982;142:2083–2086.
138. Kyle RA. Newer approaches to the management of multiple myeloma. Cancer 1993;72(suppl II):3489–3494.
139. Pasquali S, et al. Rapidly progressive renal failure (RPRF) in patients with multiple myeloma. Miner Electrol Metab 1986;12:268A.
140. Pozzi C, et al. Prognostic factors and effectiveness of treatment in acute renal failure due to multiple myeloma: a review of 50 cases. Clin Nephrol 1987;28:1–9.

141. Zucchelli P, et al. Controlled plasma exchange trial in acute renal failure due to multiple myeloma. Kidney Int 1988;33:1175–1180.
142. Johnson WJ, et al. Plasmapheresis, hemodialysis and chemotherapy in the treatment of renal failure associated with multiple myeloma. Am Soc Nephrol 1989;88A.
143. Misiani R, et al. Plasmapheresis in the treatment of acute renal failure in multiple myeloma. Am J Med 1979;66:684–688.
144. Wahlin A, Lofvenberg E, Holm J. Improved survival in multiple myeloma with renal failure. Acta Med Scand 1987;221:205–209.
145. Ganeval D, et al. Treatment of multiple myeloma with renal involvement. Adv Nephrol 1992;21:347–370.
145a. Cosio FG, et al. Severe renal failure in multiple myeloma. Clin Nephrol 1981;15: 206–210.
146. Iggo N, et al. Chronic dialysis in patients with multiple myeloma and renal failure. Q J Med 1989;270:903–910.
147. Lazarus HM, et al. Long-term survival of patients with multiple myeloma and acute renal failure at presentation. Am J Kidney Dis 1983;2:521–525.
148. Brown WW, et al. Reversal of chronic end-stage renal failure due to myeloma kidney. Ann Intern Med 1979;90:793–794.
149. Dahlberg PJ, et al. Myeloma kidney: improved renal function following long-term chemotherapy and hemodialysis. Am J Nephrol 1983;3:2422–243.
150. Randall RE, et al. Manifestations of systemic light chain deposition. Am J Med 1976;60:293–299.
151. Rao TKS, et al. Membranoproliferative glomerulonephritis (MPGN) an unusual manifestation of multiple myeloma. Kidney Int 1978;14:659A.
152. Herf S, et al. An evaluation of diabetic and pseudo-diabetic glomerulosclerosis. Am J Med 1979;66:1040–1045.
153. Gallo GR, et al. Nodular glomerulopathy associated with nonamyloidotic kappa light chain deposits and excess immunoglobulin light chain synthesis. Am J Pathol 1980;99:621–644.
154. Solling K, et al. Nonsecretory myeloma associated with nodular glomerulosclerosis. Acta Med Scand 1980;207:137–143.
155. Tubbs RR, et al. Light chain nephropathy. Am J Med 1981;71:263–269.
156. Glassock RJ, Goldstein DA. Nephrotic syndrome in a 52 year old woman with monoclonal gammopathy. Am J Nephrol 1981;1:199–205.
157. Cohen JR, Colvin R. Plasma cell dyscrasia, with systemic light-chain deposition, kappa type, widespread with renal failure. (Case records of Massachussetts General Hospital.) N Engl J Med 1981;304:33–43.
158. Gipstein RM, et al. Kappa light chain nephropathy without evidence of myeloma cells. Response to chemotherapy with cessation of maintenance hemodialysis. Am J Nephrol 1982;2:276–281.
159. Nakamoto Y, et al. IgM monoclonal gammopathy accompanied by nodular glomerulosclerosis, urine concentrating defect and hyporeninemic hypoaldosteronism. Am J Nephrol 1985;5:53–58.
160. Ganeval D, et al. Visceral deposition of monoclonal light chains and immunoglobulins: a study of renal and immunopathologic abnormalities. Adv Nephrol 1982;11: 25–63.

161. Confaloniere R, et al. Light chain nephropathy: histological and clinical aspects in 15 cases. Nephrol Dial Transplant 1988;2:150–156.
162. Sinniah R, Cohen AH. Glomerular capillary aneurysms in light-chain nephropathy. An ultrastructural proposal of pathogenesis. Am J Pathol 1985;118:298–305.
163. Heilman RL, et al. Long-term follow-up and response to chemotherapy in patients with light-chain deposition diseases. Am J Kidney Dis 1992;20:34–41.
164. Comotti C, et al. Light chain deposition nephropathy in multiple myleloma. In: Sessa A, Meroni M, Battini G, eds. Glomerulonephritis in the Elderly. Basel: Karger, Contrib Nephrol 1993;105:133–138.
165. Abt AB, Cohen AH. Newer glomerular diseases. Sem Nephrol 1996;16:501–510.
166. Fogo A, Qureshi N, Horn RG. Morphologic and clinical features of fibrillary glomerulonephritis versus immunotactoid glomerulopathy. Am J Kidney Dis 1993;22:367–377.
167. Alpers CE. Immunotactoid (microtubular) glomerulopathy: an entity distinct from fibrillary glomerulonephritis? Am J Kidney Dis 1992;19:185–191.
168. Schwartz MM. Immunotactoid glomerulopathy;the case for Occam's razor. Am J Kidney Dis 1993;22:446–447.
169. Alpers CE. Fibrillary glomerulonephritis and immunotactoid glomerulopathy: two entities, not one. Am J Kidney Dis 1993;22:448–451.
170. Brouet JC, et al. Biologic and clinical significance of cryoglobulins: a report of 86 cases. Am J Med 1987;57:775–788.
171. Monti G, et al. Cryoglobulinaemias: a multicenter study of the early clinical and laboratory manifestations of primary and secondary disease. Q J Med 1995;88: 115–126.
172. Gorevic PH, et al. Mixed cryoglobulinemia: clinical aspects and long-term follow-up of 40 patients. Am J Med 1980;69:287–308.
173. Agrafiotis A, et al. Is cryoglobulin detection of clinical significance in chronic glomerulonephritis not related to systemic diseases? Clin Nephrol 1981;16: 146–150.
174. Schifferli JA, French LE, Tissot J-D. Hepatitis C virus infection, cryoglobulinemia and glomerulonephritis. Adv Nephrol 1995;24:107–129.
175. Sinico RA, et al. Hepatitis C virus genotype in patients with essential mixed cryoglobulinemia. Q J Med 1995;88:805–810.
176. Meltzer M, et al. Cryoglobulinemia. A clinical and laboratory study. II. Cryoglobulins with rheumatoid factor activity. Am J Med 1966;40:837–856.
177. Invernizzi F, et al. A long term follow-up in essential cryoglobulinemia. Acta Haematol 1979;61:93–99.
178. Popp JW, et al. Essential mixed cryoglobulinemia without evidence for hepatitis B virus infection. Ann Intern Med 1980;92:379–383.
179. Migliorini P, et al. HLA antigens in essential mixed cryoglobulinemia. Arthritis Rheum 1981;24:932–936.
180. Tarantino A, et al. Renal disease in essential mixed cryoglobulinemia. Long-term follow-up of 44 patients. Q J Med 1981;197:1–30.
181. Maggiore Q, et al. Glomerular localization of circulating antiglobulin activity in essential mixed cryoglobulinemia with glomerulonephritis. Kidney Int 1982;21: 387–394.

182. Cordonnier D, et al. Renal diseases in 18 patients with mixed type II IgM-IgG cryoglobulinemia: monoclonal lymphoid infiltration (2 cases) and membranoproliferative glomerulonephritis. Adv Nephrol 1983;12:177–204.
183. Sinico RA, et al. Identification of glomerular immune deposits in cryoglobulinemia glomerulonephritis. Kidney Int 1988;34:109–116.
184. Frankel AH, et al. Type II essential mixed cryoglobulinaemia: presentation treatment and outcome in 13 patients. Q J Med 1992;101–124.
185. D'Amico G, et al. Renal involvement in essential mixed cryoglobulinemia. Kidney Int 1989;35:1004–1014.
186. Tsai J-F, et al. Increased IgM containing circulating immune complexes in patients co-infected with hepatitis C and hepatitis B. Medicine 1995;74:136–143.
187. Miescher PA, Huang Y-P, Izui S. Type II cryoglobulinemia. Sem Hematol 1995;32: 80–85.
188. Hamburger MI, et al. Mixed cryoglobulinemia: association of glomerulonephritis with defective reticuloendothelial system Fc receptor function. Trans Assoc Am Phys 1979;92:104–112.
189. Monga G, et al. The presence and possible role of monocyte infiltration in human chronic proliferative glomerulonephritides. Am J Pathol 1979;94:271–281.
190. Tarantino A, et al. Long-term predictors of survival in essential mixed cryoglobulinemic glomerulonephritis. Kidney Int 1995;47:618–623.
191. Misani R, et al. Interferon alfa 2 therapy in cryoglobulinemia associated with hepatitis C virus. N Engl J Med 1994;330:751–756.
192. Johnson RJ, et al. Hepatitis C virus-associated glomerulonephritis. Effect of alpha-interferon therapy. Kidney Int 1994;46:1700–1704.
193. Gettner D, et al. The effect of combination therapy (steroids, immunosuppressives and plasmapheresis) on 5 mixed cryoglobulinemia patients with renal, neurologic and vascular involvement. Arthritis Rheum 1981;24:1124–1127.
194. Germain MJ, Anderson RW, Keane WF. Renal disease in cryoglobulinemia type II: response to therapy. A case report and review of the literature. Am J Nephrol 1982;2:221–226.
195. DeVecchi A, et al. Intravenous methylprednisolone pulse therapy in essential cryoglobulinemia nephropathy. Clin Nephrol 1983;19:221–227.
196. Delaney VB, et al. Plasmapheresis as sole therapy in a patient with essential mixed cryoglobulinemia. Am J Kidney Dis 1984;4:75–77.
197. D'Amico G, et al. Renal involvement in essential mixed cryoglobulinemia: a peculiar type of immune mediated renal disease. Adv Nephrol 1988;17:219–240.
198. MacKenzie MR, Fudenberg HH. Macroglobulinemia: an analysis of forty patients. Blood 1972;39:874–889.
199. Dutcher TF, Fahey JL. The histopathology of the macroglobulinemia of Waldenström. J Natl Cancer Inst 1959;22:887–917.
200. Morel-Maroger L, et al. Pathology of the kidney in Waldenström's macroglobulinemia. Study of sixteen cases. N Engl J Med 1970;283:123–129.
201. Lin JH, et al. Waldenström's macroglobulinemia, mesangiocapillary glomerulonephritis angiitis and myositis. Nephron 1973;10:262–270.
202. Meyrier A, et al. Rapidly progressive ("crescentic") glomerulonephritis and monoclonal gammopathies. Nephron 1984;38:156–162.

203. Biava CG, et al. Crescentic glomerulonephritis associated with nonrenal malignancies. Am J Nephrol 1984;4:208–214.
204. Argani I, Kipli GF. Macroglobulinemic nephropathy. Acute renal failure in macroglobulinemia of Waldenstrom. Am J Med 1964;36:151–157.
205. Alpers CE, Cotran RS. Neoplasia and glomerular injury. Kidney Int 1986;30: 465–473.
205a. Gertz MA, Kyle RA, Noel P. Primary systemic amyloidosis: a rare complication of immunoglobulin M monoclonal gammopathies and Waldenstrom's macroglobulinemia. J Clin Oncol 1993;11:94–920.
206. Dathan JRE, Heyworth MF, Maciver AG. Nephrotic syndrome in chronic lymphocytic leukaemia. Br Med J 1974;3:655–657.
207. Cameron S, Ogg CS. Nephrotic syndrome in chronic lymphatic leukaemia. Br Med J 1974;4:164.
208. Gilboa N, et al. Immune deposit nephritis and single-component cryoglobulinemia associated with chronic lymphocyte leukemia. Clin Nephrol 1979;24:223–231.
209. Feehally J, et al. Recurrent proteinuria in chronic lymphocytic leukemia. Clin Nephrol 1981;16:51–64.
210. Stalnikowica R, et al. Hyporeninemic hypoaldosteronism associated with focal glomerular sclerosis in a patient with chronic lymphocytic leukemia. Nephron 1982;31:277–278.
211. White CA, Dillman RO, Royston I. Membranous nephropathy associated with an unusual phenotype of chronic lymphocytic leukemia. Cancer 1983;52:2253–2255.
212. Seney FD Jr, et al. A review of nephrotic syndrome associated with chronic lymphocytic leukemia. Arch Intern Med 1986;146:137–141.
213. Touchard G, et al. Nephrotic syndrome associated with chronic lymphocytic leukemia: an immunological and physiological study. Clin Nephrol 1989;31:107–116.
213a. Edgar JDM, et al. An association between ANCA positive renal disease and malignancy. Clin Nephrol 1993;40:22–25.
214. Editorial. Systemic vasculitis. Lancet 1985;1:1252–1254.
215. Alarcon-Segovia D. The necrotizing vasculitides. A new pathogenetic classification. Med Clin NA 1977;61:241–260.
216. Fauci AS, Haynes BF, Katz P. The spectrum of vasculitis. Clinical, pathologic, immunologic and therapeutic implications. Ann Intern Med 1978;89:660–676.
217. Noel L-H, et al. Antineutrophil cytoplasm antibodies: diversity and clinical applications. Adv in Nephrol 1993;22:237–267.
218. Savage COS, Lockwood CM. Antineutrophil antibodies in vasculitis. Adv Nephrol 1990;19:225–236.
219. Serra A, et al. Vasculitis affecting the kidney: presentation, histopathology and long-term outcome. Q J Med 1984;210:181–207.
220. Adu D, et al. Polyarteritis and the kidney. Q J Med 1987;239:221–237.
221. Bindi P, et al. Necrotizing crescentic glomerulonephritis without significant immune deposits: a clinical and serological study. Q J Med 1993;86:55–68.
222. Gerhardt GM, Ahmad M, Tubbs RR. Pulmonary vasculitis (Wegener's granulomatosis): immunohistochemical study of T and B cell markers. Am J Med 1983;74: 700–704.

223. Parfrey PS, et al. The spectrum of diseases associated with necrotizing glomerulonephritis and its prognosis. Am J Kidney Dis 1985;6:387–396.
224. Furlong TJ, Ibels LS, Eckstein RP. The clinical spectrum of necrotizing glomerulonephritis. Medicine 1987;66:192–201.
225. Ronco P, et al. Immunopathological studies of polyarteritis nodosa and Wegener's granulomatosis: a report of 43 patients with 51 renal biopsies. Q J Med 1983;206: 212–223.
226. Pinching AJ, et al. Wegener's granulomatosis: observations on 18 patients with severe renal disease. Q J Med 1983;208:435–460.
227. Fauci AS. Vasculitis: new insights amid old enigmas. Am J Med 1979;67:916–918.
228. Kauffman RH, et al. Circulating IgA-immune complexes in Henoch-Schonlein purpura. A longitudinal study of their relationship to disease activity and vascular deposition of IgA. Am J Med 1980;69:859–866.
229. D'Agati V, et al. Idiopathic microscopic polyarteritis nodosa: ultrastructural observations on the renal vascular and glomerular lesions. Am J Kidney Dis 1986;7:95–110.
230. Fligiel SEG, et al. Evidence for a role of hydroxyl radical in immune-complex-induced vasculitis. Am J Pathol 1984;115:375–382.
231. Patrick GB. An approach to vasculitis syndromes. Hosp Pract 1982;17:47–65.
232. Bacon PA: Evolving concepts in vasculitis. Q J Med 1985;222:609–610.
233. Hart MN, et al. Autoimmune vasculitis resulting from in vitro immunization of lymphocytes to smooth muscle. Am J Pathol 1985;119:448–455.
234. Garrett PJ, et al. Renal disease associated with circulating antineutrophil cytoplasm activity. Q J Med 1992;306:731–749.
235. Mrowka C, et al. Distribution of the granulocyte serine proteinases proteinase[3] and elastase in human glomulonephritis. Am J Kidney Dis 1995;25:253–261.
236. Wilkowski MJ, et al. Risk factors in idiopathic renal vasculitis and glomerulonephritis. Kidney Int 1989;36:1133–1141.
237. Jeffrey RF, et al. Crescentic glomerulonephritis: experience in a single unit over a five year period. Scott Med J 1992;37:175–178.
238. Gaskin G, Pusey CD: ANCA-associated renal disease. Q J Med 1993;86:138–139.
239. Fauci AS, et al. Wegener's granulomatosis: prospective clinical and therapeutic experience with 85 patients for 21 years. Ann Intern Med 1983;98:76–85.
240. Woodworth TG, et al. Severe glomerulonephritis with late emergence of classic Wegener's granulomatosis. Report of 4 cases and review of the literature. Medicine 1987;66:181–191.
241. Fauci AS, Wolf SM. Wegener's granulomatosis. Studies in eighteen patients and a review of the literature. Medicine 1973;52:535–562.
242. Shillitoe EJ, Lehner T, Lessop MH. Immunological features of Wegener's granulomatosis. Lancet 1974;1:281–284.
243. Landman S, Burgener F. Pulmonary manifestations in Wegener's granulomatosis. Arthr J Rheum 1975;122:750–757.
244. Conn DL, et al. Raised serum immunoglobulin E in Wegener's granulomatosis. Ann Rheum Dis 1976;35:377–380.
245. Baker SB, Robinson DR. Unusual renal manifestations of Wegener's granulomatosis: report of 2 cases. Am J Med 1978;64:885–889.

246. Droz D, et al. Glomerulonephritis and necrotizing angiitis. Adv Nephrol 1979;8: 343–363.
247. Stoker TC, et al. Acute fulminating intrapulmonary hemorrhage in Wegener's granulomatosis. Thorax 1982;37:315–316.
248. Novak RF, Christiansen RG, Sorensen ET. The acute vasculitis of Wegener's granulomatosis in renal biopsies. Am J Clin Pathol 1982;78:367–372.
249. Pinching AJ, et al. Wegener's granulomatosis: observations in 18 patients with severe renal disease. Q J Med 1983;208:435–460.
250. Brandwein S, et al. Wegener's granulomatosis. Clinical features and outcome in 13 patients. Arch Intern Med 1983;143:476–479.
251. tenBerge IJM, et al. Clinical and immunological follow-up of patients with severe renal disease in Wegener's granulomatosis. Am J Nephrol 1985;5:21–29.
252. DeRemee RA, McDonald TJ, Weiland LH. Wegener's granulomatosis. Observations and treatment with antimicrobial agents. Mayo Clin Proc 1985;60:27–32.
253. Weiner SR, Paulus HE, Weisbart RH. Wegener's granulomatosis in the elderly. Arthritis Rheum 1986;29:1157–1159.
254. Parry R, et al. ANCA-associated vasculitis: diagnosis and treatment in the elderly. Postgrad Med J 1996;72:423–427.
255. Appel GB, et al. Wegener's granulomatosis. Clinical-pathologic correlations and long-term course. Am J Kidney Dis 1981;1:27–37.
256. De'Oliviera J, et al. Relationship between disease activity and anti-neutrophil cytoplasmic antibody concentration in long-term management of systemic vasculitis. Am J Kidney Dis 1995;25:380–389.
257. Hind CK, et al. Prognosis after immunosuppression of patients with crescentic nephritis requiring dialysis. Lancet 1983;1:263–265.
258. Pusey CD, et al. Plasma exchange in focal necrotizing glomerulonephritis without anti-glomerular-basement membrane antibodies. Kidney Int 1991;40:757–763.
259. Reinhold-Keller E, et al. Response to trimethroprim/sulfamethoxazole in Wegener's granulomatosis. Q J Med 1996;89:15–23.
260. Stegeman CA, et al. Trimethoprim-sulfamethoxazole (cotrimoxazole) for the prevention of relapses of Wegener's granulomatosis. N Engl J Med 1996; 335:16–20.
261. Higgins RM, et al. Vasculitis and rapidly progressive glomerulonephritis in the elderly. Postgrad Med J 1996;72:41–44.
261a. Huong DLT, et al. Urogenital manifestations of Wegener's granulomatosis. Medicine 1995;74:152–161.
262. D'Agati V, et al. Idiopathic microscopic polyarteritis nodosa: ultrastructural observations in the renal vascular and glomerular lesions. Am J Kid Dis 1986; 7:95–110.
263. Lieb ES, Restivo C, Paulus HE. Immunosuppressive and corticosteroid therapy of polyarteritis nodosa. Am J Med 1979;67:941–945.
264. Cohen RD, Conn DL, Ilstrup DM. Clinical features, prognosis and response to treatment in polyarteritis. Mayo Clin Proc 1980;55:146–155.
265. Fauci AS, et al. Cyclophosphamide therapy of severe systemic necrotizing vasculitis. N Engl J Med 1979;301:235–238.

266. Klein RG, et al. Large artery involvement in giant cell (temporal) arteritis. Ann Intern Med 1975;83:806–812.
267. Balmforth GV. Temporal arteritis and renal failure. Arch Intern Med 1964;113: 230–234.
268. Von Knorring J, Erma M, Lindstrom D. The clinical manifestations of temporal arteritis. Acta Med Scand 1966;179:691–702.
269. Tallgren LG, von Knorring J. Renal vascular involvement in a case of polymyalgia rheumatica with temporal arteritis. A study of successive biopsies. Acta Med Scand 1969;185:421–425.
270. Miller LM, Galdabini JJ. Case records of Massachusetts General Hospital. N Engl J Med 1973;289:628–634.
271. Truong L, et al. Temporal arteritis and renal disease. Case report and review of the literature. Am J Med 1985;78:171–175.
272. Hamilton CR Jr, Shelley WM, Tumulty PA. Giant cell arteritis: including temporal arteritis and polymyalgia rheumatica. Medicine 1971;50:1–27.
273. Nishino H, et al. Wegener's granulomatosis associated with vasculitis of the temporal artery: report of five cases. Mayo Clin Proc 1993;68:115–121.
274. Hunder GG, et al. Daily and alternate-day cortico-steroid regimens in treatment of giant cell arteritis. Comparison in a prospective study. Ann Intern Med 1975;82: 613–618.
275. Bowers DG, Harpur JE, Turks KAD. Giant cell arteritis - the need for prolonged treatment. J Chronic Dis 1973;26:571–573.
276. Cream JJ, Gumpel JM, Peachey RDG. Schonlein-Henoch purpura in the adult. A study of 77 adults with anaphylactoid or Schonlein-Henoch purpura. Q J Med 1970;39:461–484.
277. Ballard HS, Eisinger RP, Gallo G. Renal manifestations of the Schoenlein-Henoch syndrome in adults. Am J Med 1970;49:328–335.
278. Bar-On H, Rosenmann E. Schoenlein-Henoch syndrome in adults. A clinical and histological study of renal involvement. Isr J Med Sci 1972;8:1702–1715.
279. Harrington JT, McCluskey R. Case records Massachusetts General Hospital. N Engl J Med 1983;308:267–273.
280. Roth DA, Wilz DR, Theil GB. Schoenlein-Henoch syndrome in adults. Q J Med 1985;217:145–152.
281. McKenzie PE, et al. Plasmapheresis in glomerulonephritis. Clin Nephrol 1979;12: 97–108.
282. Kiister S, et al. Contrasting clinical course of Henoch-Schonlein purpura in younger and elderly patients. In: Sessa A, Meroni M, Battini G, eds. Glomerulonephritis in the Elderly. Basel: Karger, 1993;Contrib Nephrol 105:93–97.
283. Savage COS, et al. Microscopic polyarteritis: presentation, pathology and prognosis. Q J Med 1985;220:467–483.
284. Chumbley LC, Harrison EG, DeRemee RA. Allergic granulomatosis and angiitis (Churg-Strauss syndrome). Report and analysis of 30 cases. Mayo Clin Proc 1977; 52:477–484.
285. Guillerin L, et al. Prognostic factors in polyarteritis nodosa and Churg-Strauss syndrome. Medicine 1996;75:17–28.

285a. Hogan SL, et al. Prognostic markers in patients with anti-neutrophil cytoplasmic autoantibody-associated microscopic polyangiitis and glomerulonephritis. J Am Soc Nephrol 1996;7:23–32.
285b. Nachman PH, et al. Treatment response and relapse in anti-neutrophil cysoplasmic autoantibody-associated microscopic polyangiitis and glomerulonephritis. J Am Soc Nephrol 1996;7:33–39.
286. Schwartz H, et al. Hypocomplementemic urticarial vasculitis. Association with chronic obstructive pulmonary disease. Mayo Clin Proc 1982;57:231–238.
287. Wismeski J, et al. Hypocomplementemic urticarial vasculitis syndrome: clinical and serologic findings in 18 patients. Medicine 1995;74:24–41.
288. Kellim RE, Haserick JR. Systemic lupus erythematosus. A statistical evaluation of mortality based on a consecutive series of 299 patients. Arch Intern Med 1964;113: 200–207.
289. Dimant J, et al. Systemic lupus erythematosus in the older age group: computer analysis. J Am Geriatr Soc 1979;27:58–61.
290. Hochberg MC, et al. Systemic lupus erythematosus: a review of clinicolaboratory features and immunogenetic markers in 150 patients with emphasis on demographic subsets. Medicine 1985;64:285–295.
291. Morowitz MB, Stevens MB, Shulman LE. The influence of age on the clinical pattern of systemic lupus erythematosus. Arthritis Rheum 1967;10:319–320A.
292. Wilson AH, et al. Age influences the clinical and serologic expression of systemic lupus erythematosus. Arthritis Rheum 1981;24:1230–1235.
293. Grishman E, Gerber MA, Churg J. Patterns of renal injury in systemic lupus erythematosus: light and immunofluorescence microscopic observations. Am J Kidney Dis 1982;2(suppl 1):135–141.
294. Brentjens JR, et al. Interstitial immune complex nephritis in patients with systemic lupus erythematosus. Kidney Int 1975;7:342–350.
295. McCluskey RT. Evidence for an immune complex disorder in systemic lupus erythematosus (SLE). Am J Kidney Dis 1982;2(suppl 1):119–125.
296. Baker SB, et al. Late onset systemic lupus erythematosus. Am J Med 1979;66: 727–732.
297. Cohen AS, Fries J, Masi AT. The 1982 revised criteria for the classification of systemic lupus erythematosus. Arthritis Rheum 1982;25:1271–1277.
298. Friedman S, et al. Glomerular capillary wall function in human lupus nephritis. Am J Physiol 1984;246:F580–F591.
299. Tron F, Ganeval D, Droz D. Immunologically-mediated acute renal failure of nonglomerular origin in the course of systemic lupus erythematosus (SLE). Report of two cases. Am J Med 1979;67:529–532.
300. Epstein FH, McCluskey RT. Case records of the Massachussetts General Hospital. N Engl J Med 1976;294:100–105.
301. Clinicopathologic Conference. Interstitial nephritis in a patient with systemic lupus erythematosus. Am J Med 1980;69:775–781.
302. Yeung CK, et al. Tubular dysfunction in systemic lupus erythematosus. Nephron 1984;36:84–88.
303. DeFronzo RA, Cooke CR, Goldberg M. Impaired renal tubular K secretion in systemic lupus erythematosus. Ann Intern Med 1977;86:268–271.

304. Kiley J, Zager P. Hyporeninemic hypoaldosteronism in two patients with systemic lupus erythematosus. Am J Kidney Dis 1984;4:39–43.
305. Kimberly RP, et al. High-dose intravenous methylprednisone pulse therapy in systemic lupus erythematosus. Am J Med 1981;70:817–824.
306. Boumpas DT, et al. Controlled trial of pulse methylprednisone versus two regimens of pulse cyclophosphamide in severe lupus nephritis. Lancet 1992;340:741–745.
307. Lewis EJ. Plasmapheresis for the treatment of severe lupus nephritis. Uncontrolled observations. Am J Nephrol 1982;2:182–187.
308. Lewis EJ, Lachin J. Primary outcomes in the controlled trial of plasmapheresis therapy (PTT) in severe lupus nephritis. Kidney Int 1987;31:208A.
308a. Esdaile JM, et al. The benefit of early treatment with immunosuppresive agents in lupus nephritis. J Rheumatol 1994;21:2046–2051.
308b. Fraenkel L, et al. Response to treatment as a predictor of longterm outcome in patients with lupus nephritis. J Rheumatol 1994;21:2052–2057.
308c. Ginzler E, et al. Hypertension increases the risk of renal deterioration in systemic lupus erythematosus. J Rheumatol 1993;20:1694–1700.
308d. Remuzzi G, et al. Lupus nephritis: prognostic factors and probability of maintaining life-supporting renal function 10 years after the diagnosis. Am J Kidney Dis 1992;19:473–479.
309. Cannon PJ, et al. The relationship of hypertension and renal failure in scleroderma (progressive systemic sclerosis) to structural and functional abnormalities of the renal cortical circulation. Medicine 1974;53:1–46.
310. Clements PJ, et al. The relationship of arrythmias and conduction disturbances to other manifestations of cardiopulmonary disease in progressive systemic sclerosis (PSS). Am J Med 1981;71:38–46.
311. D'Angelo WA, et al. Pathologic observations in systemic sclerosis. Am J Med 1969;46:428–440.
312. Campbell PM, Le Roy EC. Pathogenesis of systemic sclerosis: a vascular hypothesis. Sem Arthritis Rheum 1975;4:351–368.
313. Kahaleh MB, Sherer GK, Le Roy EC. Endothelial injury in scleroderma. J Exp Med 1979;149:1326–1335.
314. White B. Immunopathogenesis of systemic sclerosis. Rheum Dis Clin NA 1996;22:695–708.
315. Lee P, et al. Mortality in systemic sclerosis (scleroderma). Q J Med 1992;298: 139–148.
316. Oliver JA, et al. Renal vasoactive hormones in scleroderma (progressive systemic sclerosis). Nephron 1981;29:110–116.
317. Thurm RH, Alexander JC. Captopril in the treatment of scleroderma renal crisis. Arch Intern Med 1984;144:733–735.
318. Beckett VL, et al. Use of captopril as early therapy for renal scleroderma: a prospective study. Mayo Clin Proc 1985;60:736–771.
319. Kovalchik MT, et al. The kidney in progressive systemic sclerosis. A prospective study. Ann Intern Med 1978;89:881–887.
320. Traub YM, et al. Hypertension and renal failure (scleroderma renal crisis) in progressive systemic sclerosis. Review of a 25-year experience with 68 cases. Medicine 1983;62:335–352.

321. Steen VD. Scleroderma renal crisis. Rheum Dis Clin NA 1996;22:861–878.
322. Gavras H, et al. Is elevated plasma renin activity of prognostic importance in progressive systemic sclerosis. Arch Intern Med 1977;137:1554–1558.
323. Steen VD, Medsger TA, Rodman GP. D-Penicillamine therapy in progressive systemic sclerosis (scleroderma). Ann Intern Med 1982;97:652–659.
324. Steen VD, et al. Factors predicting development of renal involvement in progressive systemic sclerosis. Am J Med 1984;76:779–786.
325. Medsger TA, Masi AT. Survival with scleroderma II. A life-table analysis of clinical and demographic factors in 358 male U.S. veteran patients. J Chronic Dis 1973;26: 647–660.
326. Whitman HH III, Case DB. New developments in the treatment of scleroderma. Drug Ther 1981;12:85–97.
327. Simon NM, et al. Resolution of renal failure with malignant hypertension in scleroderma. Case report and review of the literature. Am J Med 1979;67:533–539.
328. Whitman HH III, et al. Variable response to oral angiotensin-converting-enzyme blockade in hypertensive scleroderma patients. Arthritis Rheum 1982;25:241–248.
329. Ichikawa I, Miele JF, Brenner BM. Reversal of renal cortical actions of angiotensin II by verapamil and manganese. Kidney Int 1979;16:137–147.
330. Cases A, et al. Captopril vs nifedipine. Clin Nephrol 1987;27:269.
331. Pope JE. Treatment of systemic sclerosis. Rheum Dis Clin NA 1996;22:893–907.
332. Ridolfi RL, Bell WR. Thrombotic thrombocytopenic purpura. Report of 25 cases and review of the literature. Medicine 1981;60:413–428.
333. Knupp CL. Thrombotic thrombocytopenic purpura in older patients. J Am Geriatr Soc 1988;36:331–338.
334. Schmidt JL. Thrombotic thrombocytopenic purpura: successful treatment unlocks etiologic secrets. Mayo Clin Proc 1989;64:956–961.
335. Editorial. Hemolytic uraemic syndrome. Lancet 1984;2:1078–1079.
336. Neild G: The haemolytic uraemic syndrome: a review. Q J Med 1987;241:367–376.
337. Grem JL, Merritt JA, Carbone PP. Treatment of mytocin-associated microangiopathic hemolytic anemia with vincristine. Arch Intern Med 1986;146:566–568.
338. Hostetter AL, et al. Chronic glomerular microangiopathy complicating metastatic carcinoma. Hum Pathol 1987;18:342–348.
339. Morel-Maroger L, et al. Prognostic importance of vascular lesions in acute renal failure with microangiopathic hemolytic anemia (hemolytic-uremic syndrome): clinicopathologic study in 20 adults. Kidney Int 1979;15:548–558.
340. Eknoyan G, Riggs SA. Renal involvement in patients with thrombotic thrombocytopenic purpura. Am J Nephrol 1986;6:117–131.
341. Thorsen CA, et al. The treatment of the hemolytic uremic syndrome with inhibitors of platelet function. Am J Med 1979;66:711–716.
342. Hakim RM, et al. Successful management of thrombocytopenia, microangiopathic anemia and acute renal failure by plasmapheresis. Am J Kidney Dis 1985;5: 170–176.
343. Myers TJ, et al. Thrombotic thrombocytopenic purpura: combined treatment with plasmapheresis and antiplatelet agents. Ann Intern Med 1980;92:149–155.

344. Brun C, et al. Renal biopsy in rheumatoid arthritis. Nephron 1965;2:65–81.
345. Samuels B, et al. Membranous nephropathy in patients with rheumatoid arthritis: relationship to gold therapy. Medicine 1977;57:319–327.
346. Helin HJ, et al. Renal biopsy findings and clinicopathologic correlations in rheumatoid arthritis. Arthritis Rheum 1995;38:242–247.
347. Schmid FR, et al. Arteritis in rheumatoid arthritis. Am J Med 1961;30:56–83.
348. Scott DGI, Bacon PA, Tribe CR. Systemic rheumatoid vasculitis. A clinical and laboratory study of 50 cases. Medicine 1981;60:288–297.
349. Meriwether JH Jr, Weinberger HJ, Gleason IO. The renal vascular lesion in rheumatoid disease. Arthritis Rheum 1967;10:298A.
350. Kuznetsky KA, et al. Necrotizing glomerulonephritis in rheumatoid arthritis. Clin Nephrol 1986;26:257–264.
350a. Harper L, et al. Focal segmental necrotizing glomerulonephritis in rheumatoid arthritis. Q J Med 1997;90:125–132.
351. McAdam LP, et al. Relapsing polychondritis: prospective study of 23 patients and a review of the literature. Medicine 1976;55:193–215.
352. Chang-Miller A, et al. Renal involvement in relapsing polychondritis. Medicine 1987;66:202–217.
353. Neild GH, et al. Relapsing polychondritis with crescentic glomerulonephritis. Br Med J 1978;1:743–745.
354. Espinoza LR, et al. Immune-complex-mediated renal involvement in relapsing polychondritis. Am J Med 1981;71:181–183.
355. Bloch KJ, et al. Sjogren's syndrome. A clinical, pathological and serological study of sixty-two cases. Medicine 1965;44:187–231.
356. Pavlidis NA, Karsh J, Motsopoulos HM. The clinical picture of primary Sjogren's syndrome: a retrospective study. J Rheumatol 1982;9:685–690.
357. Kahn M, et al. Renal concentrating defect in Sjogren's syndrome. Ann Intern Med 1962;56:883–895.
358. Whaley K, et al. Sjogren's syndrome. Q J Med 1973;167:513–548.
359. Talal N, Zisman E, Schur PH. Renal tubular acidosis, glomerulonephritis and immunologic factors in Sjogren's syndrome. Arthritis Rheum 1968;11:774–786.
359a. Eriksson P, et al. Biochemical markers of renal disease in primary Sjogren's syndrome. Scand J Urol Nephrol 1995;29:383–92.
360. El-Mallakh RS, et al. Long-term low-dose glucocorticoid therapy associated with remission of overt renal tubular acidosis in Sjogren's syndrome. Am J Med 1985;79:509–514.
361. Tu WH, et al. Interstitial nephritis in Sjogren's syndrome. Ann Intern Med 1968;69:1163–1170.
362. Motsopoulos HM, et al. Immune complex glomerulonephritis in sicca syndrome. Am J Med 1978;64:955–960.
363. Abraham PA, Keane WF. Glomerular and interstitial disease induced by nonsteroidal anti-inflammatory drugs. Am J Nephrol 1984;4:1–6.
364. Garella S, Matarese RA. Renal effects of prostaglandins and clinical adverse effects of non-steroidal anti-inflammatory agents. Medicine 1984;63:165–181.
365. Clive DM, Stoff JS. Renal syndromes associated with non-steroidal anti-inflammatory drugs. N Engl J Med 1984;310:563–572.

366. Carmichael T, Shankel SW. Effects of non-steroidal anti-inflammatory drugs on prostaglandins and renal function. Am J Med 1985;78:992–1000.
367. Cameron JS. Immunologically mediated interstitial nephritis: primary and secondary. Adv Nephrol 1989;18:207–248.
368. Radford GM, et al. Reversible membranous nephropathy associated with the use of nonsteroidal anti-inflammatory drugs. JAMA 1996;276:466–469.
369. Lamy PP. Renal effects of non-steroidal anti-inflammatory drugs. Heightened risk in the elderly? J Am Geriatr Soc 1986;34:361–367.
370. Mignon F, et al. Granulomatous interstitial nephritis. Adv Nephrol 1984;13: 219–245.
371. Warren GV, et al. Minimal change glomerulopathy associated with non-steroidal anti-inflammatory drugs. Am J Kidney Dis 1989;13:127–130.
372. Neugarten J, Gallo GR, Baldwin DS. Rifampin-induced nephrotic syndrome and acute interstitial nephritis. Am J Nephrol 1983;3:38–42.
373. Kean WF, et al. Efficacy and toxicity of D-penicillamine for rheumatoid disease in the elderly. J Am Geriatr Soc 1982;30:94–100.
374. Harkness JAL, Blake DR. Penicillamine nephropathy and iron. Lancet 1982;2: 1368–1369.
375. Hall CL, et al. Natural course of penicillamine nephropathy. A long-term study of 33 patients. Br Med J 1988;296:1083–1086.
376. Walshe JM. Management of penicillamine nephropathy in Wilson's disease: a new chelating agent. Lancet 1969;2:1401–1403.
377. Gaskin G, Thompson EM, Pusey CD. Goodpasture-like syndrome associated with anti-myeloperoxidase antibodies following penicillamine treatment. Nephrol Dial Transplant 1995;10:1925–1928.
378. Sternlieb I, Bennett B, Scheinberg HI. D-penicillamine induced Goodpasture's syndrome in Wilson's disease. Ann Intern Med 1975;82:673–676.
379. Gibson T, Burry HC, Ogg C. Goodpasture's syndrome and D-penicillamine. Ann Intern Med 1976;84:100.
380. Matloff DS, Kaplan MM. D-penicillamine-induced Goodpasture's like syndrome in primary biliary cirrhosis. Successful treatment with plasmapheresis and immunosuppressives. Gastroenterology 1980;78:1046–1049.
381. Ntoso KA, et al. Penicillamine-induced rapidly progressive glomerulonephritis in patients with progressive systemic sclerosis: successful treatment of two patients and a review of the literature. Am J Kidney Dis 1986;8:159–163.
382. Katz WA, Blodgett RC Jr, Pietrusko RG. Proteinuria in gold treated rheumatoid arthritis. Ann Intern Med 1984;101:176–179.
383. Hall CL. Gold nephropathy. Nephron 1988;50:265–272.
384. Silverberg DS, et al. Gold nephropathy. A clinical and pathologic study. Arthritis Rheumat 1970;13:812–825.
385. Wooley PH, et al. HLA-DR antigens and toxic reaction to sodium aurothiomalate and D-penicillamine in patients with rheumatoid arthritis. N Engl J Med 1980;303:300–302.
386. Grant JT, Husby G, Thorsby E. HLA-DR antigens and gold toxicity. Ann Rheum Dis 1983;42:63–66.

387. Shaw CF. The biochemistry and subcellular distribution of gold in kidney tissue: implications of chrysotherapy and nephrotoxicity. Agents Actions 1981;8(suppl): 509–528.
388. Case DB, et al. Proteinuria during long-term captopril therapy. JAMA 1980;244: 346–349.
389. Lewis EJ. Angiotensin-converting enzyme inhibitors: considerations regarding proteinuria. Am J Kidney Dis 1987;10:30–38.
390. Textor SC, et al. Membranous glomerulopathy associated with captopril therapy. Am J Med 1983;74:705–712.
391. Adler SG, Cohen AH, Border WA. Hypersensitivity phenomena and the kidney. Role of drugs and environmental agents. Am J Kidney Dis 1985;5:75–96.
392. Terpenning MS, Buggy BP, Kauffman CA. Infective endocarditis. Clinical features in young and elderly patients. Am J Med 1987;83:626–634.
393. Neugarten J, Gallo GR, Baldwin DS. Glomerulonephritis in bacterial endocarditis. Am J Kidney Dis 1984;3:371–379.
394. Beaufils M, et al. Glomerulonephritis in severe bacterial infections with or without endocarditis. Adv Nephrol 1978;7:217–234.
395. Forrest JW Jr, et al. Immune complex glomerulonephritis associated with *Klebsiella pneumoniae* infection. Clin Nephrol 1977;7:76–80.
396. Magil AB. Monocytes and glomerulonephritis associated with remote visceral infection. Clin Nephrol 1984;22:169–175.
397. Beaufils M, et al. Acute renal failure of glomerular origin during visceral abscesses. N Engl J Med 1976;295:185–189.
398. Coleman M, et al. Glomerulonephritis associated with chronic bacterial infection of a dacron arterial prosthesis. Clin Nephrol 1983;20:315–320.
399. Montseney J-J, et al. The current spectrum of infectious glomerulonephritis. Evidence with 76 patients and review of the literature. Medicine 1995;74:63–73.
400. Guillevin L, et al. Polyarteritis nodosa related to hepatitis B virus. Medicine 1995;74:238–253.
401. Mazzaro C, et al. Clinical and virological findings in mixed cryoglobulinemia. J Intern Med 1995;238:153–1660.
402. Schifferli JA, French LE, Tissot J-D. Hepatitis C virus infection, cryoglobulinemia and glomerulonephritis. Adv Nephrol 1995;24:107–129.
403. Johnson RJ, et al. Renal manifestations of hepatitis C virus infection. Kidney Int 1994;46:1255–1263.
404. Cohen AH. Renal pathology of HIV-associated nephropathy. Contemp Issues Nephrol 1995;29:155–180.
405. Hannedouche T, et al. Renal granulomatous sarcoidosis: report of six cases. Nephrol Dial Transplant 1990;5:18–24.
406. Singer DR, Evans DRJ. Renal impairment in sarcoidosis: granulomatous nephritis as an isolated cause (two case reports and a review of the literature). Clin Nephrol 1981;26:250–256.

8

Urolithiasis and Obstructive Uropathy

I. UROLITHIASIS

A. Incidence and Prevalence

Ten to nineteen percent of patients seen in a community practice for their first symptomatic kidney stone are 60 years of age or more (1–2a). Sixty three percent are between the ages of 30 and 60 years and 18% are below the age of 30 (1–3). The prevalence of renal calculi in the elderly in the United States varies geographically, increasing from north to south and from west to east (4). Males outnumber females by approximately 2.5:1. The prevalence in the United States for males aged 60–69 is 10% in Whites, 9% in Hispanics, 7% in Asians, and 5% in Blacks, and for females it is 4% in Whites, 4% in Hispanics, 3% in Blacks, and 2% in Asians. In males 70 years and older, the prevalence is 9% in Whites, 6% in Hispanics, 5% in Asians, and 4% in Blacks. The prevalence is similar among the various ethnic groups for women 70 years and older (4). In another study, White and Asian males were found to form stones more frequently than females. The reverse was noted for Blacks and Hispanics (5). This gender difference and a peak prevalence rate for individuals 60–69 years of age has also been noted in other countries (6,7).

Differences in exposure to temperature, sunlight, and liquids may contribute to the geographic variability noted in the United States (8).

B. Etiology

The etiology of kidney stones in the elderly is similar to that in younger patients. Based on stone analysis in a relatively small number (35) of well-studied patients, we found calcium oxalate in 75%, uric acid (pure or mixed) in 10%, struvite in 5%, and phosphate in the remainder. In a recent retrospective analysis of 5942 patients with urolithiasis, 12% were 65 years and older. Seventy-four percent of the stones were calcium oxalate, 11% were uric acid, 7% were calcium/uric acid, and 6% were calcium phosphate. The remaining 2 % were made of struvite, cystine, and triamterene (8a). In 40% of patients, neither metabolic nor structural abnormalities could be found. Hypercalciuria was present in 30%, with hyperuricosuria in 10%, chronic infection in 10%, hyperoxaluria in 5%, and hypocitraturia in 5%.

C. Pathogenesis

1. General

Stones form when salts present in the urine (e.g., calcium oxalate, calcium phosphate) crystallize in the renal tubule and collecting system. The different mechanisms responsible for this phenomenon include: (a) supersaturation, because a solubilizer for the constituent substances is excreted at a low rate (e.g., citrate for calcium oxalate) (9), or the volume of distribution of the constituents (in this case urine) is low, or an appropriate milieu facilitating insolubility or precipitation (e.g., low urine pH for uric acid stones) is present; (b) formation of alternative nuclei such as cell debris, uric acid, or a calcium phosphate crystal nidus that promote crystallization (a process referred to as heterogeneous nucleation) (10); (c) deficiency of naturally occurring inhibitors such as uropontin, Tamm-Horsfall proteins, nephrocalcin, or glycosaminoglyclans (glycoproteins which are capable of inhibiting the growth of calcium oxalate crystals by adsorption on their surface) (11–13). Renal epithelial cells have been found to bind and internalize calcium oxalate crystals, a process which can be inhibited by certain anionic molecules such as chondroitin sulfates A, B (13a,13b). The role of crystal adhesion in the pathogenesis of stone formation remains to be defined.

Our finding of 40% of elderly patients with no detectable abnormality is higher than the 10–25% found in the general population (14,15), but similar to the 37% reported by Gentle et al. (8a). In their study, no metabolic abnormality was found in 32% of younger patients. These patients form primarily calcium oxalate stones and it is not clear what exactly triggers the process of stone formation. The possibilities include: (a) an imbalance between urinary calcium and citrate in favor of the former (the so-called calcium-citrate index) (16); (b) an anomalous cellular transport of oxalate (17); (c) a mild degree of hyperoxaluria (18); and (d) the formation of a qualitatively defective glycoprotein inhibitor (19). It should be noted that these studies suggesting mechanisms for stone formation were performed in younger patients and may not be entirely applicable in the elderly, keeping in mind that supersaturation for calcium oxalate and calcium phosphate decreases with age in stone formers but remains the same for uric acid (19a). Early-morning crystalluria (mainly calcium phosphate) has been found in the elderly more commonly than in the general adult population (20).

2. *Hypercalciuria*

Hypercalciuria is defined as a urinary excretion of calcium greater than 140 mg/g of urinary creatinine. Hypercalciuria, which occurs either alone or combined with hyperoxaluria or hyperuricosuria, is divided into hypercalcemic and normocalcemic varieties. In our experience, hypercalcemic hypercalciuria with stone formation occurs almost exclusively in the elderly with hyerparathyroidism and sarcoidosis. In these situations the high urinary calcium is a function of an increase in filtered load (see hypercalcemia in Chapter 5). Stone formers with normocalcemic hypercalciuria have type I renal tubular acidosis (RTA), are immobilized, or have idiopathic hypercalciuria. Distal RTA (type I) is rarely a cause of lithiasis in the elderly. In these patients the hypercalciuria reflects a decrease in tubular reabsorption of calcium due to the acidosis per se (21). During acidosis there is an increase in citrate oxidation by renal cortical cell mitochondria, which lowers its urinary concentration (22). Since citrate normally binds about half of the urine calcium, more free calcium is available for crystallization with phosphate, resulting in stone formation. The high urinary concentration of phosphate is a result of the persistently alkaline urine, characteristic of this form of RTA.

Prolonged immobilization with its resulting resorptive hypercalciuria has been associated with calcium oxalate or mixed stones in younger patients and, with a lesser frequency, in the elderly (23–25).

The "idiopathic" variety is by far the most common form of hypercalciuria found in the elderly stone former; the renal type is present in 80% and the absorptive type is seen in the remaining 20% (26,27). Patients with hypercalciuria are a heterogeneous group in whom one or more of the following abnormalities are operative: (a) a decrease in the thick ascending limb of Henle calcium reabsorption, either as a primary phenomenon (28) or induced by phosphate depletion—the major defect in the latter group may be an intrinsic defect in proximal tubular phosphate reabsorption through a non-parathyroid hormone (PTH)-dependent mechanism (29); (b) accelerated intestinal calcium absorption, resulting in an increase in the postprandial serum calcium concentration, followed by suppression of PTH—the increase in jejunal calcium absorption may be secondary to an increase in the mucosal cell sensitivity to normal levels of $1,25(OH)_2$ vitamin D_3 or to an increase in sensitivity of renal 1-alpha-hydroxylase to circulating PTH (see Chapter 5) for those with elevated $1,25(OH)_2$ vitamin D_3 (30,31); (c) both an elevation of intestinal calcium absorption and a defect in renal calcium reabsorption (32,33).

The percentage of elderly patients with hypercalciuria who will form stones is not clear. For those who do, in addition to the hypercalciuria, abnormalities of the different crystal growth inhibitors are likely playing a significant role (34–36).

3. *Hyperuricosuria*

Hyperuricosuria is defined as a urine excretion of uric acid above 800 mg/day. Patients with hyperuricosuria may form pure uric acid stones, pure calcium oxalate and/or phosphate stones, or stones containing both calcium oxalate and uric acid. Patients in the last group are referred to as mixed-stone formers and usually are hypercalciuric (37). Pure uric acid stones are the most common in the elderly with hyperuricosuria, followed by mixed and calcium oxalate stones, in that order.

Uric acid stones, which are more common in the elderly than in younger subjects (8a), form when the urinary concentration of undissociated uric acid exceeds its solubility limit, which in humans is approximately 96 mg/L at 37°C (38). Because the dissociation of uric acid is pH dependent, the lower the urinary pH the higher the concentration of undissociated uric acid. In the presence of a low urine pH (5.5), the urine becomes supersaturated with free uric acid, thereby increasing the risk of stone formation (39). The impact of a change in urine pH on uric acid stone formation is greater than a change in the amount of uric acid excreted. Dietary purine excess from meat is largely responsible for the hyperuricosuria and low urinary pH. When there patients are placed on a purine-free diet, urine uric acid decreases dramatically (39). The fact that serum uric acid remains in the normal range on a high-purine diet appears to rule out a significant defect in tubular handling of urate.

Patients with mixed stones produce urine supersaturated with respect to calcium oxalate and uric acid, whereas those with either calcium oxalate or uric acid stones present an imbalance in supersaturation favoring one crystal over the other (40). The precipitation of calcium oxalate with subsequent stone formation in the hyperuricosuric patient is initiated by seed crystals of sodium hydrogen urate or uric acid through the process of heterogeneous nucleation (41). The cause for the hyperuricosuria is also dietary overindulgence in purine-rich foods. Both calcium and oxalate excretion are usually normal in these patients (42,43).

4. *Struvite Stones (Associated with Urinary Tract Infection)*

Struvite stones are made of magnesium ammonium phosphate ($MgNH_4PO_4{\cdot}6H_2O$) and form only in the presence of bacteria that possess urease, an enzyme capable of hydrolyzing urea to ammonia (urea-splitting organisms). The latter, in turn, hydrolyzes spontaneously to ammonium hydroxide, which increases urine pH. The alkaline milieu facilitates an increase in the concentration of deprotonated phosphate, and since magnesium is always present in the urine, struvite stones form. The stones grow as bacteria multiply and are found almost exclusively in women. Their occurrence in men usually means the presence of additional hypercalciuria

(44). The organisms responsible for struvite stones in the elderly are the same as those reported in younger patients, with *Proteus* species being the most common (45). Struvite stones, like uric acid stones, can become very large and are capable of filling the whole collecting system (stag-horn calculus).

5. *Hyperoxaluria*

Hyperoxaluria (urinary oxalate excretion greater than 40 mg/24 hr) may be present alone or combined with hypercalciuria or hyperuricosuria. The latter is more common in the elderly (8a). Hyperoxaluria occurs in the elderly with intestinal malabsorption and is secondary to increased oxalate absorption in the colon (46). Because of the increased oxalate excretion, the urine is supersaturated with respect to calcium oxalate, favoring crystallization (47). It has been demonstrated that an increase in urinary oxalate concentration increases supersaturation even more than an equivalent increase in calcium concentration (48). Other auxiliary factors that may be critical are low urinary output due to the presence of volume contraction in many of these patients, and low urinary citrate, a reflection of citrate malabsorption and metabolic acidosis. The latter is secondary to bicarbonate losses through the gastrointestinal tract. Since urinary pH may be persistently low in these patients, uric acid stones might also form (see earlier discussion).

6. *Hypocitraturia*

Urinary citrate inhibits crystallization and precipitation of calcium through its interaction with Tamm-Horsfall protein. Hypocitraturia (urinary citrate less than 3 mmol/L or 320 mg/day) is present in a significant number of elderly with nephrolithiasis and might be a consequence of the subclinical metabolic acidosis associated with aging (see Chapter 1). In some, it is due to the presence of mild chronic metabolic acidosis induced by carbonic anhydrase inhibitor (acetazolamide) therapy for glaucoma. Calcium phosphate stones in these patients tend to form during the first 12 months of acetazolamide therapy. Besides hypocitruria, hypermagnesiuria and perhaps an intermittent rise in urine pH due to transient decreases in bicarbonate reabsorption (at the peak of drug action) also contribute to the calcium monohydrogen phosphate supersaturation (48,49). Some patients who form stones during acetazolamide administration also have an abnormality in calcium excretion when studied after discontinuing acetazolamide (48). It should be noted that hypocitruria is not limited to calcium phosphate stone formers. Not infrequently, hypocitruria is the only metabolic abnormality in patients with calcium oxalate nephrolithiasis (50,51).

Cystinuria as a cause for nephrolithiasis practically never occurs de novo in the elderly. Since cystinuria is due to an inherited defect in the tubular transport of various dibasic amino acids (cystine, ornithine, lysine, arginine), these patients start to form stones at an earlier age.

D. Clinical Manifestations

The clinical manifestations of urolithiasis in the elderly are similar to those younger patients. Flank pain radiating to the groin, with gross or microscopic hematuria, is the most frequent presentation. Urinary infection, manifest by chills and fever and frequently associated with costophrenic angle tenderness, may be present in obstructing stone disease and is also seen in patients with struvite stones. Patients with only one functioning kidney (in some of our patients a small nonfunctioning contralateral kidney was a consequence of severe renal artery disease) may present with anuria. In a significant number of patients, particularly those with struvite stones, stones are found during the investigation for recurrent urinary tract infection or during radiological evaluation for hematuria. On requestioning, these patients will often describe having dull, persistent loin discomfort of some duration.

E. Treatment and Prognosis

Since specific therapy is dependent on the specific pathogenesis, it is important to decide which patients with urolithiasis require a metabolic workup. To answer this question, it is necessary to outline the procedure to be followed, the potential for recurrence, and the benefit(s) to be obtained from the information gained. Our initial work-up includes three 24-hr urine collections for determination of calcium, oxalate, uric acid, phosphate, citrate, pH, and volume. Blood is also taken for determination of urea, creatinine, calcium, phosphorus, total carbon dioxide, and uric acid levels. The mean values from the three collections are then determined, and, depending on the results, additional studies may be necessary, including obtaining a serum PTH and 1,25-$(OH)_2$ vitamin D_3 level, urinary cyclic AMP, and others. The median time to recurrence in the elderly (i.e., the time it takes for 50% of the patients to have a recurrence) is 11 ± 5 years, with 39% forming a second stone within 6.8 ± 0.6 years (2). There appears to be no difference in the recurrence rate between older and younger patients and between patients with and without a metabolic abnormality (8a,14). With this background information, the decision to do an extensive evaluation must be individualized, keeping in mind that diagnosis and treatment of the underlying problems are effective as well as cost effective (52), although we will try to provide some broad guidelines.

As in younger patients, our approach in the elderly patient with clinical evidence of urolithiasis is to treat the acute episode with analgesics (either with opiates or a nonsteroidal antiinflammatory drug) (53) and hydration. Patients who cannot take oral fluids because of nausea or vomiting, those with fever, and those in whom there is a strong suspicion of obstruction should be admitted to the hospital. Forty percent of our patients have been managed on an outpatient basis. Fifty percent of the elderly pass the stone spontaneously, compared to 65% of younger patients. In the remaining half, some form of urological intervention is required (54). The percentage of patients with residual stones noted with a sonogram or by X-ray in our experience is approximately 30%, with 20% having bilateral involvement. An intravenous pyelogram or a noncontrast CT scan should be obtained at some point in all elderly patients with urolithiasis and normal kidney function (55).

Once the acute episode is over, patients with organic brain syndrome, those who are frail and bedridden, and those with associated diseases with a potentially poor prognosis need not be studied metabolically. They are placed on a high-fluid intake and followed regularly with a KUB or sonogram to assess stone recurrence or growth. Urological evaluation for possible extracorporeal shock wave lithotripsy (ESWL) is advised (see later discussion) for patients with struvite stones less than 2 cm in size. Stones larger than 2 cm are best approached by percutaneous nephrolithotomy, which is relatively safe in the elderly (56), and is also the procedure of choice for lower-pole branched stones. ESWL is better for stones in the upper pole. Advanced renal insufficiency (serum creatinine > 4 mg/dl) is an absolute contraindication to ESWL. Stones located in the lower ureters are usually handled through ureteroscopy or ESWL (56a). We emphasize complete investigation in all patients with recurrences (if they have not been previously studied) (57). Stone formers with associated osteoporosis should also be fully evaluated, since the hypercalciuria noted in some is not accompanied by the usual compensatory intestinal hyperabsorption of calcium. This latter defect predisposes these patients to negative calcium balance with consequent stimulation of the parathyroids and enhanced skeletal mobilization of calcium (58).

1. Specific Therapy: Nonpharmacological

Fluid intake sufficient to ensure a urine volume above 2.5 L/day is recommended (59). Urine dilution has been found to reduce the propensity for the crystallization of calcium salts by lowering the urinary saturation of brushite (CaH_2O, which may be acting as the initial crystal nidus for certain calcium containing renal stones) and calcium oxalate and by increasing the minimum supersaturation required to elicit spontaneous nucleation of calcium oxalate (60). This approach, however, when used as the sole therapeutic modality, has not been convincingly shown to prevent stone formation (61) and might depend on the type of fluids used (62).

In patients with absorptive hyperoxaluria, beets, spinach, grapefruit, chocolate, nuts, and tea should be avoided. In addition, supplemental vitamin C should be discouraged or at least kept below 1 g/day (63). Those with uric acid and mixed stones should moderate their intake of foods rich in animal proteins. Patients with calcium oxalate stones and hypercalciuria should consider lowering their sodium intake to below 4 g/day and moderate their protein intake, if high (64–66). Dietary calcium restriction does not play a role in the management of the elderly with nephrolithiasis, as estimated calcium intake and bone mineral density are both lower in stone formers (67–68).

2. *Specific Therapy: Pharmacological*

In patients with recurrent calcium oxalate stones and no detectable urinary abnormality, we use the regimen originally proposed by Coe (14), which consists of allopurinol, 100 mg daily, and hydrochlorthiazide, 25–50 mg daily, with a 2–4 g daily sodium diet. This regimen has, in general, been well accepted and tolerated in the elderly. More recently, a combination of 42 mEq potassium, 21 mEq magnesium, and 63 mEq of citrate taken orally daily has been found to reduce significantly the risk of recurrent calcium oxalate nephrolithiasis (68a).

Hypercalciuria (both renal and absorptive) usually responds to thiazides and salt restriction (68b), although the hypocalciuric effect of the diuretic may be attenuated in time in patients with the absorptive form of the syndrome (69). The thiazides decrease urinary calcium excretion by acting directly on calcium reabsorption in the distal tubule (70), as well as by inducing a state of volume contraction (maintained by a low-sodium diet), which leads to enhanced proximal reabsorption of both sodium and calcium, thereby decreasing distal delivery. Finally, the thiazide-induced alkalosis may also contribute to the decrease in calcium excretion. We usually start with hydrochlorothiazide, 25 mg/day. In patients in whom urinary calcium excretion is not normalized, the dose is increased to 25 mg twice a day. The majority of our elderly respond to this regimen. Hypokalemia, which lowers urinary citrate, develops in 10–15% of the patients, and should be treated with potassium citrate, 15–30 mEq, twice a day. In the presence of persistent hypercalciuria despite a maximum dose of thiazide, amiloride, 2.5 mg twice a day, can be added. Since this drug increases distal tubule calcium reabsorption through a mechanism different from that of the thiazides, its hypocalciuric effect is additive (71,72).

When attenuation or loss of the hypocalciuric response to thiazides occurs in a patient with absorptive hypercalciuria, the drug may be temporarily withdrawn (for 6–10 weeks), after which there may be restoration of a normal response. Sodium cellulose phosphate, 10–15 g/day, could be substituted in the interim (73), or the slow-release form of potassium phosphate (UroPhosK), 4 tablets twice daily with meals (74), which provides 63.5 mEq of potassium a day.

In patients with uric acid stones, a low-purine diet is recommended, along with potassium citrate, 15–40 mEq twice a day, the last dose given at bedtime to assure a high overnight urine pH. The goal is to raise urine pH to 6.0. Higher levels are undesirable because they may favor secondary calcium phosphate stones (75). Allopurinol (100–300 mg/day) is added if hyperuricosuria is present. This drug is also the agent of choice for the hyperuricosuric patient who forms calcium oxalate stones (76).

Struvite stones are usually large and often associated with infection, parenchymal damage, and progressive loss of kidney function. Antibiotic therapy alone is inadequate. These patients should be referred for surgery (77) or other procedures such as ESWL for small stones (78,79). Larger stones (>2 cm) are best managed by a combination of percutaneous nephrolithothripsy and ESWL and chemical dissolution of residual infected fragments with acetohydroxamic acid, a bacterial urease inhibitor (80). Because of potential serious side effects, we believe this drug should be administered with great caution and awareness of the problems (81,82).

The ideal treatment for intestinal hyperoxaluria is control of the underlying disease, in addition to dietary restriction of oxalate-containing foods. Since this is not always feasible, other approaches have to be tried. Oral administration of large amounts of calcium, 250–1000 mg with meals, has been recommended (82). The calcium decreases gut absorption and urinary excretion of oxalate; however, because of a concurrent increase in urinary calcium excretion, there is really no significant change in the urinary state of saturation with respect to calcium oxalate. Magnesium gluconate, which binds dietary oxalate, 0.5–1.0 g every 8 hr, may be tried, as well as cholestyramine, 8–16 g/day, which can also adsorb dietary oxalate. Unfortunately, cholestyramine may interfere with the absorption of vitamin K and other drugs commonly used by the elderly (e.g., digoxin). Patients who are acidotic can be managed with potassium citrate at the usual dose outlined above. Attention should also be paid to adequate hydration (68).

In patients who form calcium phosphate stones while taking acetazolamide, the drug should be discontinued, if possible. If not, potassium citrate can be used to prevent stone formation (83). These patients should undergo metabolic evaluation to rule out abnormalities in calcium excretion.

Therapy for the hypercalcemic hypercalciuric patient who forms stones is that of the underlying cause for the hypercalcemia (see Chapter 5). Cystinuria is managed with high fluid intake, urinary alkalinization, and D-penicillamine.

The rate of recurrence of kidney stones in the elderly undergoing therapy is not known (our short follow-up and relatively small number of patients do not permit us to provide an answer). In one prospective study dealing with younger patients, the authors were able to use three characteristics to identify those patients most likely to relapse (84): (a) patients in whom there was a short interval between the time they entered the authors' program and their last episode of urolithiasis; (b) patients who had a higher urinary calcium excretion (2.79 versus 2.39 mg/kg for the nonrecurrent patients); (c) patients with a low urinary volume. Other investigators (85) have used a stepwise discriminant analysis, selecting plasma albumin, urinary pH, urinary calcium excretion, plasma phosphate, GFR, and nephrogenic cyclic AMP as the most important variables contributing to the difference between controls and recurrent stone formers. Patients with recurrent stones, despite therapy-induced "normalization" of their urinary findings, are managed symptomatically during the acute episode. We usually continue long-term therapy, since the risks associated with stone formation far exceed the risks associated with therapy (86).

II. OBSTRUCTIVE UROPATHY

As with younger patients, urinary obstruction in the elderly can be either unilateral or bilateral. In this section we discuss obstruction as a cause of renal impairment in the elderly; therefore, unless the disease process involves a patient with only one functioning kidney, our focus is mainly on bilateral obstruction.

A. Incidence and Prevalence

Obstructive uropathy is responsible for 10–15% of acute renal failure seen in the elderly (87–90). Since 4–6% of elderly patients in the hospital are evaluated for renal failure, the frequency of clinically significant obstructive uropathy will vary between 0.4% and 0.6%.

B. Etiology

Obstruction, which can be either intrinsic or extrinsic, can occur at any level of the urinary tract in the elderly. It should be considered in any patient with renal insufficiency, whether acute or chronic. The different causes for obstructive uropathy in 116 patients are outlined in Table 1. Seventy-five patients (65%) were males. Prostatic disease was the most common cause in males; in females, it was bladder involvement (either neurogenic or cancerous), followed by tumors of the pelvic organs (ovaries, uterus, cervix).

Table 1 Etiology of Obstructive Uropathy in 116 Elderly Patients

Diagnosis	Number of patients (%)
Nonmalignant causes	
Prostatic hypertrophy	41 (35)
Neurogenic bladder	18 (16)
Urolithiasis	7 (6.5)
Obstructive pyelonephritis (papillary necrosis)	7 (6.5)
Urethral stricture	4 (3)
Others (ureteropelvic junction, retroperitoneal fibrosis)	4 (3)
	Total 81 (70)
Malignant causes	
Prostatic cancer	14 (12)
Bladder cancer	9 (8)
Pelvic tumors	6 (5)
Others (colon, retroperitoneal tumors)	6 (5)
	Total 35 (30)

Source: Adapted from Kumar R, Hill CM, McGeown MG. Acute renal failure in the elderly. Lancet 1973; 1:90–91, and the authors' experience.

C. Clinical Manifestations

A significant number of patients are asymptomatic, with the diagnosis uncovered during investigation for renal insufficiency. This is particularly common in patients with neurogenic bladder or those with pelvic malignancy, in whom an elevated serum creatinine may be discovered during evaluation for chemotherapy. Symptoms are variable and include anuria (if the obstruction is complete rather than partial) pelvic discomfort, prostatism, dysuria if concomitant infection is present, new onset of enuresis, and gross hematuria (91). Thirty to forty percent of our patients were clinically uremic, with nausea, vomiting, changes in mentation, or asterixis. Evidence of sepsis (chills, fever, hypotension) may be present. Edema of the extremities, due to venous occlusive disease or lymphatic obstruction, was commonly found in patients with pelvic malignancy and lymphomas. An abdominal mass, representing an enlarged bladder, occurs in 1.7% of males evaluated for prostatic hypertrophy (92). Uterine prolapse may on occasion be responsible for obstruction (93).

The degree of renal insufficiency may vary from very mild to severe (serum creatinine 10 mg/dl or higher). Hyperkalemia and non-anion gap acidosis are found in 70% of patients, and an inappropriately elevated urine pH (>5.5) is found in 60% (94). The urine sodium may be low (<20 mEq/L) in early acute renal failure due to obstructive uropathy, mimicking the diagnosis of "prerenal" azotemia (95,96). Hematuria, either gross or microscopic, is seen in 30% of patients. The urine sediment is otherwise benign, with more than 2+ proteinuria with the dip stick present in less than 4% of patients.

The diagnosis of obstructive uropathy can be confirmed by the finding of a postvoiding residual urine greater than 150 ml and/or dilatation of the urinary collecting system on ultrasonography (or CT scan). It should be emphasized that a nondilated system does not necessarily rule out the diagnosis of obstructive uropathy (97), which occurred in 4% of our patients. This figure is similar to reports by others (98,99), in which 11 of 246 patients (4.5%) did not have upper tract dilatation, a phenomenon seen predominantly in the elderly. Therefore, in any patient in whom there is a high index of suspicion for obstruction (such as patients with a history or high probability on examination of prostatic, bladder, colon, or pelvic cancer) and in those with no obvious cause of renal failure, it is mandatory to perform retrograde pyelography even if imaging techniques do not point to obstruction. If retrograde pyelography is unsuccessful or impossible, percutaneous nephrostomy may be safely accomplished even in a nondilated collecting system (99). On postmortem examination, patients with cancer and nondilated obstructive renal failure usually have a tumor encasing both kidneys and the ureters. Patients with retroperitoneal fibrosis may also present with nondilated obstructive uropathy (100). It is postulated that the fibrotic process interferes with the normal peristaltic transport of urine from the renal pelvis to the bladder. Acute myeloma kidney or acute occlusion of the renal artery of a solitary kidney can present with anuria and a picture similar to obstructive uropathy.

D. Treatment and Prognosis

Hyperkalemia is the most common acute life-threatening complication seen in patients with obstructive uropathy. The hyperkalemia, which is a consequence of metabolic acidosis, distal renal tubular acidosis, or hyporenin- hypoaldosteronism should be treated promptly and aggressively with glucose-insulin and sodium bicarbonate prior to manipulation of the urinary tract (see Chapter 3). Antibiotics (see Chapter 9) should be administered to patients with clinical evidence of infection, adjusting the dose for the degree of renal failure and reassessing the choice of antibiotics depending on the results of the urine and/or blood cultures. We do not routinely use prophylactic antibiotics. The presence of uremic signs and symptoms are not an absolute indication for dialytic intervention prior to an attempt at relieving the obstruction. Occasionally, a patient with severe metabolic acidosis and clinical evidence of fluid overload might require dialysis with fluid removal prior to manipulation. Percutaneous nephrostomy has become the method of choice for relieving an obstruction with upper tract involvement. Patients in whom the procedure is unsuccessful can be managed either by insertion of a ureteral catheter or stent through the bladder or by open nephrostomy.

Once the obstruction is relieved, 90% of patients undergo immediate diuresis. In the remaining 10%, either superimposed volume contraction (due to poor intake, vomiting, or diarrhea) or acute tubular necrosis secondary to sepsis is responsible for the variable delay in recovery. The average time between onset of diuresis and the attainment of stable kidney function varies from 10 to 14 days (101). During the first 4–5 days, special attention should be paid to adequate replacement of urinary losses so that volume contraction resulting from the post-obstructive diuresis does not occur. The volume of losses will depend, to a certain extent, on the state of hydration at the time the obstruction is relieved. Tubular defects in salt and water reabsorption, involving the proximal tubule, the thick ascending limb of Henle, and the cortical collecting tubules, are common and may be due to metabolic alterations sustained during obstruction (102–104). Other factors that may contribute to the defect in salt and water reabsorption are atrial natriuretic peptide and medullary washout (105). Furthermore, an inability to concentrate the urine maximally due to a tubular resistance to antidiuretic hormone (ADH), at a step beyond the intracellular generation of cyclic AMP, and involving the aquaporin-2 water channels, is frequently present (103,106,106a).

The degree of recovery depends primarily on the duration of the obstruction (107). Forty percent of our patients returned to baseline kidney function, which was frequently normal, particularly in those patients who acquired the obstruction while hospitalized. In the remaining 60%, renal insufficiency was present at the time of initial hospitalization and frequently was the primary reason for hospital admission. In these patients, 6% (mainly males with prostatic disease) failed to recover at all and were placed on maintenance hemodialysis, and the remaining 54% only partially recovered renal function. Half of these patients, however, may have had underlying kidney disease related to associated medical problems (diabetic nephropathy, hypertensive nephrosclerosis, analgesic nephropathy), but specific information was not available.

Once the patient's condition stabilizes, more definitive therapy is usually necessary to manage the underlying disease (108,109). Decisions about long-term management of the patient whose obstruction results from a malignant process depend on the extent of the disease, the tumor type, and the patient's clinical status. We usually make our decision on an individual basis after discussions with the patient, the family, the urologist, and the oncologist. Patients with tumors arising outside the pelvis carry the worst prognosis. In patients with tumors arising within the pelvis the prognosis is somewhat better, with a 70% survival rate at 3 months and a mean survival of 7.6 months (110). Patients with prostatic cancer have the best prognosis and should be managed aggressively (111).

In patients with benign causes of obstruction, kidney function can remain stable for long periods of time, even in those patients with a creatinine clearance between 20 and 30 ml/min. In our experience, patients have remained stable for up to 5 years as long as the obstruction was the only cause of the renal failure. Management of these patients should be the same as that for chronic renal insufficiency of any cause (see Chapter 11).

Five to ten percent of patients remain chronic salt losers, most likely because of an intrinsic inability of the distal nephron to conserve salt (112). Clinical evidence of severe volume depletion can develop in these patients when intercurrent illnesses intervenes, which limits intake or increase losses through the gastrointestinal tract. The urinary sodium may remain high (>45 mEq/L) despite volume contraction (113). These patients are best managed chronically with either salt (NaCl tablets) supplementation or fludrocortisone, 0.1–0.3 mg daily. Patients with persistent hyperkalemic-hyperchloremic metabolic acidosis (40% of our patients) can be managed as described previously (see Chapter 3).

REFERENCES

1. Johnson CM, et al. Renal stone epidemiology: a 25-year study in Rochester, Minnesota. Kidney Int 1979;16:624–631.
2. Sutherland JW, Parks JH, Coe FL. Recurrence after a single renal stone in a community practice. Miner Electrol Metab 1985;11:267–269.
2a. Mhiri MN, et al. Lithiase urinaire en milieu geriatrique. Ann d'Urol 1995;26:382–384.

3. Scott R. Prevalence of calcified upper urinary tract stone disease in a random population survey. Report of a combined study of general practitioners and hospital staff. Br J Urol 1987;59:111–117.
4. Soucie JM, et al. Demographic and geographic variability of kidney stones in the United States. Kidney Int 1994;46:893–899.
5. Michaels EK, et al. Racial variation in gender frequency of calcium urolithiasis. J Urol 1994;152:2228–2231.
6. Kristal-Boneh E, Goffer D, Green MS. Epidemiologic features of urolithiasis among industrial employees: the Israeli CORDIS Study. J Occup Med 1994;36:1115–1119.
7. Ljunghall S: Incidence of upper tract stones. Miner Electrol Metab 1987;13:220–227.
8. Soucie JM, et al. Relation between geographic variability in kidney stones prevalence and risk factors for stones. Am J Epidemiol 1996;143:487–495.
8a. Gentle DL, et al. Geriatric urolithiasis. J Urol 1997;158:2221–2224.
9. Nicar MJ, Hill K, Pak CYC. Inhibition by citrate of spontaneous precipitation of calcium oxalate in vitro. J Bone Miner Res 1987;2:215–220.
10. Abramson PA, Smith CL. Evaluation of factors involved in calcium stone formation. Miner Electrol Metab 1987;13:201–208.
11. Steele TH. The pharmacology of renal lithiasis. Ann Rev Pharmacol Toxicol 1977; 17:11–25.
12. Bowyer RC, Brockis TS, McCulloch RK. Glycosaminoglycans as inhibitors of calcium oxalate crystal growth and aggregation. Clin Chem Acta 1979;95:23–28.
13. Daudon M, et al. Inhibitors of crystallization. Adv Nephrol 1995;24:167–216.
13a. Lieske JC, et al. Renal epithelial cells rapidly bind and internalize calcium oxalate monohydrate crystals. Proc Natl Acad Sci USA 1994;91:6987–6991.
13b. Lieske JC, Leonard R, Toback FG. Adhesion of calcium oxalate monohydrate crystals to renal epithelial cells is inhibited by specific anions. Am J Physiol 1995;268: F604–F612.
14. Coe FL. Treated and untreated recurrent calcium nephrolithiasis in patients with idiopathic hypercalciuria, hyperuricosuria and no metabolic disorders. Ann Intern Med 1977;87:404–410.
15. Pak CYC, et al. Ambulatory evaluation of nephrolithiasis. Classification, clinical presentation and diagnositic criteria. Am J Med 1980;69:19–30.
16. Parks JH, Coe FL. A urinary calcium-citrate index for the evaluation of nephrolithiasis. Kidney Int 1986;30:85–90.
17. Baggio B, et al. Raised transmembrane oxalate flux in red blood cells in idiopathic calcium oxalate nephrolithiasis. Lancet 1984;2:12–13.
18. Robertson WG, Peacock M. The cause of idiopathic calcium stone disease hypercalciuria or hyperoxaluria? Nephron 1980;26:105–110.
19. Nakagawa Y, et al. Urine glycoprotein crystal growth inhibitors. Evidence for a molecular abnormality in calcium oxalate nephrolithiasis. J Clin Invest 1985;76: 1455–1462.
19a. Goldfarb DS, Parks JH, Coe FL. Renal stone disease in older adults. Clin Geriatr Med 1998;14:367–381.
20. Moesch C, et al. Calcium oxalate crystalluria in elderly patients and treatment with naftidrofuryl oxalate. Age and Aging 1995;24:464–467.

21. Lemann J Jr, et al. Studies of the mechanism by which chronic metabolic acidosis augments urinary calcium excretion in man. J Clin Invest 1967;46:1318–1328.
22. Simpson DP. Citrate excretion: a window on renal metabolism. Am J Physiol 1983; 244:F223–F234.
23. Stewart AF, et al. Calcium homeostasis in immobilization: an example of resorptive hypercalciuria. N Engl J Med 1982;306:1136–1140.
24. Tori JA, Kewabramani LS, Orth MS. Urolithiasis in children with spinal cord injury. Paraplegia 1978;16:357–365.
25. Burr RG, Nusiebeh I. Biochemical studies in paraplegic renal stone patients. I. Plasma biochemistry and urinary calcium and saturation. Br J Urol 1985;57: 269–274.
26. Pak CYC, et al. The hypercalciurias. Causes, parathyroid functions and diagnositc criteria. J Clin Invest 1974;54:387–400.
27. Sherwood LM. Idiopathic hypercalciuria: a mixed bag of stones. J Lab Clin Med 1977;90:951–954.
28. Houillier P, et al. Calciuric response to an acute acid load in healthy subjects and hypercalciuric calcium stone formers. Kidney Int 1996;50:987–997.
29. Lau YK, et al. Proximal tubular defects in idiopathic hypercalciuria: resistance to phosphate administration. Miner Electrol Metab 1982;7:237–249.
30. Evans RA, et al. The pathogenesis of idiopathic hypercalciuria: evidence for parathyroid hyperfunction. Q J Med 1984;53:41–53.
31. Kaplan RA, et al. The role of 1α,25-dihydroxyvitamin D in the mediation of intestinal hyperabsorption of calcium in primary hyperparathyroidism and absorptive hypercalciuria. J Clin Invest 1977;59:756–760.
32. Shen FH, et al. Increased serum 1,25-dihydroxyvitamin D in idiopathic hypercalciuria. J Lab Clin Med 1977;90:955–962.
33. Coe FL, et al. Effects of low calcium diet on urine calcium excretion, parathyroid function and serum $1,25(OH)_2D_3$ levels in patients with idiopathic hypercalciuria and in normal subjects. Am J Med 1982;72:25–32.
34. Coe FL, Favus MJ. Hypercalciuric states. Miner Electrol Metab 1981;5:183–200.
35. Coe FL, et al. Urinary macromolecular crystal growth inhibitors in calcium nephrolithiasis. Miner Electrol Metab 1980;3:268–275.
36. Zerwekh JE, et al. Modulation by calcium of the inhibitor activity of naturally ocurring urinary inhibitors. Kidney Int 1988;33:1005–1008.
37. Millman S, et al. Pathogenesis and clinical course of mixed calcium oxalate and uric acid nephrolithiasis. Kidney Int 1982;22:366–370.
38. Coe FL, et al. Uric acid saturation in calcium nephrolithiasis. Kidney Int 1980;17: 662–668.
39. Coe FL, Moran E, Kavalich AG. The contribution of dietary purine overconsumption to hyperuricosuria in calcium oxalate stone formers. J Chronic Dis 1976;29:793–800.
40. Coe FL. Uric acid and calcium oxalate nephrolithiasis. Kidney Int 1983;24:392–403.
41. Pak CYC, et al. Mechanism for calcium urolithiasis among patients with hyperuricosuria. J Clin Invest 1977;59:426–431.
42. Coe FL, Kavalach KG. Hypercalciuria and hyperuricosuria in patients with calcium nephrolithiasis. N Engl J Med 1974;291:1344–1350.

43. Ito H, et al. Clinical and biochemical features of uric acid nephrolithiasis. Eur Urol 1995;27:324–328.
44. Kristensen C, et al. Reduced glomerular filtration rate and hypercalciuria in primary struvite nephrolithiasis. Kidney Int 1987;32:749–753.
45. Griffith DP, Bruce RR, Fishbein WN. Infection (Urease)-Induced Stones. In: Brenner BM, Stein JH eds. Contemporary Issues in Nephrology. Vol. 5, New York: Churchill Livingstone, 1980:231–260.
46. Dobbins JW, Binder HJ. Importance of the colon in enteric hyperoxaluria. N Engl J Med 1977;296:298–301.
47. Hodgkinson A, Wilkinson R. Plasma oxalate crystalluria and urine saturation in recurrent renal stone formers. Clin Sci 1971;40:365–374.
48. Kass MA, et al. Acetazolamide and urolithiasis. Ophthalmology 1981;88:261–265.
49. Ahlstrand C, Tiselius HG. Urine composition and stone formation during treatment with acetazolamide. Scand J Urol Nephrol 1987;31:225–228.
50. Pak CYC, Fulker C. Idiopathic hypocitraturic calcium oxalate nephrolithiasis successfully treated with potassium citrate. Ann Intern Med 1986;104:33–37.
51. Minisola S, et al. Studies in citrate metabolism in normal subjects and kidney stone patients. Miner Electrol Metab 1989;15:303–308.
52. Parks JH, Coe FL. The financial effects of kidney stone prevention. Kidney Int 1996;50:1706–1712.
53. Larsen LS, Miller A, Allegra JR. The use of intravenous ketorolac for the treatment of renal colic in emergency department. Am J Emerg Med 1993;11:197–199.
54. Elliot JS. Calcium oxalate urinary calculi: clinical and chemical aspects. Medicine 1983;62:36–43.
55. Laing FC, Jeffery RB Jr, Wing VW. Ultrasound versus excretory urography in evaluating acute flank pain. Radiology 1985;154:613–616.
56. Stoller ML, et al. Percutaneous nephrolithotomy in the elderly. Urology 1994;44: 651–654.
56a. Ehreth JT, et al. Extracorporeal shock wave lithotripsy: multicenter study. Kidney and upper ureter versus middle and lower ureter treatments. J Urol 1994;152: 1379–1385.
57. Pak CYC, et al. Is selective therapy of recurrent nephrolithiasis possible? Am J Med 1981;71:615–622.
58. Sakhaee K, et al. Postmenopausal osteoporosis as a manifestation of renal hypercalciuria with secondary hyperparathyroidism. J Clin Endocrinol Metab 1985;61:368–373.
59. Smith LH, et al. Current concepts in nutrition: nutrition and urolithiasis. N Engl J Med 1978;298:87–89.
60. Pak CYC, et al. Evidence justifying a high fluid intake in treatment of nephrolithiasis. Ann Intern Med 1980;93:36–39.
61. Ljunghall S, Fellström B, Johansson G. Prevention of renal stones by a high fluid intake? Eur Urol 1988;14:381–385.
62. Curhan GC, et al. Prospective study of beverage use and the use of kidney stones. Am J Epidemiol 1996;143:240–247.
63. Lamden MP, Chrystowskli GA. Urinary oxalate excretion by man following ascorbic acid ingestion Proc Soc Exp Biol Med 1954;85:190–195.

64. Licata AA, et al. Effects of dietary protein on urinary calcium in normal subjects and in patients with nephrolithiasis. Metabolism 1979;28:895–900.
65. Pak CYC, et al. Dietary management of idiopathic calcium urolithiasis. J Urol 1984;131:850–852.
66. Sakhaee K, et al. The potential role of salt abuse on the risk for kidney stone formation. J Urol 1993;150:310–312.
67. Jaeger P, et al. Low bone mass in idiopathic renal stone formers: magnitude and significance. J Bone Miner Res 1994;9:1525–1532.
68. Curhan GC, et al. A prospective study of dietary calcium and other nutrients and the risk of symptomatic kidney stones. N Engl J Med 1993;328:833–838.
68a. Pak CYC. Medical management of nephrolithiasis in Dallas: update 1987. J Urol 1988;140:461–467.
68b. Ettinger B, et al. Potassium, magnesium, citrate is an effective prophylaxis against recurrent calcium oxalate nephrolithiasis. J Urol 1997;158:2069–2073.
69. Preminger GM, Pak CYC. Eventual attenuation of hypocalciuric response to hydrochlorothiazide in absorptive hypercalciuria. J Urol 1987;137:1104–1109.
70. Costanzo LS, Windhager EE. Calcium and sodium transport by the distal convoluted tubule of the rat. Am J Physiol 1978;235:F492–F496.
71. Leppla D, et al. Effect of amiloride with or without hydrochlorothiazide on urinary calcium and saturation of calcium salts. J Clin Endocrinol Metab 1983;57:920–924.
72. Alon U, Constanzo LS, Chan JCM. Additive hypocalciuric effects of amiloride on hydrochlorothiazide in patients treated with calcitriol. Miner Electrol Metab 1984; 10:379–386.
73. Pak CYC. Kidney stones: various forms and treatment. Nephron 1979;23:142–146.
74. Breslau NA, et al. Physicochemical effects of a new slow-release potassium phosphate preparation (uroPhos-K) in absorptive hypercalciuria. J Bone Miner Res 1995;10:394–400.
75. Pak CYC, Sakhaee K, Fuller C. Successful management of uric acid nephrolithiasis with potassium citrate. Kidney Int 1986;30:422–428.
76. Ettinger B, et al. Randomized trial of allopurinol in the prevention of calcium oxalate calculi. N Engl J Med 1986;315:1386–1389.
77. Miller RA. Role of endoscopic surgery in management of renal and ureteric calculi: a review. J R Soc Med 1985;78:1034–1038.
78. Riehle RA Jr, Fair WR, Vaughn D Jr. Extracorporeal shock-wave lithotripsy for upper tract calculi. One year's experience at a single center. JAMA 1986;255: 2043–2048.
79. Watson GM, Wickham JEA. Initial experience with pulsed dye laser for ureteric calculi. Lancet 1986;1:1357–1358.
80. Pode D, et al. Can extracorporeal shock-wave lithotripsy eradicate persistent urinary infection associated with infected stones? J Urol 1988;140:257–259.
81. Williams JJ, Rodman JS, Peterson CM. A randomized double-blind study of acetohydroxamic acid in struvite nephrolithiasis. N Engl J Med 1984;311:792–794.
82. Barilla DE, et al. Renal oxalate excretion following oral oxalate loads in patients with ileal disease and with renal and absorptive hyppercalciurias. Effect of calcium and magnesium. Am J Med 1978;64:579–585.
83. Editorial. Citrate for calcium nephrolithiasis. Lancet 1986;1:955.

84. Strauss AL, et al. Factors that predict relapse of calcium nephrolithiasis during treatment. A prospective study. Am J Med 1982;72:17–24.
85. Thode J, et al. Simplified protocol for biochemical evaluation of recurrent renal calcium stone disease. Miner Electrol Metab 1988;14:288–296.
86. Pak CYC, Skurla C, Harvey J. Graphic display of urinary risk factors for renal stone formation. J Urol 1985;134:867–870.
87. Kumar R, Hill CM, McGeown MG. Acute renal failure in the elderly. Lancet 1973; 1:90–91.
88. Oliveira DB, Winearls CG. Acute renal failure in the elderly can have a good prognosis. Age and Ageing 1984;13:304–308.
89. Mclnnes EG, et al. Renal failure in the elderly. Q J Med 1987;64:583–588.
90. Lameire N, et al. Acute renal failure in the elderly. Chap 12:103–116, 1986. In: Oreopoulos DG, ed. Geriatric Nephrology. The Medical, Psychosocial, Nursing, Financial and Ethical Issues of Treating End-Stage Renal Disease in the Elderly. Boston: Martinus Nijhoff, 103–116.
91. Jones DA, O'Reilly PH, George NJR. Reversible hypertension associated with unrecognized high pressure chronic retention of urine. Lancet 1987;1:1052–1054.
92. Mukamel E, et al. Occult progressive renal damage in the elderly male due to benign prostatic hypertrophy. J Am Geriatr Soc 1979;27:403–406.
93. Elkin M, Goldman SM, Meng CH. Ureteral obstruction in patients with uterine prolapse. Radiology 1974;110:289–294.
94. Battle DC, Arruda JAL, Kurtzman NA. Hyperkalemic distal renal tubular acidosis associated with obstructive uropathy. N Engl J Med 1981;304:373–380.
95. Hoffman LM, Suki W. Obstructive uropathy mimicking volume depletion. JAMA 1976;236:2096–2097.
96. Miller TR, et al. Urinary diagnostic indices in acute renal failure. A prospective study. Ann Intern Med 1978;89:47–50.
97. Spital A, Valvo JR, Segal AJ. Nondilated obstructive uropathy. Urology 1988;31: 478–482.
98. Naidich JB, et al. Nondilated obstructive uropathy. Percutaneous nephrostomy performed to reverse renal failure. Radiology 1986;160:653–657.
99. Maillet PJ, et al. Nondilated obstructive acute renal failure: diagnostic procedures and therapeutic management. Radiology 1986;160:659–662.
100. Lalli A. Retroperitoneal fibrosis and inapparent obstructive uropathy. Radiology 1977;122:339–342.
101. Nadig PW, Valk WL. Recovery from obstructive disease. J Urol 1982;88:470–472.
102. Buerkert J, Head M, Klahr S. Effects of acute bilateral ureteral obstruction on deep nephron and terminal collecting duct function in the young rat. J Clin Invest 1977;59:1055–1065.
103. Hanley MJ, Davidson K. Isolated nephron segments from rabbit models of obstructive uropathy. J Clin Invest 1982;69:165–174.
104. Nito H, et al. Effect of unilateral ureteral obstruction on renal cell metabolism and function. J Lab Clin Med 1978;91:60–71.
105. Solez K, et al. Inner medullary plasma flow in the kidney with ureteral obstruction. Am J Physiol 1976;231:1315–1321.

106. Fine LG, et al. Functional profile of the isolated uremic nephron. J Clin Invest 1978;61:1519–1527.
106a. Nielsen S, et al. The aquaporin family of water channels in kidney: an update on physiology and pathophysiology of aquaporin-2. Kidney Int 1996;49:1718–1723.
107. Sarmina J, Resnick MI. Obstructive uropathy in patients with benign prostatic hyperplasia. J Urol 1989;141:866–869.
108. Herr HW. Intermittent catheterization in neurogenic bladder disorders. J Urol 1975;113:477–479.
109. Applebaum SM. Pharmacologic agents in micturitional disorders. Urology 1980;16:555–568.
110. Bodner D, Kursh ED, Resnick MI. Palliative nephrostomy for relief of ureteral obstruction secondary to malignancy. Urology 1984;24:8–10.
111. Khan AV, Utz DL. Clinical management of cancer of prostate with bilateral ureteral obstruction. J Urol 1975;113:816–819.
112. Bishop MC. Diuresis and renal functional recovery in chronic retention. Br J Urol 1985;57:1–5.
113. Uribarri J, Oh MS, Carroll HJ. Salt-losing nephropathy. Clinical presentation and mechanisms. Am J Nephrol 1983;3:193–198.

9

Urinary Infection

I. INCIDENCE AND PREVALENCE

It is now well established that significant bacteriuria, as defined by Kass (10^5 organisms/ml of a midstream urine) (1), increases with age. The higher prevalence in the elderly occurs in both sexes, and the higher ratio of females to males seen in younger patients decreases with aging (2). In 1996 patients 70 years of age or older screened for bacteriuria by Nordenstam et al. (3), the frequency of positive cultures ($>10^5$ organisms/ml) was 9.0% among women and 2.4% among men. Even higher prevalence rates (10–16% in ambulatory men and 17–37% in ambulatory women) have been found by others (4–7). For the elderly living in nursing homes or extended care facilities, the incidence of bacteriuria is 15–37% in men and 17–55% in women (2,8,9). It is estimated that, in elderly hospitalized patients, 30–33% of the men and 32–50% of the women either have or will subsequently develop bacteriuria (2).

II. PATHOGENESIS

There are several reasons why the elderly are more prone to develop a urinary tract infection.

A. Colonization

In general, vaginal and periurethral colonization with the offending organism precedes the onset of cystitis in women with recurrent urinary tract infection (10). Both increasing age and debilitation are associated with increased colonization of the skin and mucous membranes by gram-negative organisms (11). Fecal incontinence, a common occurrence in the elderly with dementia, results in colonization of the urinary tract by organisms usually localized to the gastrointestinal tract (11a).

B. Adherence

Even though increased susceptibility to perineal and periurethral colonization with gram-negative bacteria has been found in women with recurrent urinary infections, the infection need not be with the colonizing organism (12). Moreover, infection does not necessarily follow colonization (13), suggesting that other factors must be operative. Bacterial adherence, which represents an interaction between organisms and uroepithelial cells, appears to be important (14). For instance, the bacteria which are more likely to cause infection and are more often associated with infection have a higher adherence rate to squamous epithelium than do less virulent strains isolated from the vaginal introitus (15). Although adherence appears to play a role, it is not a completely independent risk factor in the increased incidence of urinary tract infection in the elderly (16). Other variables modulate the degree of adherence of a given microorganism to the uroepithelium (17), including (a) the ability of the uroepithelial cell to produce local antibody (18), (b) the genetic susceptibility of the host (19), and (c) intravaginal pH. Only the latter has been specifically studied in a small number of postmenopausal women. A high intravaginal pH (>5.2) was found to be associated with increased bacterial adherence, which was reversed once the pH was brought to normal with continuous low-dose intravaginal estrogen therapy (20). This beneficial effect of estrogen for some reason has been found to benefit only those women who previously had a hysterectomy (21).

C. Urine Stasis

Vesical emptying and high urine flow have been shown by Cox and associates (10,22) to play an important preventive role in urinary tract infection. Bladder emptying is frequently impaired in the elderly, with problems such as prostatic enlargement in the male and changes in bladder function and pelvic musculature in the female. Also, difficulty in micturition arising from neuromuscular disorders, dementia, and concomitant use of drugs such as the anticholinergics is common in the elderly. Postvoiding residual volume is increased in both elderly men and elderly woman (23,24). A high (>50 ml) residual, however, seems to represent more of a risk for developing urinary incontinence than for infection (25). Finally, recent studies by Parsons and Mulholland (26) have provided strong evidence for the role of bladder surface glycosaminoglycans in protecting against infection. It is quite probable that with advancing age there are either quantitative or qualitative changes in this substance.

D. Urinary Tract Instrumentation

It is estimated that 40–60% of hospitalized elderly or those living in nursing homes and other institutions and 10–20% of community-dwelling elderly are incontinent (27,28). Despite the fact that incontinence is transient in as many as 50% of these patients and that two-thirds of the remainder can be cured or markedly improved (29), physicians often resort to catheterization. In one study, only 27.5% of catheterized patients had been adequately evaluated as to the cause of their incontinence (30). The presence of an indwelling catheter is guaranteed to cause bacteriuria within a few days. The incidence is 100% within 4 days when an open system is used and 50% with a closed system. In general, catheter-associated urinary infections increase approximately 8–10% per day with a closed system (31). The use of condom catheters is also associated with a high rate of urinary tract infection after prolonged use (32,33).

Bacteria are usually introduced at time of catheterization or enter the bladder either by extraluminal migration from the urethral meatus or by intraluminal migration following contamination of the drainage bag. The bacteria may originate from the patient's normal flora (e.g., *Escherichia coli*) or by cross-contamination from external sources (e.g., *Serratia marcescens*) (34). A transient increase in the adherence of gram-negative bacteria to bladder epithelial cells has been shown to be an important early event in the development of catheter-associated bacteriuria (35).

E. Alteration in Host Defense Mechanisms

There is evidence that old rats have more difficulty than younger rats in clearing bacteria introduced into their urinary tract (36). Whether this factor is operative in humans remains to be shown; however, evidence for local urinary immune and inflammatory responses, as assessed by the presence in the urine of antibodies to the infecting organism and/or increased urinary levels of interleukins-1α or -6, is found in 25–50% of the elderly with asymptomatic bacteriuria (37,38). A 10-fold decrease in antigen processing, a defective primary response to mitogens, and increased intensity of delayed hypersensitivity reactions as well as diminished bactericidal activity and altered oxygen metabolism have been reported in the elderly, and these changes may increase susceptibility to infection (39–41). Anergy and depressed cell-mediated immunity are frequently associated with a variety of disease states as well as with malnutrition, so it is possible that some of the immunological defects observed in the elderly are related to underlying diseases rather than old age per se (42).

Once the bladder is invaded by bacteria, the patient is at risk of developing a kidney infection. This process might start with bacteria adhering to the ureteral mucosa. Endotoxin produced by these bacteria alters ureteral motility, causing it to act as if mechanically obstructed and in turn causing changes in the shape of the renal papillae. Intrarenal reflux of bacteria ensues, with subsequent adherence to the renal tubular epithelium. This sequence of events is then followed by complement activation, an inflammatory response in the kidneys, and subsequent phagocytosis of the microorganisms (43). In a minority of patients, bacteria gain access to the kidneys by hematogenous seeding from a distant pyogenic focus.

III. CLINICAL MANIFESTATIONS

Asymptomatic bacteriuria is associated with leukocyturia far more commonly in the elderly (both males and females) than in younger subjects (8,44), although leukocyturia may be present in a significant number of institutionalized, nonbacteriuric elderly (9). Nonspecific urinary symptoms such as incontinence, frequency, urgency, and suprapubic pain are usually of little diagnostic importance, since they are found with equal frequency in subjects with or without bacteriuria (45,46), and should not be used as the only indications for therapy in the elderly with bacteriuria. In our experience, approximately 5% of bacteriuric patients present with significant dysuria and 8% have symptomatic upper tract infection (pyelonephritis).

The clinical presentation of acute pyelonephritis is similar in older and younger patients. However, changes in mentation are more common in the elderly. The diagnosis should be considered in any patient who presents with fever and rigors following manipulation of an indwelling bladder catheter (46a). Other symptoms, such as dysuria and flank pain with costovertebral angle tenderness, are commonly present. Pyuria, defined as more than 10 polymorphonuclear leukocytes per high-power field, is a universal finding (47). Leukocytosis is present in 76% of patients. In 15%, neither fever nor leukocytosis is present (48). Blood cultures are positive in 58% of patients, and shock is present in 33%, both values being significantly higher than for younger patients (49,49a). In fact, the urinary tract is the most common source of gram-negative bacteremia in the elderly, accounting for as much as 32% of community-acquired cases (50) and probably more for those with an indwelling catheter (51–54). The presence of other medical problems (cerebrovascular disease, pulmonary disease, decubitus ulcers) may occasionally direct the clinician's attention away from the urinary tract and delay proper diagnosis (55).

IV. NATURAL HISTORY AND TREATMENT

A. Asymptomatic Bacteriuria

1. Noncatheterized Patients

As already noted, asymptomatic bacteriuria is very common in the elderly. Suntharalingham and colleagues (56), using the bladder washout method of Fairley et al. (57) in 31 elderly female patients with bacteriuria, were able to locate the site of infection to the upper tract in 17 (55%) and to the lower in the remaining 14 (45%). Using a similar technique, Nicolle and associates (58) found a 67% incidence of upper tract infection in elderly institutionalized females. Unfortunately, no data were provided on the therapeutic outcome in either of these two studies. These rates of upper tract infection in the elderly are higher than the 32% found by Rubin et al. (59) using the antibody-coated bacteria technique in younger patients. In a study of 36 elderly institutionalized men with bacteriuria, 20 were not treated and remained bacteriuric. Sixteen were treated, and although they had fewer months of bacteriuria, only 1 of the 16 remained free of bacteriuria during the 2-year study period (8). No differences were found in mortality rate nor in infectious morbidity in this study. Similar data have also been reported in elderly institutionalized women (60). Furthermore, spontaneous resolution of bacteriuria appears to be rather common in the elderly, occurring in up to 33% of the patients (46,61,62). Based on these data and also on the fact that antimicrobial therapy might be associated with significant adverse effects (63), the present recommendation is not to treat the elderly patient (male or female) with asymptomatic bacteriuria, even in the presence of pyuria and/or urinary incontinence (9,63–66). Furthermore, more than 50% of the treated patients develop bacteriuria again within 4 weeks of discontinuing antibiotic treatment (9). A reduction in survival has been found by some in the bacteriuric elderly (symptomatic or nonsymptomatic), particularly in those patients who have a positive antibody-coated bacteria test compared to nonbacteriuric subjects (67,69), although others have not confirmed this finding (70). It is possible that bacteriuria constitutes a marker for a worse outcome in some elderly patients (71).

2. Catheterized Patients

There is a very high incidence of bacteriuria in patients catheterized for more than 4 days (72). Recent studies have shown that a bacterial count of greater than 10^2 organisms/ml represents a more valid index of infection in the catheterized patient compared to the usual 10^5 organisms/ml (midstream specimen) used for the noncatheterized patient (73). Attempts to reduce the incidence of bacteriuria through such measures as meatal care, antibiotic catheter coating, frequent bag changing, catheter irrigation, and antibiotic prophylaxis have all proved unsuccessful (74–76).

It is generally accepted that antimicrobial therapy for patients with long-term indwelling catheters should be reserved for those who develop symptoms such as fever or severe suprapubic pain, or for prophylaxis if an invasive genitourinary procedure (e.g., cystoscopy) is undertaken (75,77). The same approach is recommended for patients requiring intermittent catheterization (78). One exception might be the patient with asymptomatic bacteriuria seen after a prostatectomy (79). In these patients the bacteriuria tends to persist (except when *Staphylococcus epidermidis* is the organism), even after the indwelling catheter has been removed. A 7- to 10-day course of antibiotic therapy is indicated, based on the organism isolated and sensitivity results.

The rationale for not treating asymptomatic bacteriuric catheterized patients is that the incidence of upper tract infection is low in these patients, and the bacterial flora changes rapidly, a process which might be enhanced by antimicrobial therapy (80). Also, the emergence of drug-resistant organisms will be promoted, making the treatment of subsequent infections more difficult (81). The incidence of symptomatic infection has been estimated to be 10–30% in the elderly with bacteriuria following short-term catheterization (≤30 days) and 1 episode per 100 days in patients with bacteriuria following long-term catheterization (>30 days) (9). There is also a higher incidence of chronic pyelonephritis and other inflammatory changes in the kidneys at autopsy in the elderly subjected to long-term catheterization (82). As noted by some authors for noncatheterized patients, an increase (threefold) in mortality has been found among hospitalized bacteriuric patients with indwelling bladder catheters (83). The significance of this association is yet to be determined.

B. Symptomatic Bacteriuria

The management of acute dysuria in the elderly is similar to that in younger patients (84), although the optimal approach in the elderly is not well defined. The following has been our practice. At the initial visit, a complete history and physical examination are performed, paying special attention to the pelvic and urethrovaginal areas in the female and the prostate in the male. Part of a midstream urine specimen is examined microscopically, and the rest is sent to the laboratory for culture, since, in contrast to younger patients, older patients with urinary tract infection are more likely to experience a uropathogen other than *E. coli,* the organism most commonly isolated in the former (85). Therapy is then started with trimethoprim-sulfamethoxazole, one double-strength tablet twice a day, or a fluoroquinolone (86). A 7- to 10-day course is recommended, rather than the 3-day course used in younger patients, because of a higher rate of failure and relapse (9,87). This regimen has been shown to be quite effective even when upper tract infection is present (88). Other antibiotics useful in the therapy of urinary tract infection and their dosages in the elderly are listed in Table 1. Fosfomycin tromethamine in a single 3-g dose can eradicate bacteriuria in a large number of elderly patients with uncomplicated urinary tract infections (88a). However, the

Table 1 Antibiotic Therapy for the Elderly with Urinary Tract Infection

Indication	Antimicrobial agent	Administration route	Frequency of administration according to GFR (ml/min)		
			>50	50–10	<10
Cystitis	Trimethoprim-sulfamethoxazole, double strength	Oral	q12hr	q18hr	q18hr
	Nitrofurantoin microcrystals, 100 mg	Oral	q6hr	Avoid	Avoid
	Ciprofloxacin, 100–250 mg	Oral	q12hr	q18hr	q24hr
	Norfloxacin, 200–400 mg	Oral	q12hr if GFR >30	q24hr for GFR <30	
	Ofloxacin, 200–300 mg	Oral	q12hr	q12hr	q24hr
	Fosfomycin 3 g	Oral	one dose × 1 day		
Acute bacterial pyelonephritis					
In ambulatory patients	(Same as above)				
In nursing home, patients, patients, with indwelling catheters, complicated pyelonephritis	Cefotaxime, 1–2 g	IV	q6–8hr if GFR >20	q12–16hr if GFR <20	
	Ceftazidime, 500 mg	IV	q8–12hr	q24hr	q48hr
	Aztreonam, 1g	IV	q12hr	q24hr following an initial loading dose of 1 gm	250 mg q12hr
	Ofloxacin, 200–400 mg	IV	See above	See above	See above
	Gentamicin, 1 mg/kg	IM/IV	q8hr	q12–72hr	q72hr
	Tobramycin, 1 mg/kg	IM/IV	q24–72hr		q72hr
	Amikacin, 7.5 mg/kg	IV	q12hr	q72–240hr	q240hr
Other infections of the urinary tract	Vancomycin, 15–20 mg/kg	IV	q24hr	q24–48hr	q240hr
	Ethambutol, 15 mg/kg	Oral	q24hr	q24–36hr	q48hr
	Isoniazid, 300 mg	Oral	q24hr	q24hr	q24hr
	Rifampin, 600 mg	Oral	q24hr	q24hr	q24hr
	Amphotericin B, 0.4–0.6 mg/kg	IV	q24hr	q24hr	q24–36hr
	Ketoconazole, 200–400 mg	Oral	q6hr	q24hr	q24–36hr
	Flucytosine, 25–100 mg/kg	Oral	100 mg q24hr	q12–24hr	q24–48hr
	Fluconazole, 200 mg loading	Oral	q12hr	50 mg q24hr	50 mg q24hr
	Methenamine hippurate, 1 g	Oral	q12hr	Avoid	Avoid

drug is expensive, and how it will compare with the standard 7- to 10-day course with trimethoprim-sulfamethoxazole or a fluoroquinolone remains to be determined (88b). The patient is always seen for follow-up confirmation of bacteriological and symptomatic cure, since in the female the bacteriuria might be coincidental and the dysuria due to desiccation of the urethra or vaginal mucosa secondary to estrogen deficiency (89), various forms of vaginitis (90), or noninfectious cystitis (91). The incidence of nonbacterial (e.g., chlamydia, trachomatis) causes of acute dysuria in the elderly is not known.

We usually do a postvoiding residual in every male, diabetic female, and any patient with evidence of peripheral neuropathy who presents with symptomatic urinary tract infection. If a significant residual volume is found (>150 ml), the patient is referred for urological evaluation. Intravenous pyelogram and cystoscopy are recommended for males with acute dysuria not due to prostatitis and for females with relapsing (bacteriuria with the same organism within 2 weeks following antibiotic-induced bacteriologic cure) or recurrent infections (3 or more infections in a 1-year period with the same organism) (84). There are no studies, however, indicating what the yield of these procedures is in the elderly. Similar investigations should also be undertaken in both males and females with pyelonephritis.

Women with a normal genitourinary tract and recurrent symptomatic infection should be considered for a 6-month course of 40 mg of trimethoprim and 200 mg of sulfamethoxazole, nitrofurantoin macrocrystals, 100 mg, or norfloxacin, 200 mg, orally at bedtime (92). This approach has been found to be both efficient and cost effective (93). For patients who cannot tolerate these agents, methenamine hippurate, 1 g every 12 hr can be tried (94). It should be noted, however, that prophylaxis does not prevent recurrences after therapy has been discontinued (95). When that occurs, a longer (5-year) course of trimethoprin-sulfamethoxazole, 40-200 mg three times weekly at bedtime, may be tried (96). Also, recurrent urinary tract infection in men may require a long course of therapy (6–12 weeks) (97,98). Since chronic prostatitis is responsible for the bacteriuria in a great many of these patients, either a quinolone such as norfloxacin, 800 mg/day, or ciprofloxacin, 250–750 mg twice a day, is an effective alternative (99,100). These antibiotics have been found to have good prostatic tissue penetration (101) (see Table 1).

C. Acute Pyelonephritis

In all elderly patients presenting with symptoms and signs of acute pyelonephritis, a urinary Gram stain should be done and treatment with an intravenous antibiotic should be started after all the cultures (urine and blood) are taken. In the noncatheterized patient, gram-negative organisms are isolated in 81% and gram-positive in 19%. *E. coli* is found in approximately 45%, followed by *Proteus mirabilis*, *Pseudomonas aeruginosa*, *Klebsiella pneumoniae*, and *Providencia* species. *Staphylococcus aureus* is the most commonly isolated gram-positive organism (14%), and *Streptococcus faecalis* is next (4%) (48,49). For the chronically catheterized patient, gram-negative organisms (*E. coli*) still predominate, but the probability of a polymicrobial infection is greater; 40% in patients catheterized for less than 30 days, 68% in those catheterized for more than 30 days, and 86% in those catheterized for more than 1 year (53,82).

In patients with community-acquired infection, treatment can be initiated with either a fluoroquinolone or a trimethoprim-sulfamethoxazole, since *E. coli,* the most commonly isolated organism, is usually sensitive to both drugs (102), keeping in mind that the resistance rate to trimethoprim-sulfamethoxazole is 5–15% and increasing, whereas resistance to fluoroquinolones remains below 5% (87). Ofloxacin is associated with a cure rate of 90–92% compared to the 78–83% with ciprofloxacin therapy, and is considered the drug of choice in this group (87a). (Table 1). Aminoglycosides can be used, with the maintenance dose calculated by determining the GFR from the formulas reviewed in Chapter 1. Given the marked interindividual variations and the narrow therapeutic range of these drugs, it is mandatory that serum drug and creatinine levels be monitored carefully (103,104). Therapy is usually continued for a full 14 days.

For catheterized patients or for those confined to a nursing home, treatment with an aminoglycoside alone may be started, unless the urinary Gram stain shows the presence of a gram-positive organism. Our preference is tobramycin, since *P. aeruginosa* was isolated in 47% of our cultures. Third generation cephalosporins such as cefotaxime, ceftizoxime, or a fluoroquinolone can also be used (9,48). The dose and scheduling for tobramycin are the same as that used for gentamicin (105). If the organism is sensitive to a less toxic drug, we switch accordingly. If not, tobramycin is continued, with the dose altered according to serum levels or the patient's GFR. The dose of amikacin, another aminoglycoside reserved for more resistant organisms, should also be adjusted in the elderly according to the measured or estimated GFR (106). Aztreonam is an alternative to the aminoglycosides (Table 1). For suspected gram-positive infections, vancomycin is used initially, along with a loading dose of an aminoglycoside until culture results become available. With early and adequate antibiotic administration, the outcome is generally good for the elderly with acute bacterial pyelonephritis. Most patients become afebrile within 48–96 hr, and death due to sepsis is rare. The patients who die usually have other associated life-threatening illnesses. Antibiotic therapy is usually administered for a total of 2 weeks.

Persistence of fever and generalized toxicity, despite an adequate antibiotic regimen, or the development of acute renal failure, should lead to a vigorous search for one of the following complications.

1. Pyonephrosis

Pyonephrosis is the most common complication of pyelonephritis in elderly patients when ureteral obstruction is present. A calculus is usually responsible for the obstruction, although a sloughed papilla or other obstructing lesion may occasionally be found. The diagnosis is made by either ultrasonographic examination or CT scan of the kidneys. An intravenous pyelogram (IVP) can also be used if renal function is normal or near normal and the patient is properly prepared. On confirmation of the diagnosis, a urologist should be consulted for early drainage.

2. *Renal Papillary Necrosis*

Fifty-one percent of elderly patients who develop renal papillary necrosis also have acute pyelonephritis (107–109). Sixty-seven percent of elderly patients with pyelonephritis and renal papillary necrosis are diabetic. When the entire papillary surface is destroyed, it sloughs into the pelvis and may cause obstruction. Management consists of early drainage. In the absence of obstruction, antibiotic therapy alone may be adequate.

3. *Perinephric Abscess*

Perinephric abscess usually results from rupture of a corticomedullary abscess into the perinephric space, a consequence of retrograde spread of infection from the lower urinary tract. Fortunately, this complication is not common. The diagnosis is made either by IVP, ultrasound, or CT scan. The latter is the diagnostic technique of choice because it identifies the lesion and best defines its extent and surrounding anatomy (110,111). In addition to antibiotics, percutaneous drainage under sonographic guidance is usually necessary. Patients with multiple abscesses and a poorly functioning kidney often require a nephrectomy, debridement, and postoperative drainage.

4. *Emphysematous Pyelonephritis*

The emphysematous form of pyelonephritis is associated with the presence of gas in the collecting system (emphysematous pyelitis) or within the renal parenchyma (emphysematous pyelonephritis). The gas is produced by the infecting bacteria. This complication occurs primarily in diabetics, often in association with ureteral obstruction. The diagnosis can be confirmed by CT scan, which will accurately depict the position and pattern of the gas. Since the mortality rate is high, immediate urological intervention is necessary when obstruction is present. In the absence of ureteral obstruction, good results have been reported in patients with pyelitis treated with antibiotics alone (112–114). Forty-one percent of the patients with emphysematous pyelitis and 37% of those with emphysematous pyelonephritis reported by Evanoff et al. (113) were over the age of 60.

V. SPECIAL FORMS OF PYELOCYSTITIS IN THE ELDERLY

A. Tuberculosis

In the majority of patients, urinary tuberculosis represents a reactivation of a dormant focus from earlier hematogenous spread during the primary infection. Originally, the mycobacterium lodges in the preglomerular capillary bed. Because of acquired cellular immunity, bacterial multiplication stops and healed granulomata form. During reactivation, these granulomata enlarge and coalesce while new foci are initiated within the renal pyramids, followed by caseous necrosis. This process, if left untreated, will eventually destroy the kidney.

The exact incidence of renal tuberculosis in the elderly is not known, but it is known that 10–16% of reported cases of genitourinary tuberculosis occur in this age group (115). Females are more commonly affected than males.

In most patients, no past history of tuberculosis can be elicited, and dysuria is usually the most common initial presentation. In 5 (33%) of our 15 patients, there were no symptoms at all. The disease was found during investigation of sterile ``pyuria'' or during evaluation for unrelated problems. Systemic symptoms such as fever, weight loss, and cachexia are rare (116). Pyuria is a universal finding, and hematuria is present in one-third of the patients. An old lesion can be identified on chest X-ray in 25% of patients. The purified protein derivative (PPD) is positive in over 90% of patients.

Renal failure due to bilateral kidney involvement is rare (one of our patients had had nephrectomy for tuberculosis 10 years earlier, and the disease was destroying the remaining kidney). The findings on IVP vary in severity from calyceal dilatation with scarring to obstruction and destructive dilatation of the pyelocalyceal system. Occasionally, the appearance is that of a space-occupying lesion secondary to a large cortical abscess. Calcification is common.

The diagnosis of renal tuberculosis is based on the isolation of the organism in the urine. It is recommended that first morning specimens be obtained and cultured three times. On occasion, the diagnosis may be established by biopsy material obtained at the time of cystoscopy.

The initial therapy is usually medical, consisting of isoniazid (INH), 300 mg orally once a day, together with 50 mg daily of pyridoxine supplementation to prevent neuropathy. Kinetic data concerning the disposition of INH in a large group of elderly are lacking (117). It is recommended that serum transaminases be monitored monthly during treatment, and if any value exceeds three times normal the drug should be temporarily discontinued. The sensation of hyperexcitability, occasionally reported by the elderly taking this drug, can be avoided by using a divided-dose regimen of 100 mg every 8 hr (118). In all instances, a second drug should be given; either ethambutol, 25 mg/kg per day for the first 2 months followed by 15 mg/kg per day thereafter, or rifampin, 600 mg daily (see Table 1). Ophthalmological evaluation is routinely necessary in the elderly prior to treatment with ethambutol. Side effects of rifampin are mainly hepatic, and no dosage alteration is necessary in the elderly (119). Some authors recommend adding streptomycin for the first 6 months in advanced cases (116). Our practice is to perform a yearly sonogram (or IVP) to detect the presence of obstructive uropathy, usually secondary to the development of a ureteral stricture. The prognosis for cure with a 24-month course of double antibiotic therapy is generally good. Although this is the approach recommended by the authors, good results have also been reported with a course of daily rifampin and INH for 2 months, switching to either a twice-a-week regimen for 7 additional months or a three-times-a-week regimen for 2 additional months (120). Five of our patients died from cardiovascular causes, and autopsy was performed in three with no residual active disease found.

In some patients surgery may be necessary. The indications include intractable pain, persistent bleeding, suspicion of malignancy in a nonfunctioning kidney (121), and refractory hypertension associated with a poorly functioning kidney. For the latter, nephrectomy is the treatment of choice after demonstrating that the offending kidney is renin producing (122).

B. Xanthogranulomatous Pyelonephritis

Xanthogranulomatous pyelonephritis is a severe, chronic form of renal parenchymal infection characterized by the accumulation of large numbers of lipid-laden macrophages in the inflamed areas. These foamy macrophages may be mistaken for the clear cells of renal carcinoma when closely packed. This progressive granulomatous reaction generally results from prolonged, low-grade suppuration in a kidney in which urine flow is retarded by either a calculus or other abnormality affecting the ureteropelvic junction (123). The disease is usually unilateral. The peak incidence is in the 6th and 7th decades, with 45% of reported patients older than 60 years, mainly females (124–126). Fever, flank pain, and chills are the most common presenting manifestations. Malaise, weight loss, and lower urinary tract complaints have also been reported (127). Physical examination usually reveals abdominal distention and a palpable mass on the involved side. The erythrocyte sedimentation rate is usually elevated, leukocytosis is common, and the urine culture is positive in 70% of patients, with *E. coli* and *P. mirabilis* being the predominant organisms. On X-ray examination of the abdomen, an upper tract calculus (plain or staghorn) is found in 71% of patients. The IVP reveals either a nonfunctioning (76%) or poorly functioning kidney. An abdominal CT scan is the most useful diagnostic test, since the extent of perirenal involvement as well as the details of the intrarenal lesions (caliculi, necrosis, hydronephrosis, abscesses) can be seen with the greatest detail. Cure is possible only with surgical treatment (usually complete nephrectomy) (128).

C. Fungal Infections

Urinary fungal infections in the elderly present either as a primary infection or as a manifestation of a systemic infection. In nonhospitalized patients, the incidence of fungal urinary tract infection (defined as $>10^3$ organisms/ml) is not known, but it is rather unusual in our experience and occurs most often in diabetics and in patients who had been treated with a broad-spectrum antibiotic. The asymptomatic patient may be monitored carefully with periodic reassessment, as most cases resolve once the underlying risk factors are addressed (129,129a). In the presence of diabetes mellitus, good glycemic control should be attempted first. In the symptomatic patient (with urgency or hematuria) or in the patient with two positive consecutive cultures, oral flucytosine, 25–100 mg/kg daily in divided doses, has been used (130, 131). The duration of treatment is not well established. Relapses have been noted after 2 weeks of therapy; however, in one study the initial response rate with this regimen was 94% (132). This drug should probably not be used in the elderly with renal insufficiency. Ketoconazole, 200–400 mg orally, has also been found effective in a small number of patients (133) (Table 1). Fluconazole, a better choice, can be used with a loading dose of 200 mg followed by 4 days of a maintenance dose, according to GFR (see Table 1) (129a). It is recommended that an investigation for an anatomical genitourinary tract abnormality be carried out in a previously healthy patient with persistent funguria (133a).

In hospitalized patients, funguria (most commonly due to *Candida albicans*) is not uncommon in elderly patients who have been on systemic antibiotic therapy, particularly with intravenous and/or bladder catheters inserted. In the absence of any evidence of systemic fungal infection (such as a rising serum *Candida* antibody titer or retinal lesions), all catheters should be removed and, if possible, antibiotics discontinued. The fungus generally disappears from the urine in 4–5 days with this approach. If the organism persists, the bladder may be irrigated continuously with a solution of 200–300 ml of sterile water containing 1 mg/dl of amphotericin B. The double-lumen catheter used for this purpose should be cross-clamped for 60–90 min at regular intervals (134). This regimen is usually continued for 5–7 days, and cultures then repeated (134a). In one prospective study this approach was found to be associated with a prompt but short-lived clearance of the fungus (134b). Oral fuconazole at the dose outlined above represents a better alternative.

Urinary infection through the hematogenous route (fungemia) can occur with any of the fungi known to produce clinically important disease in humans. In some instances (e.g., histoplasmosis), the patient may first seek medical attention because of urinary complaints (135). Therapy consists of parenteral administration of amphotericin B. It is recommended that 0.3 mg/kg be used as an initial dose, gradually increasing to 0.4–0.6 mg/kg/day, while monitoring kidney function closely (136) (see Table 1). Duration of therapy depends on the clinical response, the fungus involved, and the site of involvement (135). The role of one of the currently available triazole (itraconazole, fluconazole, fluconazole) as consolidation therapy following induction therapy with amphotericin B is yet to be determined in controlled randomized trials (136a).

VI. ANTIBIOTIC PROPHYLAXIS FOR UROLOGICAL SURGERY

A detailed analysis of prophylactic use of antibiotics for urological surgery in the elderly is beyond the scope of this discussion. The reader is referred elsewhere (137). In general, antibiotic prophylaxis is considered beneficial for (a) transrectal biopsy, (b) cystoscopy in patients with chronic indwelling catheters, (c) transurethral prostatectomy, particularly in patients with preexisting bacteriuria and indwelling catheters, with some controversy regarding the benefits of prophylaxis in other patients (138–140). For these patients, ciprofloxacin, 250 mg twice daily, has been found to be superior to sulfadiazine-trimethoprim, 500 mg/160 mg twice daily, in one study (141); The drug was started on the evening preceding the intervention and continued up to the day following removal of the indwelling catheter. Other indications include (d) ureteral and renal stone surgery and (e) penile prosthesis insertion. In general, the choice of antibiotic should be based on the results of urine culture in patients with chronic catheters. For the others, any antibiotic with broad gram-negative coverage can be used. The drug should be given 1 or 2 hr prior to surgery and continued for 24 hr postoperatively, noting that the renal clearance of many of the commonly used antibiotics is reduced in the elderly (142).

REFERENCES

1. Kass EH. Bacteriuria and the diagnosis of infection in the urinary tract. Arch Intern Med 1957;100:709–713.
2. Kaye D. Urinary tract infections in the elderly. Bull NY Acad Med 1980;56: 209–220.
3. Nordenstam GR, et al. Bacteriuria and mortality in an elderly population. N Engl J Med 1986;314:1152–1156.
4. Dean NC, Yamamura R, Yoshikawa TT. Pyuria: its predictive value of asymptomatic bacteriuria in ambulatory elderly man. J Urol 1986;135:520–522.
5. Wolfson SA, et al. Epidemiology of bacteriuria in a predominantly geriatric male population. Am J Med 1965;250:168–173.
6. Dontas AS, et al. Bacteriuria and survival in old age. N Engl J Med 1981;304: 939–943.
7. Norman DC, Yoshikawa TT. Frequency of asymptomatic bacteriuria in ambulatory elderly males. Clin Res 1988;36:96A.
8. Nicolle LE, et al. Bacteriuria in elderly institutionalized men. N Engl J Med 1983;309:1420–1425.
9. Yoshikawa TT, Nicolle LE, Norman DC. Management of complicated urinary tract infection in older patients. J Am Geriatr Soc 1996;44:1235–1241.
10. Cox CE, Lacy SS, Hinman F Jr. The urethra and its relationship to urinary infection II. The urethral flora in the female with recurrent urinary infection. J Urol 1968;99: 632–634.

11. Johnson WG, Pierce AK, Sanford JP. Changing pharyngeal bacterial flora of hospitalized patients. N Engl J Med 1969;281:1137–1140.
11a. Lara LL, et al. The risk of urinary tract infection in bowel incontinent men. J. Gerontol Nurs 1990;16:24–26.
12. Brumfitt W, Gargan RA, Hamilton-Miller JMT. Periurethral enterobacterial carriage preceding urinary infection. Lancet 1987;1:824–826.
13. Kunin CM, Polyach F, Posted F. Periurethral bacterial flora in women. Prolonged intermittent colonization with *E. coli.* JAMA 1980;243:143.
14. Fowler JE, Samey TA. Studies on introital colonization in women with recurrent urinary infections. VIII: The role of bacterial adherence. J Urol 1977;117:472–476.
15. Schaeffer AJ, et al. Variable adherence of uropathogenic *E. coli* to epithelial cells from women with recurrent urinary tract infection. J Urol 1982;128:1227–1230.
16. Sobel JD, Muller G. Pathogenesis of bacteriuria in elderly women: the role of *E. coli* adherence to vaginal epithelial cells. J Gerontol 1984;39:682–685.
17. O'Hanley P, et al. Gal-Gal binding and hemolysin phenotypes and genotypes associated with uropathogenic *E. coli.* N Engl J Med 1985;313:414–420.
18. Stamey TA, et al. The immunologic basis of recurrent bacteriuria. Medicine 1978;57: 47–56.
19. Schaeffer AJ, Jones JM, Dunn JK. Association of in-vitro *E. coli* adherence to vaginal and buccal epithelial cells with susceptibility of women to recurrent urinary tract infections. N Engl J Med 1981;304:1062–1066.
20. Parsons CL, Schmidt JD. Control of recurrent lower urinary tract infection in the post-menopausal women. J Urol 1982;128:1224–1226.
21. Orlander JD, et al. Urinary tract infections and estrogen use in older women. J Am Geriatr Soc 1992;40:817–820.
22. Cox CE. The urethra and its relationship to urinary tract infection: the flora of the normal female urethra. South Med J 1966;59:621–623.
23. Andersen JT, et al. Bladder function in healthy elderly males. Scand J Urol Nephrol 1978;12:123–127.
24. Brocklehurst JC, Dillane JB. Studies of the female bladder in old age. I. Cystometrograms in non-incontinent women. Gerontol Clin (Basel) 1966;8:285–305.
25. Grosshans CL, Passadori Y, Peter B. Urinary retention in the elderly: a study of 100 hospitalized patients. J Am Geriatr Soc 1993;41:633–638.
26. Parsons CL, Mulholland SG. Bladder surface mucin: its antibacterial effect against various bacterial species. Am J Pathol 1978;93:423–432.
27. Resnick NM, Yalla SV. Management of urinary incontinence in the elderly. N Engl J Med 1985;313:800–805.
28. Ouslander JG, et al. Incontinence among elderly community-dwelling dementia patients. Characteristics, management, and impact on caregivers. J Am Geriatr Soc 1990;38:440–445.
29. Chutka DS, et al. Urinary incontinence in the elderly population. Mayo Clin Proc 1996;71:93–101.
30. Ribeiro BJ, Smith SR. Evaluation of urinary catheterization and urinary incontinence in a general nursing home population. J Am Geriatr Soc 1985;33:479–482.
31. Garibaldi RA, et al. Factors predisposing to bacteriuria during indwelling urethral catheterization. N Engl J Med 1974;291:215–218.

32. Johnson ET. The condom catheter: urinary tract infection and other complications. South Med J 1983;76:579–582.
33. Ouslander JG, Greengold B, Chen S. External catheter use and urinary tract infections among incontinent male nursing home patients. J Am Geriatr Soc 1987;35: 1063–1070.
34. Maki DG, et al. Nosocomial urinary tract infection with S. marcescens: an epidemiologic study. J Infect Dis 1973;128:579–587.
35. Daifukee R, Stamm WE. Bacterial adherence to bladder uroepithelial cells in catheter-associated urinary tract infection. N Engl J Med 1986;314:1208–1213.
36. Freedman LR. Experimental pyelonephritis XV: increased susceptibility to *E. coli* infection in old rats. Yale J Biol Med 1969;42:30–38.
37. Nicolle LE, Brunka J. Urinary IgG and IgA antibodies in elderly institutionalized subjects with bacteriuria. Gerontology 1990;36:345–355.
38. Nicolle LE, et al. Urinary immunoreactive interleukin-1 alpha and interleukin-6 in bacteriuric institutionalized elderly subjects. Urology 1993;149:1049–1053.
39. Gross JS. Infections in the elderly. Med Times 1985;113:93–104.
40. Kaack MB, et al. Immunology of pyelonephritis VIII. *E. coli* causes granulocytic aggregation and renal ischemia. J Urol 1986;136:1117–1122.
41. Saltzman RL, Peterson PK. Immunodeficiency in the elderly. Rev Infect Dis 1987; 9:1127–1139.
42. Kniker WI, et al. Multitest MCI for the standardized measurement of delayed cutaneous hypersensitivity and cell-mediated immunity. Ann Allergy 1984;52: 75–82.
43. Roberts JA. Pathogenesis of pyelonephritis. J Urol 1983;129:1102–1106.
44. Boscia JA, et al. Pyuria and asymptomatic bacteriuria in elderly ambulatory women. Ann Intern Med 1989;110:404–405.
45. Brocklehurst JC, et al. Dysuria in old age. J Am Geriatr Soc 1971;19:582–592.
46. Boscia JA, et al. Lack of association between bacteriuria and symptoms in the elderly. Am J Med 1986;81:979–982.
46a. Pfilzenmeyer P, et al. Predicting bacteremia in older patients. J Am Geriatr Soc 1995;43: 230–235.
47. Norman DC, Yamamura R, Yoshikawa TT. Pyuria: its predictive value of asymptomatic bacteriuria in ambulatory elderly man. J Urol 1986;135:520–522.
48. Ackermann RJ, Monroe PW. Bacteremic urinary tract infection in older people. J Am Geriatr Soc 1996;44:927–9332.
49. Gleckman R, et al. Community-acquired bacteremic urosepsis in elderly patients: a prospective study of 34 consecutive episodes. J Urol 1982;128:79–81.
49a. Armitage KB, Salata RA, Landefeld CS. Urosepsis in the elderly: clinical and microbiologic characteristics. Infect Dis Clin Pract 1993;2:260–266.
50. Whitelaw DA, Rayner BL, Willcox PA. Community-acquired bacteremia in the elderly: a prospective study of 121 cases. J Am Geriatr Soc 1992;40:996–1000.
51. Stamm WE, Martin SM, Bennett JV. Epidemiology of nosocomial infections due to gram-negative bacilli: aspect relevant to development and use of vaccines. J Infect Dis 1977;136:S151–S160.
52. Esposito AL, et al. Community-acquired bacteremia in the elderly: analysis of one hundred consecutive episodes. J Am Geriatr Soc 1980;28:315–319.

53. Gleckman R, et al. Catheter-related urosepsis in the elderly: a prospective study of community-derived infections. J Am Geriatr Soc 1982;30:255–257.
54. Rudman D, et al. Clinical correlates of bacteremia in a Veterans Administration extended care facility. J Am Geriatr Soc 1988;36:726–732.
55. Milnes JP, Swain DG. Severe renal sepsis in the very elderly. Postgrad Med 1986; 62:643–645.
56. Suntharalingam M, Seth V, Moore-Smith B. Site of urinary tract infection in elderly women admitted to an acute geriatric assessment unit. Age and Aging 1983;12: 317–322.
57. Fairley KF, et al. Simple test to determine the site of urinary tract infection. Lancet 1967;2:427–428.
58. Nicolle LE, et al. Localization of urinary tract infection in elderly institutionalized women with asymptomatic bacteriuria. J Infect Dis 1988;157:65–70.
59. Rubin RH, et al. Single-dose amoxicillin therapy for urinary tract infection. JAMA 1980;244:561–564.
60. Nicolle LE, Mayhew WJ, Bryan L. Prospective randomized comparison of therapy and no therapy for asymptomatic bacteriuria in institutionalized elderly women. Am J Med 1987;83:27–33.
61. Abrutyn E, et al. Epidemiology of asymptomatic bacteriuria in elderly women. J Am Geriatr Soc 1991;39:388–393.
62. Monroe M, et al. Epidemiologic and diagnostic aspects of bacteriuria: a longitudinal study in older women. J Am Geriatr Soc 1995;43:618–622.
63. Boscia JA, et al. Therapy versus no therapy for bacteriuria in elderly ambulatory non-hospitalized women. JAMA 1987;257:1067–1071.
64. Abruytyn E, Boscia JA, Kaye D. The treatment of asymptomatic bacteriuria in the elderly. J Am Geriatr Soc 1988;36:473–475.
65. Ouslander JG, et al. Does eradicating bacteriuria affect the severity of chronic urinary incontinence in nursing home residents? Ann Intern Med 1995;122:749–754.
66. Abrutyn E, et al. Does treatment of asymptomatic bacteriuria in older ambulatory women reduce subsequent symptoms of urinary tract infection? J Am Geriatr Soc 1996;44:293–295.
67. Sourander LB, Kasanen A. A 5-year follow-up of bacteriuria in the aged. Gerontol Clin 1972;14:274–281.
68. Dontas AS, et al. Bacteriuria and survival in old age. N Engl J Med 1981;304: 939–943.
69. Nicolle LE, et al. Asymptomatic bacteriuria, urinary antibody, and survival in the institutionalized elderly. J Am Geriatr Soc 1992;40:607–613.
70. Nicolle LE, et al. The association of bacteriuria with resident characteristics and survival in elderly institutionalized men. Ann Intern Med 1987;106:682–686.
71. Nordenstam GR, et al. Bacteriuria and mortality in an elderly population. N Engl J Med 1986;314:1152–1156.
72. Gleckman RA. The chronically catheterized elderly patient. A selective review. J Am Geriatr Soc 1985;33:489–491.
73. Stark RP, Maki DG. Bacteriuria in the catheterized patient. What quantitative level of bacteriuria is relevant? N Engl J Med 1984;311:560–564.

74. Reid RI, et al. Comparison of urine bag- changing regimens in elderly catheterized patients. Lancet 1982;2:754–756.
75. Warren JW, et al. Sequelae and management of urinary infection in the patient requiring chronic catheterization. J Urol 1981;125:1–8.
76. McFarlane DE. Prevention and treatment of catheter-associated urinary tract infection. J Infection 1985;10:96–106.
77. Siler WO, Stahclin HB. Practical management of catheter-associated urinary tract infections. Geriatrics 1988;43:43–50.
78. Mohler JL, Cowen DL, Flanigan RC. Suppression and treatment of urinary tract infection in patients with an intermittently catheterized neurogenic bladder. J Urol 1987;138:336–340.
79. Gordon DL, et al. Diagnostic criteria and natural history of catheter-associated urinary tract infections after prostatectomy. Lancet 1983;2:1269–1271.
80. Stovall CW, Mihaldzic N, Lloyd FA. Incidence of renal bacteriuria in the presence of long standing bladder infections. In: Proc 16th V.A. Spinal Cord Injury Conf, 1967: 172–176.
81. Breitenbucher RB. Bacterial changes in the urine samples of patients with long-term indwelling catheters. Arch Intern Med 1984;144:1585–1589.
82. Warren JW, et al. Long-term urethral catheterization increases risk of chronic pyelonephritis and renal inflammation. Am J Geriatr Soc 1994;42:1286–1290.
83. Platt R, et al. Mortality associated with nosocomial urinary tract infection. N Engl J Med 1982;307:637–642.
84. Komaroff AL. Acute dysuria in women. N Engl J Med 1984;310:368–375.
85. Yoshikawa TT. Unique aspects of urinary tract infections in the geriatric population. Gerontology 1984;30:339–344.
86. Stamm WE, et al. Diagnosis of coliform infection in acutely dysuric women. N Engl J Med 1982;307:463–468.
87. Stamm WE, Hooton TM. Management of urinary tract infections in adults. N Engl J Med 1996;329:1328–1334.
87a. Neu HC. Quinolone antimicrobial agents. Annu Rev Med 1992;43:465–486.
88. Stamm WE, McKevitt M, Counts GW. Acute renal infection in women. Treatment with trimethoprim-sulfamethoxazole or ampicillin for two or six weeks. Ann Intern Med 1987;106:341–345.
88a. Janknegt R, et al. Urinary concentrations of fosfomycin after a single 3g dose of fosfomycin to elderly nursing home patients. Pharm World Sci 1994;16:149–153.
88b. Fosfomycin for urinary tract infections. The Medical Letter 1997;39:66–68.
89. Fihn S, Stamm WE. Management of women with acute dysuria. In: Rund DA, ed. Emergency Medicine Annual 1983. Norwalk, CT: Appleton-Century-Crofts, 1983: 225–246.
90. Komaroff AL, et al. Management strategies for urinary and vaginal infections. Arch Intern Med 1978;138:1069–1073.
91. Tauscher JW, Shaw DC. Eosinophilic cystitis. Clin Pediatr 1981;20:741–743.
92. Stamm WE, et al. Antimicrobial prophylaxis of recurrent urinary tract infections. A double-blind, plecebo-controlled trial. Ann Intern Med 1980;92:770–775.
93. Stamm WE, et al. Is antimicrobial prophylaxis of urinary tract infections cost effective? Ann Intern Med 1981;94:251–255.

94. Cronberg S, et al. Prevention of recurrent acute cystitis by methanamine hippurate: double-blind controlled cross-over long term study. Br Med J 1987;294:1507–1508.
95. Kunin CM. Duration of treatment of urinary tract infections. Am J Med 1981;71:849–854.
96. Nicolle LE, et al. Efficacy of five years of continuous, low dose trimethoprim-sulfamethoxazole prophylaxis for urinary tract infection. J Infect Dis 1988;157: 1239–1242.
97. Smith JW, et al. Recurrent urinary tract infections in men. Characteristics and response to therapy. Ann Intern Med 1979;91:544–548.
98. Lipsky BA. Urinary tract infections in men. Epidemiology, pathophysiology, diagnosis and treatment. Ann Intern Med 1989;110:138–150.
99. Childs SJ, Goldstein EJC. Ciprofloxacin as treatment for genitourinary tract infection. J Urol 1989;141:1–5.
100. Sant GR, Weinstein BS. Therapy of urinary tract infections in the elderly: role of fluoroquinolones. Urol 1990;35(Suppl):19–21.
101. Hamus PM, Danziger LH. Treatment of chronic bacterial prostatitis. Clin Pharm 1984;3:49–55.
102. Johnson JR, Stamm WE. Urinary tract infections in women. Diagnosis and treatment. Ann Intern Med 1989;111:906–917.
103. Bauer LA, Blovin RA. Gentamicin pharmacokinetics: effects of aging in patients with normal renal function. J Am Geriatr Soc 1982;30:309–311.
104. Zaske DE, et al. Wide interpatient variations in gentamicin dose requirements for geriatric patients. JAMA 1982;248:3122–3126.
105. Bauer LA, Blouin RA. Influence of age on tobramycin pharmacokinetics in patients with normal renal function. Antimicrob Agents Chemother 1981;20:587–589.
106. Bauer LA, Blouin RA. Influence of age on amikacin pharmacokinetics in patients without renal disease. Eur J Clin Pharmacol 1983;24:639–642.
107. Eknoyan G, et al. Renal papillary necrosis: an update. Medicine 1982;61:55–73.
108. Harvald B. Renal papillary necrosis. A clinical survey of sixty-six cases. Am J Med 1963;35:481–486.
109. Faubert PF, Porush JG. Unpublished observations, 1987.
110. Sheinfeld J, et al. Perinephric abscess. Current concepts. J Urol 1987;137:191–194.
111. Edelstein H, McCabe RE. Perinephric abscess: modern diagnosis and treatment in 47 cases. Medicine 1988;67:118–131.
112. Ahlering TE, et al. Emphysematous pyelonephritis: a 5-year experience with 13 patients. J Urol 1985;134:1086–1088.
113. Evanoff GV, et al. Spectrum of gas within the kidney. Am J Med 1987;83:149–154.
114. Koh KB, Lam HS, Lee SH. Emphysematous pyelonephritis: drainage or nephrectomy? Br J Urol 1993;71:609–611.
115. Alvarez S, McCabe WR. Extrapulmonary tuberculosis revisited. A review of experience at Boston City and other hospitals. Medicine 1984;63:25–55.
116. Simon HB, et al. Genitourinary tuberculosis. Clinical features in a general hospital population. Am J Med 1977;63:410–420.
117. Advemeier C, et al. Pharmacokinetics of isoniazide in the elderly [letter]. Br J Clin Pharmacol 1980;10:167–169.

118. Yoshikawa TT, Nagami PH. Adverse drug reactions in tuberculous therapy. Risks and recommendations. Geriatrics 1982;37:61–66.
119. Advenier C, et al. Pharmacokinetic studies of rifampicin in the elderly. Ther Drug Monit 1983;5:61–65.
120. Weinberg AC, Boyd SD. Short-course chemotherapy and role of surgery in adult and pediatric genitourinary tuberculosis. Urol 1988;31:95–102.
121. Lattimer JK, Wechsler MW. Editorial comment. J Urol 1980;124:191.
122. Flechner SM, Gow JC. Role of nephrectomy in the treatment of non-functioning or very poorly functioning unilateral tuberculous kidney. J Urol 1980;123:822–825.
123. McDonald GSA. Xanthogranulomatous pyelonephritis. J Pathol 1981;133:203–213.
124. Tolia BM, et al. Xanthogranulomatous pyelonephritis: detailed analysis of 29 cases and a brief discussion of atypical presentations. J Urol 1981;126:437–442.
125. Petronic V, Buturovic J, Isvaneski M. Xanthogranulomatous pyelonephritis. Br J Urol 1989;64:336–338.
126. Chuang CK, et al. Xanthogranulomatous pyelonephritis: experience in 36 cases. J Urol 1992;147:333–336.
127. Grainger RG, Longstaff AJ, Parsons MA. Xanthogranulomatous pyelonephritis: a reappraisal. Lancet 1982;1:1398–1401.
128. Malek RS, Elder JS. Xanthogranulomatous pyelonephritis. A critical analysis of 26 cases and of the literature. J Urol 1978;119:589–593.
129. Schonebeck J. Studies on Candida infection of the urinary tract and on the antimycotic drug 5-fluorocytosine. Scand J Urol Nephrol 1972;11(suppl):7–48.
129a. Jacobs LG: Fungal urinary tract infections in the elderly: treatment guidelines. Drugs Aging 1996;8:89–96.
130. Fisher J, et al. Fungus balls of the urinary tract. South Med J 1979;72:1281–1284.
131. Rohner TJ Jr, Tuliszewski RM. Fungal cystitis: awareness, diagnosis and treatment. J Urol 1980;124:142–143.
132. Wise GJ, Kozinn PJ, Goldberg P. Fluocytosine in the management of genitourinary candidiasis: 5 years of experience. J Urol 1980;124:70–72.
133. Gaybill JR, et al. Ketoconazole therapy for fungal urinary tract infections. J Urol 1983;129:68–70.
133a. Fisher JF, Newman CL, Sobel JD. Yeast in the urine: solutions for a budding problem. Clin Infect Dis 1995;20:183–189.
134. Fisher JF, et al. Urinary tract infections due to *Candida albicans.* Rev Infect Dis 1982;4:1107–1118.
134a. Jacobs LG, et al. Oral fluconazole compared with bladder irrigation with amphotericin B for treatment of fungal urinary tract infections in elderly patients. Clin Infect Dis 1996;22:30–35.
134b. Leu H-S, Huang C-T. Clearance of funguria with short-course antifungal regimens: a prospective, randomized, controlled study. Clin Infect Dis 1995;20:1152–1157.
135. Frangos DN, Nyberg LM Jr. Genitourinary fungal infections. South Med J 1986; 79:455–459.
136. Bennett JE. Chemotherapy of systemic mycosis. N Engl J Med 1974;290:30–31.
136a. Kauffman CA: The role of systemic triazoles in the treatment of fungal infections. Formulary 1997;32:806–819.

137. Larsen EH, Gasser TC, Madsen PO. Antimicrobial prophylaxis in urologic surgery. Urol Clin NA 1986;13:591–604.
138. Coptcoat MJ, et al. Is antibiotic prophylaxis necessary for routine urodynamic investigations? A controlled study in 100 patients. Br J Urol 1988;61:302–303.
139. Grabe M. Antimicrobial agents in transurethral prostatic resection. J Urol 1987; 138:245–252.
140. Te Slaa E, et al. Urinary tract infections following laser prostatectomy: is there a need for antibiotic prophylaxis? Br J Urol 1996;77:228–232.
141. Lukkarinen O, et al. Prospective randomized open study between ciprofloxacin and a combination of sulfadiazine and trimethoprim in antibiotic prosphylaxis in connection with transurethral prostatectomy. Scand J Urol Nephrol 1996;30:33–36.
142. Ljungberg B, Nilsson-Ehle I. Pharmacokinetics of antimicrobial agents in the elderly. Rev Infect Dis 1987;9:250–264.

10

Acute Renal Failure

Acute renal failure (ARF), defined as an increase in the BUN or serum creatinine, can be due to prerenal, renal, or postrenal causes. Postrenal (or obstructive) uropathy is discussed in Chapter 8. In this chapter the discussion involves mainly acute prerenal and renal failure, complications that occur in approximately 8% of admissions of patients over 60 years of age at our hospital. Among this group, prerenal failure occurred in 52% of the patients, similar to the 47% reported by Pascual et al. (1) and 55% reported by Mclnnes et al. (2). The remaining 48% had acute tubular necrosis (ATN). The incidence of the latter form of ARF in the elderly has increased significantly during the past decade (3). For instance, in a series of ARF due to ATN in adult patients reported prior to 1980, 24–46% of the patients were elderly (4–6), compared to 48–76% in more recent studies (6–11). Our experience is similar, a phenomenon that cannot be explained solely by a higher percentage of elderly patients occupying hospital beds. The population of our hospitalized elderly patients has increased by only 30% over this same period.

I. PRERENAL FAILURE (PRERENAL AZOTEMIA)

A. Etiology

The etiology of prerenal azotemia in our hospitalized elderly patients, in order of decreasing frequency, includes volume contraction, congestive heart failure, and drugs such as nonsteroidal antiinflammatory drugs (NSAIDs), converting enzyme inhibitors, diuretics, and antibiotics.

B. Pathogenesis and Clinical Manifestations

Volume contraction is the most common cause of prerenal azotemia in the elderly (1). The typical patient is admitted for congestive heart failure, given a diuretic, and put on a low-sodium diet. Frequently, aggressive diuresis is continued after the patient has attained euvolemia, leading to volume contraction with an increase in BUN and serum creatinine (the latter often disproportionately less). In elderly patients with congestive heart failure, the diuresis may be so aggressive that acute prerenal azotemia ensues even though the patient is not dehydrated. This phenomenon is seen more frequently in patients receiving a loop diuretic in combination with a thiazide (12). Other groups at risk include elderly patients with mild preexisting renal insufficiency who are hospitalized for either elective surgery or other acute illnesses and placed on a salt-restricted diet or a diuretic for hypertension. Symptoms vary from nonspecific complaints such as generalized weakness to those related to a decrease in circulating plasma volume, such as increased thirst and postural lightheadedness or vertigo. On physical examination, poor skin turgor and an orthostatic drop in blood pressure may be noted.

The sensitivity of the physical examination as outlined above, in concert with the history and chart review, in the diagnosis of volume contraction in the elderly is not very high. Indeed, in one prospective study involving adult patients of various ages, the sensitivity was found to be only 49% and specificity was 51% (13). Besides the disproportionate rise in the BUN compared to the serum creatinine, hyponatremia is present in 30% of the patients. Hypernatremia may be seen in confused, bed-ridden elderly without access to water. Unless there is concomitant preexisting renal disease, the urine sediment may be benign. In 50 elderly patients with prerenal azotemia seen by the authors, urinary indices revealed a urine/plasma creatinine of 34 ± 8 (which is generally compatible with prerenal azotemia). The urine sodium (Na) concentration, which is expected to be low in prerenal azotemia (<10 mEq/L), when assessed by the renal failure index (RFI) (UNa ÷ Ucreatinine/Pcreatinine) or fractional excretion of Na (FE_{Na}) (UNa/PNa ÷ Ucreatinine/Pcreatinine), was 1.5 ± 0.8. In prerenal azotemia the RFI or FE_{Na} is usually less than 1.0%. The prerenal azotemia accompanying diuretic use is frequently associated with a high urinary sodium concentration and thus is not helpful. When prerenal azotemia occurs in the setting of metabolic alkalosis with bicarbonaturia, the urinary Na concentration may be relatively high (>40 mEq/L), and the urinary chloride is more diagnostic (<10 mEq/L) (14). Both proximal and distal nephron segments participate in the enhanced salt reabsorption seen with volume contraction, the stimulus including renal factors such as a decreased glomerular filtration rate (GFR), peritubular physical factors related to an elevated filtration fraction and a decrease in papillary plasma flow (15), and humoral factors including catecholamines, angiotensin, aldosterone, and vasopressin (16). In addition to the hemodynamic factors, the decrease in kidney function seen in these patients may also be related to a decrease in the glomerular ultrafiltration coefficient (17).

In patients with ARF due to uncontrolled congestive heart failure, the diagnosis is not difficult because dyspnea, distended neck veins, S_3 gallop, or hepatic congestion is usually present. The RFI and FE_{Na} are low (below 1.0%), occasionally even in patients receiving diuretic therapy. A combined decrease in transcapillary hydraulic pressure and glomerular ultrafiltration coefficient appears to be responsible for the decline in kidney function seen in these patients (18). In general, the reduction in GFR tends to be more severe in the elderly, which possibly reflects an age-associated hemodynamic pattern governing GFR in this age group (19).

The ARF secondary to NSAID is usually of the prerenal variety and is a complication encountered almost exclusively in the elderly, since over 80% of reported patients have been over the age of 60 (20,21). Males are affected as frequently as females. The agents most commonly responsible are indomethacin, ibuprofen, zomepirac, sulindac, naproxen, and salicylates. The acute worsening in kidney function tends to occur early after initiation of the drug (11), usually during the first 3–5 days, and does not depend on dose (see section on drug-induced hyperkalemia in Chapter 3). It develops in patients with an "ineffective" circulatory volume (congestive heart failure, liver cirrhosis, sepsis, dehydration) and chronic renal insufficiency. The degree of the renal failure varies in severity, with some patients developing symptoms and signs of uremia (22). Most patients (71%) with NSAID-induced ARF are nonoliguric. Hyperchloremic metabolic acidosis as well as a rise in serum potassium (K) occur in virtually every patient. The severity of the hyperkalemia depends on the preexisting K level and the rate of urine formation. Findings suggestive of acute interstitial nephritis (another complication of NSAID, see below), such as skin rash, eosinophilia, eosinophiluria, and proteinuria, are usually absent. The urinary sediment is benign, and the RFI or FE_{Na} is less than 1% in more than 80% of patients. Histological examination of the kidney in two of our patients who died (one from a cardiac arrhythmia and the other from a massive pulmonary embolus) failed to show any significant abnormalities. Both prostaglandin E_2 (PGE_2) and 6-keto-PGF_1a (a stable breakdown product of prostacyclin or PG_2) have been found to be significantly decreased in such patients. Renal function appears to decline in parallel with the decrease in 6-keto-PGF_1a rather than PGE_2 (23,24). Glomerular and vascular prostaglandins, mainly PGE_2 and PGI_1, play an important homeostatic role in modulating or antagonizing the vasoconstriction induced by angiotensin II and activation of the renal autonomic nervous system. Thus, the administration of NSAID to patients with the risk factors noted earlier induces renal failure by removing the negative feedback or modulatory role of vasodilatory prostaglandins (mainly prostacyclin), thereby accentuating renal vasoconstriction (25).

ARF secondary to the angiotensin-converting enzyme inhibitors (ACEi) occurs in 27% of patients taking captopril and in 17% of those taking enalapril with bilateral renal artery stenosis or renal artery stenosis in a solitary kidney (26,27). The rise in serum creatinine can be attributed to the decrease in blood pressure and efferent glomerular arteriolar tone, which decreases transglomerular hydraulic pressure and, thereby, GFR. The fact that 25% of patients on captopril and 23% of those on enalapril with unilateral renal artery stenosis and a normally functioning contralateral kidney also develop ARF suggests that factor(s) other than angiotensin II blockade might be responsible for the effects of these agents on kidney function (26). The urinary sediment in these patients is usually benign, with the RFI and FE_{Na} suggesting prerenal azotemia. Serum creatinine may also rise in patients with advanced congestive heart failure and preexisting chronic mild to moderate renal insufficiency (serum creatinine 1.5–2.0 mg/dl) following the administration of captopril, enalapril, or any other ACEi (28). The renal failure in this situation may be the result of excessively rapid diuresis, since lowering the dose of the diuretic without changing the dose of the ACEi may return kidney function to baseline. The long-acting enalapril, however, might be detrimental to renal function in some patients, regardless of their extracellular volume status. In these instances the relative hypotension induced may be responsible for the decrease in kidney function (29).

ARF has been reported in elderly with preexisting renal insufficiency receiving potassium-sparing diuretics (30). In this study, involving 19 elderly patients, the drug most commonly used was amiloride in combination with hydrochlorothiazide (10 patients), followed by triamterene with hydrochlorothiazide (8 patients) and amiloride alone (1). Six patients were taking other diuretics, and 5 were using NSAIDs. Hypovolemia might have been a contributing factor in some of these patients. The renal insufficiency was reversible upon discontinuing the involved drugs in 17 patients, suggesting that a functional rather than a structural abnormality was responsible for the renal failure. Of the remaining 2 patients, 1 did not improve and 1 died with renal failure. It is clear that renal function must be monitored regularly in these patients.

Finally, the use of demeclocycline for correction of hyponatremia (mainly in patients with preexisting liver disease) can be associated with prerenal azotemia due to increased urinary salt losses (see Chapter 2).

C. Treatment and Prognosis

The prognosis is usually good in elderly with prerenal azotemia due to volume contraction. Unless sepsis develops, exposure to nephrotoxic agents occurs, or other problems arise to alter the course of the prerenal azotemia by producing acute tubular necrosis (a complication seen in 2–3% of our patients), recovery is the rule. Patients who are symptomatic with orthostatic hypotension and those with uremic symptoms should receive fluid parenterally, the rate of infusion being adjusted according to the quantity and electrolyte content of the fluid lost. In the others, a more gradual approach can be used, changing the diet to a regular-salt diet and liberalizing oral fluid intake. Diuretics should be discontinued. Weight and kidney function should be monitored frequently. The dosage of all drugs excreted by the kidneys (e.g., digoxin) should be reassessed regularly and altered according to the GFR.

Most patients with declining kidney function secondary to congestive heart failure per se will improve with a low-salt diet, bed rest, judicious use of inotropic agents, vasodilators, and diuretic administration. Furosemide or other loop diuretics are the most widely used in these patients, with the intravenous method of administration preferred because of the altered pharmacodynamics seen in these patients (31). In the elderly, 30–50% less furosemide reaches the renal tubules compared to younger subjects with normal renal function (32). In general, doses of 160–200 mg of furosemide, 3–5 mg of bumetanide, or 50–100 mg of torsemide are sufficient to produce a maximum diuretic response (33). If necessary, hydrochlorothiazide, 50–100 mg/day, or metolazone, 5–10 mg/day orally, can be added to the loop diuretic (12,34). If all else fails, dialysis or continuous arteriovenous hemofiltration (CAVH) may be necessary (35,36). The mortality rate is high in those patients who fail to respond to diuretics and vasodilator therapy; however, the chances of recovering baseline kidney function in those patients in whom the heart failure is controlled are good except for diabetics, in whom the incidence of irreversible losses of function of varying degree is well above 30% in our experience. For patients in whom CAVH was necessary, 25% died during the course of treatment and 46% improved. In the remaining 29%, cardiac function improved but renal function worsened (36).

In approximately 85% of patients with ARF secondary to NSAIDs, kidney function returns to baseline within 5–6 days of discontinuing the drug. Dialysis may be required in the remaining 15%, but eventually these patients recover sufficient kidney function to allow discontinuation of dialysis. In this latter group of patients, FE_{Na} was greater than 1%, suggesting that they may have developed ATN. The reason for this more severe form of the ARF is not clear.

The renal insufficiency precipitated by ACEi usually reverses upon discontinuing therapy. In patients in whom the impairment in kidney function is mild (a rise in serum creatinine of 1–1.5 mg/dl), creatinine clearance stabilizes over time or might even increase despite continuing the drug (26).

II. ACUTE TUBULAR NECROSIS

A. Etiology

The etiology of acute renal failure due to ATN in 466 elderly patients is outlined in Table 1, showing that hypovolemic, septic shock, and nephrotoxic agents are

Table 1 Etiology of Acute Tubular Necrosis in 466 Elderly Patients

	No. of patients	Percentage
Medical		
Hypovolemic shock	153	32.8
Septic shock	93	20.0
Nephrotoxic agents	41	8.8
Cardiovascular catastrophes	41	8.8
Hepatobiliary diseases	10	2.2
Pigments (myoglobin, hemoglobin)	5	1.1
	Total 343	73.7
Surgical	123	26.3

Source: Refs. 37–39, and the authors' experience.

responsible for 53% of the cases (37–39). Multiple etiological factors including systemic inflammatory response syndrome and multiple organ dysfunction syndrome are found in over 44% of elderly patients with ATN (1).

B. Clinical Manifestations

In the elderly, as in younger patients, ATN is manifested by a rise in BUN of 10–20 mg/dl/day and in creatinine of 0.5–2 mg/dl/day. Prior to the 1980s, the reported incidence of oliguria, defined as a daily urine output less than 400 ml, was in the range of 60–75% with ATN (5). In more recent reports, however, oliguria is reported in only 30–45% (40). Our experience has been about the same, both in the general population and in the elderly. Anuria, defined as a urinary output less than 100 ml/day, occurs in 8–12%. Hyperkalemia is seen almost exclusively in the oliguric group, more so in patients with increased muscle and other tissue breakdown. Acidosis is generally mild, with a serum bicarbonate concentration of 18–20 mEq/L in 80% of the patients. RFI and FE_{Na} are usually greater than 3%, similar to that reported in younger patients with ATN (38,41). Defects in the inner medullary collecting duct sodium reabsorption appear to play an important role in the increased FE_{Na} seen in ATN (42). Five to ten percent of elderly patients, however, have a low FE_{Na} in the presence of ATN. This phenomenon is most often seen in the early stages of radiocontrast nephropathy (43), myoglobinuric renal failure, and sepsis in which spasm of the glomerular capillaries may be playing a role. The urinary sodium in ATN may also be misleadingly low in patients in shock and those who have congestive heart failure or the hepatorenal syndrome. The measurement of urinary osmolality is usually of limited value in differentiating prerenal azotemia from ATN in the elderly, given the diminished ability to concentrate the urine that is generally present in the aged (44). Microscopic examination of the urine may reveal large numbers of tubular cells, tubular cell casts, and coarsely granular pigmented casts. Such a characteristic urinary sediment was present in approximately 60% of our patients with ATN.

C. Specific Forms of Acute Tubular Necrosis

1. Ischemic ATN

This form of ATN is due to inadequate renal perfusion which occurs with hypovolemia, sepsis, or cardiogenic shock accounts for 61.6% of all cases of ATN in the elderly, a somewhat higher rate than the 50% reported in the general population (45). In the initiation phase of this form of ARF, adenosine triphosphate (ATP) is depleted following the ischemic episode, resulting in inactivity of the Na-K-ATPase pump with subsequent water uptake by the cell and cell swelling, erythrocyte aggregation, congestion, and stasis (46). Reactive inflammatory response following the ischemic injury also plays a role (47). In general, the metabolic and functional severity is related to the degree of loss of residual nucleotides during the ischemic episode (48). The decrease in cortical blood flow resulting from vascular congestion could induce vasoconstriction of the afferent artery of the glomerular capillary and medullary ischemia (49,49a), which is responsible for intraluminal tubular obstruction and a decrease in the glomerular ultrafiltration coefficient (50,51). These factors, together with tubular backleak of glomerular ultrafiltrate and activation of the tubulo-glomerular feedback loop, contribute to the maintenance phase of ATN (52–54). The predominance of one mechanism over the other may vary significantly among individual patients and may help to explain why some patients are oliguric and others not and why some have a protracted course and others a shorter one.

The biochemical changes responsible for cell injury during the maintenance phase of ATN are still unsettled. Several pathways are involved, including the accumulation of free radicals and free fatty acids, a decrease in phospholipids, and an increase in membrane permeability with subsequent increased intracellular calcium (55), the end point being mitochondrial and plasma membrane damage (56). In patients with sepsis, it is not unusual for a drop in urinary output to precede by hours the temperature spike and hypotension. This phenomenon represents endotoxin-induced renal ischemia due to renal nerve activation (57) and increased release of platelet-activating factor (58), thromboxane A_2, and leukotrienes (59). It is therefore prudent for a clinician facing a sudden, otherwise unexplained drop in urinary output in an elderly patient at risk (those with respiratory failure or an indwelling catheter) to start adequate antibiotic coverage after all the appropriate cultures are taken.

2. Nephrotoxin-Induced ATN

Nephrotoxin-induced ATN accounts for 8.8% of cases seen in the elderly (Table 1). The agents responsible for this disorder are outlined in Table 2.

Table 2 Agents Responsible for Nephrotoxin-Induced ATN

Agent	Frequency (%)
Antibiotics	40
Nonsteroidal antiinflammatory drugs	22
Contrast media	18
Cancer chemotherapy	9
Other drugs or a combination of nephrotoxic drugs	11
	100

a. Antibiotics. Aminoglycoside-induced nephrotoxicity occurs in 8–20% of the patients receiving any one of the three commonly used drugs: gentamicin, tobramycin, and amikacin (60–63). The incidence is particularly high in the elderly, since these drugs are handled mainly through glomerular filtration, which tends to decrease with age. The usually recommended dose not infrequently is associated with higher peak and rough levels as well as abnormal proximal tubular cell accumulation of the antibiotic in the elderly (64). Therefore, the best approach when using aminoglycosides in the elderly is to measure serum concentrations and individually calculate each patient's dosage requirement early during treatment. By so doing the incidence of nephrotoxicity can be lowered significantly (65). The incidence of nephrotoxicity is not lower with the once-a-day dosage regimen when compared to the more conventional twice-a-day schedule (66). Data similar to that existing for the general population, comparing the relative nephrotoxicity of one aminoglycoside over the other, are not available in the elderly (67,68). Besides age, other factors associated with an increased risk of nephrotoxicity include: preexisting renal insufficiency, liver disease, concomitant drug administration such as furosemide or a cephalosporin, volume depletion, hypokalemia, and long duration of therapy (69–71). As in younger patients, the elderly with aminoglycoside-induced nephrotoxicity present with a progressive increase in BUN and creatinine, starting around the second week of therapy. Nonoliguria is the rule. Since a vasopressin-resistant concentrating defect as well as an increase in FE_{Na} generally precede the rise in BUN and creatinine (72), 70–80% of our patients also showed evidence of volume contraction at time of diagnosis. The defect in Na reabsorption appears to involve both the proximal and distal tubules. Renal tubular epithelial casts are frequently found on examination of the urine sediment. Enzymuria and proteinuria (usually less than 1 g/24 hr) are frequently observed. The exact mechanisms responsible for the ARF in aminoglycoside-induced nephrotoxicity are not clear. The final common pathway, as in ischemic ATN, is renal tubular cell injury, including binding by the drug to cell membrane phospholipids, provoking changes in renal phospholipid content and in plasma membrane permeability and transport, as well as direct effects on cell mitochondrial and lysosomal functions (69).

Besides the aminoglycosides, the cephalosporins can also induce nephrotoxicity, particularly when the two are used in combination (73,74). ATN due to cephalothin or cephalexin has been reported in the elderly (75–77). The clinical picture is identical to that of the aminoglycoside toxicity. Renal failure is more common with high doses, occurring anytime between the 3rd and 14th day of therapy, and can be severe enough to require dialysis. Changes compatible with ATN are seen on examination of kidney tissue (78). The mechanisms by which these antibiotics induce renal tubular cell necrosis are not clear. It should be noted that cefoxitin can interfere with the creatinine assay, thereby causing a false elevation in serum creatinine levels, more so in patients with preexisting chronic renal insufficiency (79).

An increase in BUN and serum creatinine occurs in virtually every elderly patient receiving the antifungal agent amphotericin B. No correlation seems to exist between the degree of renal failure and the total dose of drug administered. Although renal function improves when the drug is discontinued, a certain percentage of elderly patients (more so than younger patients) end up with a persistent reduction in creatinine clearance compared to pretreatment values (80). The usual recommendation is that therapy be withheld when the serum creatinine exceeds 3 mg/dl (81). The renal failure is generally nonoliguric. Proteinuria is minimal, and tubular casts are frequently found in the urine sediment. Histologically, necrosis of proximal and distal tubule epithelial cells with intracellular and intratubular calcium deposits are seen, with the severity correlating with the degree of renal insufficiency (82,83). Besides ATN, patients receiving amphotericin B may also develop various forms of tubular dysfunction manifested by hypokalemia, nephrogenic diabetes insipidus, and renal tubular acidosis. These complications result from direct tubular epithelial cell damage by the drug (84).

ATN, not always reversible, has been reported in elderly with preexisting renal insufficiency given a tetracycline other than doxycycline. The exact mechanism responsible for the worsening of kidney function is unclear. It is therefore recommended that other antibiotics be used in these patients whenever feasible (85).

b. NSAIDs. Histologically proven ATN has been reported in elderly taking these drugs (86). The overall clinical picture is similar to that found in patients who develop prerenal azotemia, except that renal indices are compatible with ATN and the course is more prolonged after the offending agent is withdrawn. Some patients, as discussed earlier, may even require dialysis, and recovery of 100% of baseline kidney function may not take place.

c. Contrast Media. Eighteen percent of nephrotoxin-induced ATN in the elderly is due to radio-contrast agent administration (see Table 2) and occurs almost exclusively in patients with underlying kidney disease. This form of ATN may develop after any intravascular injection of contrast media, whether it is for angiography, intravenous pyelography, computed tomography (CT), or intravenous cholangiography. The incidence of ATN, however, appears to be highest among patients undergoing arteriography (87). Patients with serum creatinine greater than 1.5 mg/dl should receive a nonionic, low-osmolality contrast agent, since these appear to lower the risk of nephrotoxicity in these specific patients (88,88a). Of 151 patients reported with contrast media-induced ATN, 115 (76%) were over the age of 60. One or several of the proposed risk factors (Table 3) were present in 94% of the older patients and 89% of the younger ones (87,89–99). Therefore, it seems unlikely that old age per se, in the absence of any risk factor, increases the likelihood of a patient developing ARF following contrast dye administration.

The BUN and creatinine start to rise within 24–48 hr after injection of the radiocontrast, reaching a peak by the 3rd to 4th day (97). Most of the patients are nonoliguric, with oliguria present in only 16–20% (89–99). In our experience, renal tubular epithelial cell or muddy-brown casts in the urinary sediment are unusual. In general, FE_{Na} is greater than 1%, but values of less than 1% have been reported (96,100). The pathogenesis of radiocontrast-induced ATN is probably multifactorial, with direct tubular toxicity and renal ischemia due to a dye-induced vasoconstriction playing roles. The latter may lead to disruption of the medullary oxygen balance, possibly contributing to the initiating insult (101,102). Tubular obstruction caused by Tamm-Horsfall protein precipitation with contrast media and perhaps a decrease in the glomerular ultrafiltration coefficient have been implicated in the maintenance phase (103–105). As a rule, if dye has to be given to a patient with underlying renal insufficiency, it is prudent to make sure the patient is neither volume contracted nor in congestive heart failure. We routinely administer furosemide (dose in mg = 4000 ÷ creatinine clearance, either measured or calculated) or 250 ml of 20% mannitol at the time of dye infusion. This regimen has been associated with a 75% decrease in the incidence of dye-induced ATN at our institution (106). These results have not been confirmed in a recent study (107); however, there were many issues in this study which cast doubt on the findings. It has also been suggested that administering an amount of dye

Table 3 Risk Factors Associated with Dye-Induced ATN

Preexisting renal insufficiency (due mainly to nephrosclerosis)
Diabetic nephropathy, with or without renal insufficiency
''Ischemic'' kidney due to either volume contraction or congestive heart failure
Multiple myeloma
Prior contrast-induced ATN
Contrast volume >200 ml
Serum albumin <3.5 g/dl

estimated by the following formula [5 ml of contrast × body weight (kg) ÷ serum creatinine (mg/dl), up to a maximum of 300 ml] could significantly lower the risk of developing ATN with radiocontrast media use (108).

d. Chemotherapy. As in younger patients, drugs such as methotrexate, streptozotocin, mitomycin (see section on hemolytic uremic syndrome in Chapter 7), and cisplatin can induce ATN in the elderly (109). With methotrexate, intratubular precipitation of the drug occurs in concentrated and acid urines, resulting in obstruction. This complication is now seen with less frequency because hydration and alkalinization are routinely carried out prior to therapy (110). The nephrotoxicity of streptozotocin is dose related, occurring most frequently at doses exceeding 1.5 g/m^2/week. The renal failure, which is oliguric, is usually preceded by clinical evidence of tubular damage, manifested by proteinuria, Fanconi's syndrome, or nephrogenic diabetes insipidus (111). Cisplatin is the anticancer drug most frequently associated with renal failure in the elderly. Age per se, despite the decrease in GFR, is not a risk factor as long as the dose is kept at or below 60 mg/m^2/month (112). The nephrotoxicity, which is dose related, results in direct damage to the S_3 segment of the proximal tubule. A reduction in renal blood flow and transglomerular hydrostatic pressure, accounting for the decrease in GFR, has been demonstrated in animals (113). Hypomagnesemia and nephrogenic diabetes insipidus may develop. Acute uric acid nephropathy, a consequence of intratubular urate deposition, which was originally described in patients with lymphoproliferative disorders undergoing chemotherapy, has become a rarity nowadays, since preventive measures such as volume expansion and allopurinol administration are routine (114).

e. Other. Anesthetic agents such as methoxyflurane may be associated with nonoliguric ATN. The pathogenesis is not clear. ATN may be seen in patients taking paracetamol at either excessive or therapeutic doses (115,116). Clinical evidence of hepatotoxicity may not be present. Finally, several other drugs have been associated with ATN (117); however, in many of these reports it is not clear whether one is dealing with ATN or acute interstitial nephritis, since histological examination of kidney tissue was not included in the report.

It is not uncommon for elderly with preexisting renal disease to develop a rise in serum creatinine while receiving a $histamine_2$ blocker such as cimetidine (118). The kidney function in these patients is unchanged. The increase in serum creatinine is secondary to the inhibition of creatinine secretion in the proximal tubule. An unchanged BUN is a clue to the diagnosis. The creatinine returns to baseline once the drug is discontinued.

3. Hepatobiliary Disease

Hepatobiliary diseases are responsible for 2.2% of cases of ATN in the elderly (Table 1). The renal failure associated with acute cholecystitis, acute cholangitis, and acute hepatitis is oliguric in 57% of patients and tends to occur early, although in patients with acute cholangitis or cholecystitis it can manifest itself during the postoperative period. The FE_{Na} is usually greater than 1%. A lower value should suggest the possibility of hepatorenal syndrome. Several mechanisms, acting singly or in concert, contribute to the high incidence of ATN seen with hepatobiliary diseases; these include sepsis, hypotension related to the cardiodepressor or the natriuretic effect of cholemia, circulating endotoxin, and changes in vascular reactivity (119–124). Bailey (125) has reported a high correlation between the presence of circulating endotoxin and decrease in creatinine clearance seen in patients with obstructive jaundice. These high levels of endotoxin may be derived from increased gut absorption due to the absence of bile salts in the intestinal lumen. Bile salts apparently exert an inhibitory effect on endotoxin absorption.

ATN complicates acute pancreatitis in 1.4% of elderly patients (126). In our experience, oliguria is present in approximately 65% of the patients. Blood pressure is usually in the normotensive range, although it is lower compared to that seen following recovery (by 10–20 mmHg in every patient). The incidence of hypocalcemia is similar to that observed in other forms of ATN. The studies of Levy et al. (127) suggest that hypovolemia induced by the release of specific enzymes from the inflamed pancreas with subsequent loss of protein-rich plasma from the vascular space appears to be responsible for the renal damage.

4. Pigment-Induced ATN

Pigment-induced ATN occurs less frequently in the elderly compared to younger patients (38). The nontraumatic form of rhabdomyolysis secondary to influenza-like illness, seizures, alcoholism, immobilization, hyperosmolar state, and muscle necrosis associated with gangrene due to vascular occlusion (128) are more prevalent in the elderly compared to the posttraumatic variety and is present in 0.8% of hospitalized elderly (129). Also, ARF associated with hemolysis is far less common than that associated with rhabdomyolysis in our experience. As in younger patients with these complications, volume contraction is almost universally present. Oliguria is present in 40% and hypocalcemia in 65% (130). The exact mechanisms by which myoglobin or hemoglobin induce renal failure are not clear. Since both substances contain iron, it is quite possible that intracellular formation of toxic oxygen radicals and the generation of potentially cytotoxic fatty acids are involved (131). Furthermore, by binding to nitric oxide, hemoglobin and myoglobin promote medullary vasoconstriction and hypoxia (49). Since volume contraction plays a significant role in pigment-induced nephropathy, it is suggested that an alkaline solute diuresis be immediately instituted in these patients (132).

5. Acute Tubular Necrosis in Surgical Patients

ATN complicates the course in 26.3% of elderly surgical patients (see Table 1). Except in abdominal aortic aneurysmectomy and intervention in the jaundiced patient (see previous section on hepatobiliary disease), in our experience the rate of ATN does not depend on the type of procedure being performed. Hypotension, particularly in patients who are volume contracted (owing to continuation of diuretics and a low-salt diet during the preoperative period in a patient with preexisting chronic renal insufficiency), and sepsis secondary to abscess formation or a perforated viscous are responsible for most of the cases occurring during the preoperative period. At various times during the recovery period, cardiovascular catastrophies or sepsis due to wound, lung, or genitourinary infections become the predominant factors. Multiple factors were present in 78% of our patients.

The overall incidence of ATN in the elderly undergoing abdominal aortic surgery varies between 14% and 24% (133,134). In this group, the majority (68% in one study) (135) had undergone emergency surgery for a ruptured aneurysm. Hypotension, prolonged ischemia time in patients who needed suprarenal aortic clamping, and atheroembolic disease (see Chapter 13), are primarily responsible for the renal failure (136,137), which is nonoliguric in the majority of patients, reflecting current practice of rapid fluid replacement and intraoperative use of mannitol. Since the presence of ARF alters the outcome unfavorably, Swan-Ganz catheterization and volume loading should be undertaken whenever feasible before, during, and after surgery. In one study, in which fluid balance was carefully monitored and the pulmonary artery wedge pressure kept at 10 mmH_2O, the occurrence of ARF was decreased by one-third (134). There is also some evidence that isovolemic hemodilution can also preserve renal function (138).

D. Treatment

Therapy for ATN is supportive. Attention should be paid to fluid homeostasis, particularly in the oliguric patient. In our experience, volume overload in an elderly patient with preexisting cardiac disease and/or multiple organ failure is the most common indication for initiating dialytic therapy (8%). Uncontrolled hyperkalemia and acidosis also necessitate dialysis.

Furosemide, 200–1000 mg (100 mg/5 min), should be administered to oliguric patients in an attempt to increase urine output in order to make fluid management easier (139–141a). Using this approach, 40% of patients can be converted from an oliguric to a nonoliguric form of ATN, which does not change the mortality rate but does hasten recovery and decrease the need for dialysis (40). We usually start with 200 mg of furosemide administered intravenously and increase the dose every 2–3 hr if there is no response, up to a maximum single dose of 1000 mg. There is no evidence that the use of either dopamine or atrial natriuretic peptide (ANP) improves renal function or outcome in elderly with established acute renal failure (142,143). ANP, however, may improve dialysis-free survival in very severe, oliguric acute renal failure (143).

1. Dialysis

All three dialytic interventions presently available, including peritoneal dialysis, hemodialysis, and continuous arteriovenous hemofiltration with dialysis (CAVHD), have been used successfully in the elderly (144–148). In general, these modalities are as well tolerated in the elderly as in younger patients. The choice of one over another is dictated by the treating physician's experience. For elderly patients with severe hyperkalemia (serum K > 6.5 mEq/L) accompanied by acidosis and marked catabolism, hemodialysis is preferred, using biocompatible membranes (polyacrylonitrile or polymethylmethacrylate) (148a). Patients with multiple organ failure and those requiring the removal of large amounts of fluids, those with recent or old abdominal surgical scars, and those requiring large amounts of fluid for nutritional purposes can be treated by CAVHD (147,148). The latter might eventually become the therapeutic modality of choice for the elderly with acute renal failure. So far it appears that the delivered dialysis dose rather the dialytic procedure per se determines the outcome (149,150).

2. Nutrition

In the critically ill elderly patient, attention should be paid to providing adequate nutrition. The gastrointestinal tract remains the optimal route for the delivery of nutrients and should be used first unless there are clear contraindications. In patients who are unable to ingest food normally, a nasogastric tube may be necessary. If this situation is prolonged, a feeding gastrostomy or jejunostomy may be necessary (150a,151). Once the method of delivery has been chosen, a continuous infusion of any of the available feeding mixtures can be used. We generally start with a half-strength mixture as well as half the usual infusion rate, increasing both gradually, depending on the patient's tolerance, until the desired volume and caloric requirements are achieved. Formulas for calculating caloric requirements in the basal as well as in the stressed state are available (152–154). For patients in whom enteral feeding is not possible, peripheral vein total parenteral nutrition or central venous hyperalimentation should be used. We prefer the latter approach in the postoperative patient. Glucose remains the primary source of calories, not to exceed 2.5 g/kg, or approximately 30–40% of total caloric intake. Insulin is added to the solution if necessary. Protein (in the form of both mixed essential and nonessential amino acids), 0.6–1.5 g/kg/day, should be administered, according to the degree of catabolism (155). The use of specific nutritional support does provide marginal improvement in nitrogen balance and reduces catabolism, but, in general, does not change the course or the outcome of ATN in the elderly.

Finally, several new therapeutic modalities targeted toward the basic pathophysiological alterations seen in acute renal failure are now being studied. Although they are still in the experimental phase, the possibilities remain strong that they will eventually alter in a positive way the natural history of acute renal failure (155a).

E. Prognosis

A higher mortality was found in older patients with ATN compared with younger patients in most series published prior to 1980 (156,157). Since 1980, age as a risk factor for increased mortality in patients with ATN has been found in only a few studies (3,7,8,158,158a). Based on our personal experience and that of many others (1,5,6,9,37–39,135,159–162), age per se does not have any bearing on the prognosis of the patient with ATN, except in those who develop renal failure following aortic aneurysmectomy. In this group, patients over 70 years of age definitely have a statistically higher mortality than younger patients (134,136). Most studies suggest (as does our personal experience) that the concomitant presence of pulmonary complications such as respiratory failure, jaundice, cardiovascular complications, sepsis, and oliguria are associated with a poor outcome in the elderly with ATN (1,3,38,39,163).

Forty-nine percent of elderly with ischemic ATN die during the maintenance phase of the renal failure, and 12% die despite recovery of kidney function. The average recovery time for those who survive varies between 16 and 20 days and follows a pattern similar to the B pattern described by Myers and Moran (164). Of those who survive, 59% will have complete recovery of kidney function, 38% will remain with varying degree of renal impairment, and 3% will require maintenance hemodialysis (39,165). The long-term outcome in the latter group has generally been poor (166).

Mortality in our population of elderly patients with nephrotoxic ATN is less than 10%. The overall incidence in the adult population is approximately 13% (3,167), 7% at 14 days and 10% at 21 days in one study (167a). Dialytic intervention is required in 20% of patients, with permanent renal damage ensuing in 8%, mainly diabetics. In general, the recovery period tends to be significantly longer in the elderly.

As noted, the serum creatinine in patients with ATN secondary to contrast nephropathy usually peaks on the 3rd or 4th day, and recovery is usually complete by 10–14 days, with the great majority of patients returning to the pretreatment level of kidney function (97). Dialysis is rarely necessary except in diabetics, who occasionally are left with a persistently lower level of kidney function that only rarely requires maintenance dialysis. The mortality rate among patients undergoing a contrast-media study is higher in those who develop acute renal failure. Respiratory failure, mental status changes, and sepsis are the most common complications in these patients (97a).

Mortality in the elderly with ARF associated with liver disease is high, approaching 100% in those with the hepatorenal syndrome. The recovery rate in patients with biliary tract disease and renal failure varies between 44% and 76% (119,120,123). With acute pancreatitis, no specific data is available, but all of our elderly patients recovered kidney function.

Most elderly patients with pigment-induced ATN do well, particularly those with non-trauma-related rhabdomyolysis.

The mortality rate in patients with ARF following aortic aneurysm repair is between 63% and 77% and is higher in patients over 70 years of age. Mortality is only 12% in patients who do not develop renal failure (134,136). A significant number of patients who survive have residual chronic renal insufficiency, which may be severe enough to require maintenance dialysis. This complication is particularly common in patients with preexisting renovascular disease and is usually a result of cholesterol embolization (136).

F. Differential Diagnosis

The diagnosis of ATN is usually made on the basis of history, physical examination, and routine laboratory data. Once the diagnosis has been established, patients follow a fairly predictable course. In 5–15% of elderly with ARF in whom the findings are confusing, particularly when no precipitating event is evident or in whom the clinical course is atypical, other diagnostic steps such as a percutaneous kidney biopsy or a renal angiogram are needed (1,3,39). In this group of patients, ATN is found in 15%, acute interstitial nephritis in 30%, acute atheroembolic disease in 30%, acute glomerulonephritis in 19%, and other diseases in 6% (38,168–170).

Extracapillary glomerulonephritis and IgA nephropathy is found in the majority of patients with ARF due to a glomerulonephritis. Other disorders, such as multiple myeloma, amyloidosis, scleroderma, and hemolytic uremic syndrome, can induce ARF (Chapter 7).

III. ACUTE INTERSTITIAL NEPHRITIS

Acute interstitial nephritis (AIN) is a disorder characterized on biopsy by diffuse infiltration of the renal interstitium by mononuclear inflammatory cells and eosinophils, tubulitis, and, on occasion, scattered noncaseating granulomas with multinucleated giant cells (170). A cell-mediated immune mechanism involving T cells, mediated by a release of lymphokines and eosinophil chemostatic factors, appears to be primarily responsible for the renal findings (171,172). Eosinophil activation and degranulation with release of the eosinophil basic protein, a known epithelial toxin, are also of pathogenetic importance (Fig. 1) (173,174).

AIN may be idiopathic or related to an infection or drug (175). The idiopathic and infectious varieties occur infrequently in the elderly in our experience. Drug-induced AIN is the most common form seen in the elderly. Its true incidence in this age group is not known, but it was present in 15–30% of the patients in whom renal biopsies were performed and 7% of all the cases of ARF in the elderly (38,39,176,177).

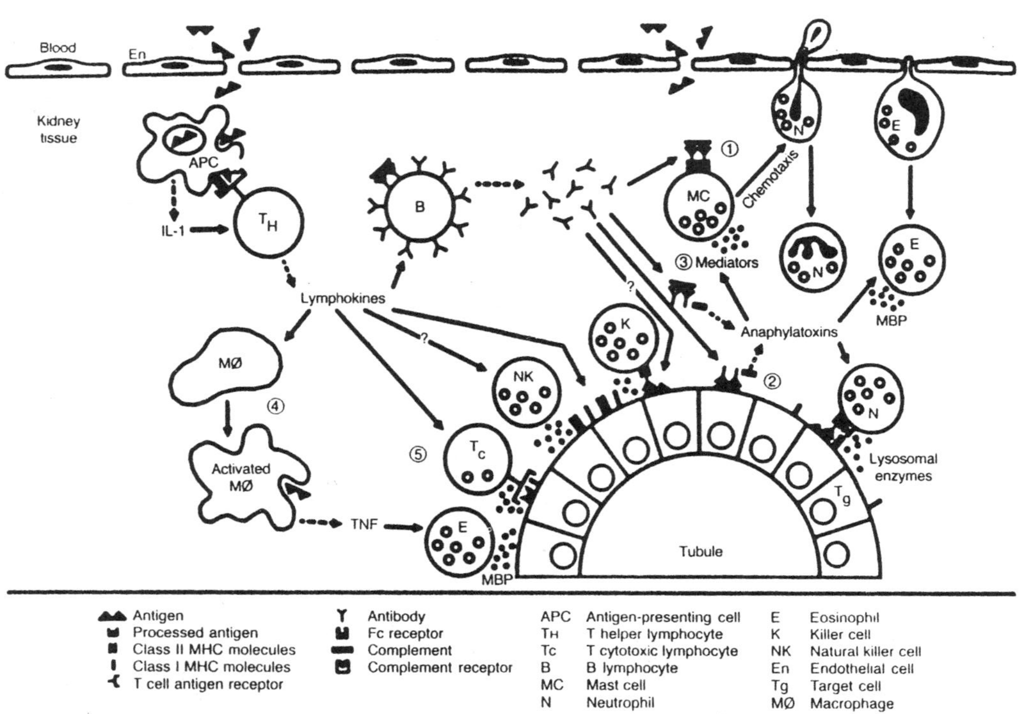

Figure 1 Schematic representation of humoral and cell-mediated immune mechanisms in pathogenesis of acute interstitial nephritis. 1 = type 1 hypersensitivity; 2 = type 2 hypersensitivity; 3 = type 3 hypersensitivity; 4 and 5 = cell-mediated hypersensitivity; IL-1 = interleukin-1; MBP = eosinophilic major basic protein; MHC = major histocompatibility complex; TNF = tumor necrosis factor. (From Ten RM, et al. Acute interstitial nephritis: immunologic and clinical aspects. Mayo Clin Proc 1988; 63:921–930.)

The list of drugs implicated in the etiology of AIN is quite extensive (175), but in the elderly the major offenders are NSAIDs (fenoprofen and meclofenamate more so than the others), antibiotics (penicillins, cephalosporins, sulfonamides, rifampin ciprofloxacin), diuretics (furosemide, potassium-sparing agents), and others (allopurinol, cimetidine, captopril). Acute deterioration of renal function is the most common manifestation of AIN, which can occur anytime from hours to months after the offending drug has been started (164,178). Skin rash, fever, and eosinophiluria were found in less than one-third of our patients. The urine indices (U_{Na}, RFI, and FE_{Na}) are similar to those characteristic of patients with ATN and therefore are not specifically helpful diagnostically (179). Eosinophiluria, defined as eosinophils constituting more than 1% of urinary leukocytes, is a very helpful sign when detected (this may require Hansel's stain) but is present in only a minority of patients and may also be seen in patients with rapidly progressive glomerulonephritis, a relatively common cause of ARF in the elderly (180). Hematuria is uncommon. Proteinuria is common, usually less than 1 g/24 hr, but may reach nephrotic range when AIN is due to an NSAID (see Chapter 7). The value of the gallium scan of the kidneys has been limited in our experience (181). The urinary level of eosinophilic major basic protein, as measured by radioimmunoassay, has been found to be elevated in patients with AIN compared to those with other forms of kidney disease (174). Further experience with this test is necessary before its value in the diagnosis of AIN can be assessed.

Since the definitive diagnosis of AIN can be made only on kidney biopsy, which may not be immediately feasible in all patients in whom the disease is suspected, it is prudent to discontinue the suspected drug if the diagnosis is entertained. In patients taking multiple drugs, we usually start with the one with the highest probability of inducing AIN. Withdrawal of the offending drug usually leads to resolution over a variable period of time (days to weeks). Glucocorticoids (prednisone, 60 mg/day given orally, with rapid tapering once kidney function stabilizes or returns to baseline) can be used. The beneficial effect of this therapy is supported by several retrospective studies (175). The prognosis of AIN is good in the elderly, with the majority of patients recovering baseline kidney function. In some patients (less than 5% in our experience), permanent loss of kidney function may occur, particularly in diabetics.

REFERENCES

1. Pascual J, et al. Incidence and prognosis of acute renal failure in older patients. J Am Geriatr Soc 1990; 38:25–30.
2. McInnes EG, et al. Renal failure in the elderly. Q J Med 1987;243:583–588.
3. Turney JH, et al. The evolution of acute renal failure. 1956–1988. Q J Med 1990;273: 83–104.
4. Scott RB, et al. Why the persistently high mortality in acute renal failure? Lancet 1972;2:75–79.

5. Minuth AN, Terrell JB Jr, Suki WN. Acute renal failure: a study of the course and prognosis of 104 patients and of the role of furosemide. Am J Med Sci 1976;271:317–324.
6. Abreo K, Moarthy A, Osborne M. Changing patterns and outcome of acute renal failure requiring hemodialysis. Arch Intern Med 1986;146:1338–1341.
7. Lien J, Chan V. Risk factors influencing survival in acute renal failure treated by hemodialysis. Arch Intern Med 1985;145:2067–2069.
8. Bullock ML, et al. The assessment of risk factors in 462 patients with acute renal failure. Am J Kidney Dis 1985;2:97–103.
9. Rosenfeld JB, et al. Acute renal failure: a disease of the elderly? Adv Nephrol 1987;16:159–168.
10. Liaño F, et al. Epidemiology of acute renal failure: a prospective, multicenter, community-based study. Kidney Int 1996;50:811–818.
11. Evans JMM, et al. Non-steroidal anti-inflammatory drugs and hospitalization for acute renal failure. Q J Med 1995;88:551–557.
12. Wollam GL, et al. Diuretic potency of combined hydrochlorothiazide and furosemide therapy in patients with azotemia. Am J Med 1982;72:929–938.
13. Chung HM, et al. Clinical assessment of extracellular fluid volume in hyponatremia. Am J Med 1987;83:905–908.
14. Anderson RJ, Gabow PA, Gross PA. Urinary chloride concentration in acute renal failure. Miner Electrol Metab 1984;10:92–97.
15. Chou, SY, et al. Inner medullary hemodynamics in chronic salt-depleted dogs. Am J Physiol 1984;246:F146–F154.
16. Shapiro JI, Anderson RJ. Sodium depletion states. In: Contemporary Issues in Nephrology. Vol. 16. New York: Churchill Livingston, 1987:246–276.
17. Steiner RW, Tucker BJ, Blantz RC. Glomerular hemodynamics in rats with chronic sodium depletion. J Clin Invest 1979;64:503–512.
18. Myers BD, et al. Dynamics of glomerular ultrafiltration following open-heart surgery. Kidney Int 1981;20:366–374.
19. Cody RJ, et al. Relation of glomerular filtration rate in chronic congestive heart failure patients. Kidney Int 1988;34:361–367.
20. Blackshear JL, Davidman M, Stillman T. Identification of risk for renal insufficiency from nonsteroidal anti-inflammatory drugs. Arch Intern Med 1983;143:1130–1134.
21. Corwin HL, Bonventre JV. Renal insufficiency associated with non-steroidal anti-inflammatory agents. Am J Kidney Dis 1984;4:147–152.
22. McCarthy JT, et al. Acute intrinsic renal failure induced by indomethacin. Role of prostaglandin synthetase inhibition. Mayo Clin Proc 1982;57:289–296.
23. Cinotti GA, et al. Effects of sulindac and ibuprofen in patients with chronic glomerular disease. Evidence of the dependence of renal function on prostacyclin. N Engl J Med 1984;310:279–283.
24. Abraham PA, Stillman TM. Salsalate exacerbation of chronic renal insufficiency. Relation to inhibition of prostaglandin synthesis. Arch Intern Med 1987;147:1674–1676.
25. Horton R, Zipser R, Fichman M. Prostaglandins, renal function and vascular regulation. Med Clin N Am 1981;64:891–914.

26. Franklin SS, Smith RD. Comparison of effects of enalapril plus hydrochlorothiazide versus standard triple therapy on renal function in renovascular hypertension. Am J Med 1985;79(suppl 3C):14–23.
27. Hollenberg NK. The treatment of renovascular hypertension: surgery, angioplasty and medical therapy with converting-enzyme inhibitors. Am J Kidney Dis 1987;10(suppl 1):52–60.
28. Packer M, et al. Functional renal insufficiency during long term therapy with captopril and enalapril in severe chronic heart failure. Ann Intern Med 1987;106:346–354.
29. Packer M, et al. Comparison of captopril and enalapril in patients with severe chronic heart failure. N Engl J Med 1986;315:847–853.
30. Lynn KL, Bailey RR, Swainson CP. Renal failure with potassium-sparing diuretics. N Z Med J 1985;98:629–633.
31. Brater DC, et al. Bumetanide and furosemide in heart failure. Kidney Int 1984;26: 183–189.
32. Kerremans ALM, et al. Furosemide kinetics and dynamics in aged patients. Clin Pharm Ther 1983;34:181–189.
33. Voelker JR, et al. Comparison of loop diuretics in patients with chronic renal insufficiency. Kidney Int 1987;32:572–578.
34. Oster JR, Epstein M, Smoller S. Combined therapy with thiazide-type and loop-type diuretic agents for resistant sodium retention. Ann Intern Med 1983;99:405–406.
35. Bartlett RH, et al. Continuous arteriovenous hemofiltration for acute renal failure. Trans Am Soc Artif Intern Organs 1988;34:67–77.
36. Canand B, et al. Slow isolated ultra-filtration for the treatment of congestive heart failure. Am J Kidney Dis 1996;28(suppl 3):S67–S73.
37. Kumar R, Hill CM, McGeown MG. Acute renal failure in the elderly. Lancet 1973; 1:90–91.
38. Lameire N, et al. Acute renal failure in the elderly. In: Oreopoulos DG, ed. Geriatric Nephrology. Boston: Martinus Nijhoff, 1986;103–116.
39. Druml W, et al. Acute renal failure in the elderly. Clin Nephrol 1994;41:342–349.
40. Anderson RJ, et al. Non-oliguric acute renal failure. N Engl J Med 1977;296: 1134–1138.
41. Oken DE. On the differential diagnosis of acute renal failure. Am J Med 1981;71: 916–920.
42. Wilson DR, Honrath U. Inner medullary collecting duct function in ischemic acute renal failure. Clin Invest Med 1988;11:157–166.
43. Fang LS, et al. Low fractional excretion of sodium with contrast media-induced acute renal failure. Arch Intern Med 1980;140:531–533.
44. Sporm NI, Lancestremere RG, Papper S. Differential diagnosis of oliguria in aged patients. N Engl J Med 1962;267:130–132.
45. Dixon BS, Anderson RJ. Non-oliguric acute renal failure. Am J Kidney Dis 1985; 6:71–80.
46. Mason J. The pathophysiology of ischemic acute renal failure. A new hypothesis about the initiation phase. Renal Physiol 1986;9:129–147.
47. Rabb H, et al. Role of CD 11a and CD 11b in ischemic acute renal failure in rats. Am J Physiol 1994;267:F1052–F1058.

48. Stromski ME, et al. Metabolic and functional consequences of inhibiting adenosine deaminase during renal ischemia in rats. J Clin Invest 1988;82:1694–1699.
49. Brezis M, Rosen S. Hypoxia of the renal medulla—its implications for disease. N Engl J Med 1995;332:647–655.
49a. Alejandro V, et al. Mechanisms of filtration failure during postischemic injury of the human kidney. J Clin Invest 1995;95:820–831.
50. Moran SM, Myers BD. Pathophysiology of protracted acute renal failure in man. J Clin Invest 1985;76:1440–1448.
51. Oken DE. Hemodynamic basis for human acute renal failure (vasomotor nephropathy). Am J Med 1984;76:702–710.
52. Myers BD, et al. Pathophysiology of hemodynamically mediated acute renal failure in man. Kidney Int 1980;18:495–504.
53. Meyers BD, et al. Glomerular and tubular function in non-oliguric acute renal failure. Am J Med 1982;72:642–649.
54. Thurau K, Boylan JW. Acute renal success: the unexpected logic of oliguria in acute renal failure. Am J Med 1976;61:308–315.
55. McCoy CE, et al. Adenosine triphosphate depletion induces a rise in cytosolic free calcium in canine renal epithelial cells. J Clin Invest 1988;82:1326–1332.
56. Epstein FH. Acute renal failure: a collection of paradoxes. Hosp Pract 1988;1: 171–194.
57. Henrich WL, et al. Dissociation of systemic and renal effects of endotoxemia. Prostaglandin inhibition uncovers an important role of renal nerves. J Clin Invest 1982;69:691–699.
58. Wang J, Dunn MJ. Platelet-activating factor mediates endotoxin-induced acute renal insufficiency in rats. Am J Physiol 1987;253:F1283–F1289.
59. Badr KF, Kelley VE, et al. Roles for thromboxane A_2 and leukotrienes in endotoxin induced acute renal failure. Kidney Int 1986;30:474–480.
60. Law WK, et al. Comparative efficacy and toxicity of amikacin/carbenicillin versus gentamicin/carbenicillin in leukopenic patients. Am J Med 1977;62:959–966.
61. Smith CR, et al. Controlled comparison of amikacin and gentamicin. N Engl J Med 1977;296:349–353.
62. Smith CR, et al. Double-blind comparison of the nephrotoxicity and auditory toxicity of gentamicin and tobramycin. N Engl J Med 1980;30:1106–1109.
63. Lane AZ, Wright GE, Blair DC. Ototoxicity and nephrotoxicity of amikacin. An overview of phase II and phase III in the United States. Am J Med 1977;62:911–918.
64. Schentag JJ, et al. Gentamicin tissue accumulation and nephrotoxic reactions. JAMA 1978;240:2067–2069.
65. Zaske DE, et al. Wide interpatient variations in gentamicin dose requirements for geriatric patients. JAMA 1982;248:3122–3126.
66. Koo J, et al. Comparison of once-daily versus pharmacokinetic dosing of aminoglycosides in elderly patients. Am J Med 1996;101:177–183.
67. Kumin GD. Clinical nephrotoxicity of tobramycin and gentamicin. A prospective study. JAMA 1980;244:1808–1810.
68. Whelton A, Solez K. Aminoglycoside nephrotoxicity. A tale of 2 transports. J Lab Clin Med 1982;99:148–155.

69. Humes HD, Weinberg JM, Knauss TC. Clinical and pathophysiologic aspect of aminoglycoside nephrotoxicity. Am J Kidney Dis 1982;2:5–29.
70. Moore RD, Smith CR, Lietman PS. Increased risk of renal dysfunction due to interaction of liver disease and aminoglycosides. Am J Med 1986;80:1092–1097.
71. Smith CR, Moore RD, Lietman PS. Studies of risk factors for aminoglycoside nephrotoxicity. Am J Kidney Dis 1986;8:308–313.
72. HSU CH, et al. Renal tubular sodium and water excretion in antibiotic-induced nephrotoxicity. Renal function in antibiotic nephrotoxicity. Nephron 1978;20: 227–234.
73. Player JE. Association of renal injury combined with cephalothin-gentamicin therapy among patients severely ill with malignant disease. Cancer 1976;37:1937–1941.
74. Foord D. Cephaloridine, Cephalothin and the kidney. J Antimicrob Chemother 1975;1(suppl 1):119–133.
75. Burton JR, et al. Acute renal failure during cephalothin therapy. JAMA 1974;229: 679–682.
76. Carling PC, et al. Nephrotoxicity associated with cephalothin administration. Arch Intern Med 1975;135:797–801.
77. Fung-Herrera CG, Mulvaney WP. Cephalexin nephrotoxicity. Reversible nonoliguric acute renal failure and hepatotoxicity associated with cephalexin therapy. JAMA 1974;229:318–319.
78. Barientos A, Bello I, Gutierrez-Millet V. Renal failure and cephalothin. Ann Intern Med 1976;84:612.
79. Saah AJ, Koch TR, Drusano GL. Cefoxitin falsely elevates creatinine levels. JAMA 1982;247:205–206.
80. Miller RP, Bates JH. Amphotericin B toxicity. A follow-up report of 53 patients. Ann Intern Med 1969;71:1089–1095.
81. Terrell CL, Hermans PE. Antifungal agents used for deep-seated mycotic infections. Mayo Clin Proc 1987;62:1116–1128.
82. Iovine G, et al. Nephrotoxicity of amphotericin B. Arch Intern Med 1963;112: 853–862.
83. Wertlake PT, et al. Nephrotoxic tubular damage and calcium deposition following amphotericin B therapy. Am J Pathol 1963;43:449–457.
84. Andreoli TE. On the anatomy of amphotericin B-cholesterol pores in lipid bilayer membranes. Kidney Int 1973;4:337–345.
85. Phillips ME, et al. Tetracycline poisoning in renal failure. Br Med J 1974;2:149–151.
86. Adams DH, et al. Non-steroidal antiinflammatory drugs and renal failure. Lancet 1986;1:57–60.
87. Rich MW, Crecelius CA. Incidence, risk factors and clinical course of acute renal insufficiency after cardiac cathetherization in patients 70 years of age or older. A prospective study. Arch Intern Med 1990;150:1237–1242.
88. Barrett QJ, Carlise EJ. Meta-analysis of the relative nephrotoxocity of high and low osmolality iodinated contrast media. Radiology 1993;188:171–178.
88a. Rudnick MR, et al. Nephrotoxicity of ionic and nonionic contrast media in 1196 patients: a randomized trial. Kidney Int 1995;47:254–261.
89. Swartz RD, et al. Renal failure following major angiography. Am J Med 1978;65: 31–37.

90. Carvallo A, et al. Acute renal failure following drip infusion pyelography. Am J Med 1978;65:38–45.
91. Van Zee B, et al. Renal injury associated with intravenous pyelography in non-diabetic and diabetic patients Ann Intern Med 1978;89:51–54.
92. Byrd L, Sherman RL. Radiocontrast-induced acute renal failure: a clinical and pathophysiologic review. Medicine 1979;58:268–279.
93. Ansari Z, Baldwin DS. Acute renal failure due to radio-contrast agents. Nephron 1976;17:28–40.
94. Krumlovsky FA, et al. Acute renal failure. Association with administration of radiographic contrast material. JAMA 1978;239:125–127.
95. Alexander RD, Berkes SL, Abuelo JG. Contrast media-induced oliguric renal failure. Arch Intern Med 1978;138:381–384.
96. Fang LST, et al. Low fractional excretion of sodium with contrast media-induced acute renal failure. Arch Intern Med 1980;140:531–533.
97. Shafi T, et al. Infusion intravenous pyelography and renal function. Effects in patients with chronic renal insufficiency. Arch Intern Med 1978;138:1218–1221.
97a. Levi EM, Viscoli CM, Horwitz RIL. The effect of acute renal failure on mortality: a cohort analysis. JAMA 1996;275:1516–1517.
98. Arkonen S, Kjellstrand CM. Intravenous pyelography in nonuremic diabetic patients. Nephron 1979;24:268–270.
99. Anto HR, et al. Infusion intravenous pyelography and renal function. Effects of hypertonic mannitol in patients with chronic renal insufficiency. Arch Intern Med 1981;141:1652–1656.
100. D'Elia JA, et al. Inadequacy of fractionnal excretion of sodium test. Arch Intern Med 1981;141:818.
101. Norby LH, DiBona GF. The renal vascular effects of meglumine diatrizoate. J Pharmacol Exp Ther 1975;193:932–940.
102. Brazis M, Epstein FH. A closer look at radiocontrast-induced nephropathy. N Engl J Med 1989;320:179–181.
103. McKenzie JK, Patel R, McQueen EG. The excretion rate of Tamm-Horsfall urinary mucoprotein in normals and in patients with renal disease. Austral NZ J Med 1964;13:32–39.
104. Vari RC, et al. Induction, prevention and mechanisms of contrast media-induced acute renal failure. Kidney Int 1988;33:699–707.
105. Berns AS. Nephrotoxicity of contrast media. Kidney Int 1989;36:730–740.
106. Porush JG, et al. Infusion intravenous pyelography and renal function: effects of hypertonic mannitol and furosemide in patients with chronic renal insufficiency. In: Eliahou HE, ed. Acute Renal Failure. London: John Libbey, 1982:161–167.
107. Solomon R, et al. Effects of saline, mannitol, and furosemide on acute decreases in renal function induced by radiocontrast agents. N Engl J Med 1994;331:1416–1420.
108. Cigarroa RG, et al. Dosing of contrast material to prevent contrast nephropathy in patients with renal disease. Am J Med 1989;86:649–652.
109. Schilsky RL. Renal and metabolic toxicities of cancer chemotherapy. Semin Oncol 1982;9:75–83.
110. Ries F, Klastersky J. Nephrotoxicity induced by cancer chemotherapy with special emphasis on cisplatin toxicity. Am J Kidney Dis 1986;8:368–379.

111. Sadoff I. Nephrotoxicity of streptozotocin (NSC-85998). Cancer Chemother Res 1979;54:457–459.
112. Hrushesky WJM, Shimp W, Kennedy BJ. Lack of age-dependent cisplatin nephrotoxicity. Am J Med 1984;76:579–584.
113. Safirstein R, et al. Cisplatin nephrotoxicity. Am J Kidney Dis 1986;8:356–367.
114. Klinenberg JR, et al. Urate deposition disease. How is it regulated and how can it be modified. Ann Intern Med: 1973;78:99–111.
115. Kleinman JG, Breitenfield RV, Roth DA. Acute renal failure associated with acetaminophen ingestion: report of a case and review of the literature. Clin Nephrol 1980;14:201–205.
116. Gabriel R, et al. Acute renal failure following therapeutic dose of paracetamol (acetaminophen). In: Eliahou HE, ed. Acute Renal Failure. London: John Libbey, 1982;125–128.
117. Roxe DM. Toxic nephropathy from diagnostic and therapeutic agents. Review and commentary. Am J Med 1980;69:759–774.
118. Dubb J, et al. Effect of cimetidine on renal function in normal man. Clin Pharmacol Ther 1978;24:76–83.
119. Anderson JB, Sorensen FH, Skjoldborg H. Acute renal failure in association with choledocholithiasis. Acta Clin Scand 1971;137:81–86.
120. Bismuth H, Kuntziger H, Corlette MB. Cholangitis with acute renal failure. Priorities in therapeutics. Ann Surg 1975;181:881–887.
121. Green J, et al. The "jaundiced heart": a possible explanation for postoperative shock in obstructive jaundice. Surgery 1986;100:14–20.
122. Better OS. Renal and cardiovascular dysfunction in liver disease. Kidney Int 1986;29:598–607.
123. Wait RB, Kahng K. Renal failure complicating obstructive jaundice. Am J Surg 1989;157:256–263.
124. Coratelli P, Passovanti G. Pathophysiology of renal failure in obstructive jaundice. Miner Electrol Metab 1990;16:61–65.
125. Bailey ME. Endotoxin, bile salts and renal function in obstructive jaundice. Br J Surg 1976;63:774–778.
126. Park J, Fromkes J, Cooperman M. Acute pancreatitis in elderly patients. Pathogenesis and outcome. Am J Surg 1986;152:638–642.
127. Levy M, Guller R, Hymovitch S. Renal failure in dogs with experimental acute pancreatitis: role of hypovolemia. Am J Physiol 1986;251:F969–F977.
128. Haimovici H. Muscular, renal and metabolic complications of acute arterial occlusions: myonephropathic-metabolic syndrome. Surgery 1979;85:461–468.
129. Marcus EL, Rudensky B, Sonnenblick M. Occult elevation of CK as a manifestation of rhabdomyolysis in the elderly. J Am Geriatr Soc 1992;40:454–456.
130. Gabow PA, Kaehny WD, Kelleher SP. The spectum of rhabdomyolysis. Medicine 1982;61:141–152.
131. Peller MS. Hemoglobin and myoglobin-induced acute renal failure in rats: role of iron in nephrotoxicity. Am J Physiol 1988;255:F539–F544.
132. Ron D, et al. Prevention of acute renal failure in traumatic rhabdomyolysis. Arch Intern Med 1984;144:277–280.

133. McComb's PR, Brooke R. Acute renal failure following resection of abdominal aortic aneurysm. Surg Gynecol Obstet 1979;148:175–178.
134. Hesdorffer CS, et al. The value of Swan Ganz catheterization and volume loading in preventing renal failure in patients undergoing abdominal aneurysmectomy. Clin Nephrol 1987;28:272–276.
135. Beaman M, et al. Changing pattern of acute renal failure. Q J Med 1987;237:15–23.
136. Gornick CC, Kjellstrand CM. Acute renal failure complicating aortic aneurysm surgery. Nephron 1983;35:145–157.
137. Myers BD, et al. Nature of renal injury following total renal ischemia in man. J Clin Invest 1984;73:329–341.
138. Welch M, et al. The preservation of renal function by isovolemic hemodilution during aortic operations. J Vasc Surg 1993;18:858–866.
139. Kleinknecht D, et al. Furosemide in acute oliguric renal failure. A controlled trial. Nephron 1976;17:51–58.
140. Brown CB, Ogg CS, Cameron JS. High dose furosemide in acute renal failure. A controlled trial. Clin Nephrol 1981;15:90–96.
141. Lindner A, et al. Dopamine and furosemide in acute renal failure. In: Eliahou HE, ed. Acute Renal Failure. London: John Libbey, 1982:174–175.
141a. Thadhani R, Pascual M, Bonventre JV. Acute renal failure. N Engl J Med 1996;334:1448–1460.
142. Denton MD, Chertow GM, Brady HR. Renal dose dopamine for the treatment of acute renal failure: scientific rationale, experimental studies and clinical trials. Kidney Int 1996;49:4–14.
143. Allgren RL, et al. Anaritide in acute tubular necrosis. N Engl J Med 1997;336:828–834.
144. Sonnenblick M, et al. Acute renal failure in the elderly treated by one-time peritoneal dialysis. J Am Geriatr Soc 1988;36:1039–1044.
145. Gibney NRT, et al. Continuous arteriovenous hemodialysis: an alternative therapy for acute renal failure with critical illness. Can Med Assoc J 1988;139:861–866.
146. Peachey TD, et al. Pump control of continuous arteriovenous haemodialysis. Lancet 1988;2:878.
147. Mault JR, et al. Continuous arteriovenous filtration: an effective treatment for surgical acute renal failure. Surgery 1987;101:478–484.
148. Bellomo R, Farmer M, Boyce N. The outcome of critically ill elderly patients with severe acute renal failure treated by continuous hemodiafiltration. Int J Artif Organs 1994;17:466–472.
148a. Hakim RM, et al. A multicenter comparison of biocompatible membranes in the treatment of acute renal failure. J Am Soc Nephrol 1994;5:394a.
149. Kierdorf HP, Sieberth HG. Continuous renal replacement therapies versus intermittant hemodialysis in acute renal failure: What do we know? Am J Kidney Dis 1996;28(suppl 3):S90–S96.
150. Paganini EP, et al. Establishing a dialysis therapy/patient outcome link in intensive care unit acute dialysis for patients with acute renal failure. Am J Kidney Dis 1996;28(suppl 3):S81–S89.

150a. Delaney HM, et al. Postoperative nutritional support using needle catheter feeding jejunostomy. Ann Surg 1977;186:165–170.
151. Ponsky JL. Percutaneous endoscopic gastrostomy: a closer look. Endoscopy Rev 1984;24–29.
152. Anderson CF, Loosbrook LM, Moxness KE. Nutrient intake in critically ill patients: too many or too few calories? Mayo Clin Proc 1986;61:853–858.
153. Staats BA, Gastineau CF, Offord KP. Predictive equations for basal caloric requirement derived from the data of Boothby, Berkson and Dunn. Mayo Clin Proc 1988; 63:409–410.
154. Miller LS, et al. Enteral and parenteral nutrition in the critically ill patient. Hosp. Formul 1986;21:672–682.
155. Sponsel H, Conger JD. Is parenteral nutrition therapy of value in acute renal failure patients? Am J Kidney Dis 1995;25:96–102.
155a. Humes HD: Acute renal failure: prevailing challenges and prospects for the future. Kidney Int 1995;48:S26–S32.
156. Balslov JT, Jorgenson HE. A survey of 499 patients with acute anuric renal insufficiency. Causes, treatment, complications and mortality. Am J Med 1963;34:753–764.
157. Scott RB, et al. Why the persistently high mortality in acute renal failure? Lancet 1972;2:75–79.
158. Wheeler DC, Feehally J, Walls J. High risk acute renal failure. Q J Med 1986;234: 977–984.
158a. Brivet FG, et al. Acute renal failure in intensive care units. Causes, outcome and prognostic factors of hospital mortality. A prospective, multicenter study. Crit Care Med 1996;24:192–198.
159. Rasmussen HH, et al. Prediction of outcome in acute renal failure by discriminant analysis of clinical variables. Arch Intern Med 1985;145:2015–2018.
160. Corwin HL, et al. Prediction of outcome in acute renal failure. Am J Nephrol 1987;7:8–12.
161. Menashe PI, Ross SA, Gottlieb JE. Acquired renal insufficiency in critically ill patients. Crit Care Med 1988;16:1106–1109.
162. Oliveira DBG, Winearls CG. Acute renal failure in the elderly can have a good prognosis. Age and Ageing 1984;13:304–308.
163. Amerio A, et al. Prognosis in acute renal failure accompanied by jaundice. Nephron 1981;27:152–154.
164. Myers BD, Moran SM. Hemodynamically mediated acute renal failure. N Engl J Med 1986;314:97–105.
165. Faubert PF, Porush JGP. Unpublished observations, 1996.
166. Bhandari S, Turney JH. Survivors of acute renal failure who do not recover renal function. Q J Med 1996;89:415–421.
167. Kleinknecht D, Landais P, Goldfarb B. Drug-associated acute renal failure. A prospective multicenter report. Kidney Int 1985;28:226A.
167a. Weisberg LS, et al. Cause of acute tubular necrosis affects its prognosis. Arch Intern Med 1997;157:1833–1838.
168. DeMarco S, et al. Acute renal failure in the elderly: a retrospective clinicopathological analysis of 17 cases. Miner Electrol Metab 1986;12:259A.

169. Tanter Y, et al. Acute renal failure secondary to glomerular disease in patients over 65 years. Miner Electrol Metab 1986;12:273A.
170. Mignon F, Méry JP, Morel-Maroger L. Granulomatous tubulointerstitial nephritis. Adv Nephrol 1984;13:219–245.
171. Husby G, Tungksk, Williams RC Jr. Characterization of renal tissue lymphocytes in patients with interstitial nephritis. Am J Med 1981;70:31–38.
172. Finkelstein A, et al. Fenoprofen nephropathy: lipoid nephrosis and interstitial nephritis. A possible T-lymphocyte disorder. Am J Med 1982;72:81–87.
173. Ten RM, et al. Localization of eosinophil major basic protein (MBP) in kidney disease. Kidney Int 1987;31:339A.
174. Ten RM, et al. Acute interstitial nephritis: immunologic and clinical aspects. Mayo Clin Proc 1988;63:921–930.
175. Cameron JS. Allergic interstitial nephritis: clinical features and pathogenesis. Q J Med 1988;250:97–115.
176. Preston RA, et al. Renal biopsy in patients 65 years of age or older: an analysis of the results of 334 biopsies. J Am Geriatr Soc 1990;38:669–674.
177. Modesto-Segondo A, et al. Renal biopsy in the elderly. Kidney Int 1990;38:1237A.
178. Linton AL, et al. Acute interstitial nephritis due to drugs. Review of the literature with a report of nine cases. Ann Intern Med 1980;93:735–741.
179. Lins RL, et al. Urinary indices in acute interstitial nephritis. Clin Nephrol 1986;26: 131–133.
180. Nolan CR 3rd, Auger MS, Kelleher SP. Eosinophiluria. A new method of detection and definition of the clinical spectrum. N Engl J Med 1986;315:1516–1519.
181. Linton AL, et al. Gallium^{67} scintigraphy in the diagnosis of acute renal disease. Clin Nephrol 1985;24:84–87.

11

Chronic Renal Failure

In general, renal failure is defined as an elevation of the BUN or serum creatinine, the latter being a more reliable parameter. In younger patients, a significant loss of kidney function (up to 50% or more) may be present without producing an abnormal BUN or serum creatinine. In the elderly, detection of renal failure is even more of a problem because they frequently eat less protein or have a decreased muscle mass, either of which can significantly lower the BUN and/or serum creatinine. As noted in Chapter 1, there are formulas that can be used to derive the creatinine clearance from the serum creatinine level and the weight and age of the patient. In patients with an abnormal urinalysis or other suggestions of kidney disease, a creatinine clearance [or other more accurate measurement of glomerular filtrate rate (GFR)] should be obtained, because the formula for deriving the creatinine clearance provides only an approximation. For the purpose of this discussion, an elevated BUN or serum creatinine (particularly the latter) is used as the definition of renal insufficiency; however, in the elderly, when contemplating the use of a nephrotoxic drug or a drug that is excreted renally, a creatinine clearance should be obtained or derived from the Cockcroft and Gault formula to make appropriate dose adjustments, if necessary.

I. INCIDENCE AND PREVALENCE

Chronic renal failure (CRF) is a relatively common problem in the elderly. Among patients admitted to three geriatric units, 4.5–8.3% had an elevated BUN

Table 1 Annual Percentage Increase in Patients Entering the ESRD Program in the United States (1985–1990)

Year	All age groups	65–74 yrs old	75+ yrs old
1985–1986	7.0	11.3	16.1
1986–1987	7.9	10.7	17.0
1987–1988	7.8	8.8	13.7
1988–1989	9.9	11.7	16.1
1989–1990	1.7	14.2	17.3
5-year average	8.9	11.3	16.0

Source: Agodoa L, Eggers PW. Renal replacement therapy in the United States: data from the United States Renal Data System. Am J Kidney Dis 1995; 25:119–133.

or serum creatinine, with intrinsic renal disease apparent in 30–40% (1). Renal failure was the final diagnosis in 201 (15.3%) of 1310 hospitalized elderly patients reported by Llera and Gregorio (2). Fifty percent of the patients evaluated by us during a 6-year period (1985–1990) for CRF were 60 years or older. Since, as noted, the BUN and serum creatinine are rather insensitive parameters for detecting a decrease in renal function (particularly in the elderly), it is clear that the actual incidence of renal insufficiency in this group of patients must be significantly higher than the literature suggests. At the present time the highest rate of new patients entering the end-stage renal disease (ESRD) program in the United States is in the age group 65 years or older (Table 1) Similar trends are also noted in Canada (3) and Europe (4). Forty-five percent of patients treated in the United States for ESRD during 1989–1993 were older than 64 years (5).

II. ETIOLOGY

We evaluated 467 elderly patients with an elevated serum creatinine (>1.5 mg/dl) over a 6-year period. As noted by others (6), nephrosclerosis and diabetic nephropathy were the two most common causes of CRF in these patients (Table 2). These two entities are also responsible for CRF in more than 70% of patients 64 years and older entering the U.S. ESRD program during the period 1989–1993 (5), keeping in mind that in a significant number of these patients renovascular disease (ischemic nephropathy, Chapter 13) might have been the cause or contributed to the renal insufficiency (7). In fact, ischemic nephropathy was diagnosed in 22% of the patients we studied who were originally diagnosed as having nephrosclerosis. Fifty-eight percent of these 467 patients were male, similar to the percentage of males in our overall ESRD population.

In general, it is possible to classify patients with CRF into broad diagnostic categories on the basis of a 24-hr urinary protein excretion rate.

Table 2 Etiology of CRF in 467 Elderly Patients Seen at the Brookdale University Hospital and Medical Center over a 6-Year Period (1985–1990)

Diagnosis	Number of patients (%)
Nephrosclerosis	217 (46.5)
Diabetic nephropathy	125 (26.8)
Tubulointerstitial disorders	45 (9.6)
Glomerular diseases	40 (8.6)
Obstructive uropathy	34 (7.2)
Hereditary: polycystic kidney disease	6 (1.3)
	Total 467 (100.0)

1. Glomerular disease (either primary or secondary): proteinuria of greater than 3 g/24 hr.
2. Tubulointerstitial disease: proteinuria between 1 and 2 g/24 hr.
3. Vascular (either major arterial or arteriolar) disease and obstructive uropathy: proteinuria less than 1 g/24 hr.

It is important to note that this classification is not inclusive and that overlap does exist. Obstructive uropathy should be ruled out either by sonography or by computed tomography (CT) in every patient with renal insufficiency. An intravenous pyelogram should be avoided in patients with CRF. Small kidneys reflect chronic advanced disease, with minimal chance of reversibility. Obviously, it may be necessary to do a kidney biopsy in order to make a definitive diagnosis, particularly for the glomerulopathies.

III. PATHOGENESIS AND CLINICAL MANIFESTATIONS

Unless the GFR is very low (usually less than 10 ml/min), symptoms attributable to chronic renal disease per se are either nonspecific (e.g., nocturia) or completely, absent. Therefore, it is not surprising that most patients with CRF are discovered during the evaluation of a systemic disease known to be associated with kidney involvement or during a visit to the physician's office or hospitalization for a completely unrelated problem.

IV. SPECIFIC DISEASE ENTITIES

Nephrosclerosis, ischemic nephropathy, diabetic nephropathy, obstructive uropathy, and glomerular disease are reviewed in separate chapters, as are myeloma kidney and staghorn calculi, which are the two most common forms of tubulointerstitial disease in the elderly. In this section we specifically address other chronic tubulointerstitial disorders and hereditary nephropathies.

A. Tubulointerstitial Disorders

Chronic tubulointerstitial diseases can be due to (a). drugs (analgesics, lithium); (b) metabolic disturbances (urate and oxalate nephropathy); (c) heavy metals (lead); (d) physical factors (radiation nephritis); or (e) other (sarcoidosis, chronic idiopathic interstitial nephritis).

1. Drugs

The risk of developing CRF may be increased in daily users of phenacetin and acetaminophen, the combination of ASA-acetaminophen, acetylsalicylic acid-acetaminophen combined (especially when taken with caffeine), and perhaps other nonsteroidal antiinflammatory drugs as well (8,9). The true incidence of chronic tubulointerstitial disease in the elderly is not known, but probably varies widely according to geographic area (10,11). We systematically take a history of analgesic use in our elderly patients and on only very few occasions have been able to attribute their renal disease to analgesic abuse. Females are more commonly affected than males. Renal insufficiency of varying degree, proteinuria less than 2 g/day, sterile pyuria, and inability to concentrate urine are present in most patients. Severe volume contraction and papillary necrosis are not uncommon complications (12). Morphologically, the early lesions consist of patchy areas of necrosis of interstitial cells, loops of Henle, and capillaries (a consequence of drug accumulation in the renal medulla), which interfere with medullary blood flow and result in medullary tissue ischemia (13). Late findings consist of glomerular sclerosis, tubular atrophy, and interstitial as well as periglomerular fibrosis. Discontinuing the analgesic may result in stabilization or even improvement in kidney function (14,15). The risk of developing renal pelvic cancer appears to be higher in patients with phenacetin-induced nephropathy (16).

Tubular atrophy, interstitial fibrosis, and sclerotic glomeruli have been reported in patients on chronic therapeutic doses of lithium carbonate (17). In a recent critical evaluation of the available evidence, it was concluded that the danger of chronic renal damage from lithium per se is quite small in patients on well-controlled therapy (18). Rather, it seems that the incidence of tubulointerstitial damage is higher in psychiatric patients taking drugs other than lithium (19). It is recommended that a creatinine clearance be performed in every patient taking lithium prior to starting the drug and at yearly intervals thereafter. Decreasing kidney function is an indication for discontinuing the drug. Lithium has also been associated with polyuria by interfering with the effect of antidiuretic hormone (ADH) on the cortical collecting tubule. Patients with this form of nephrogenic diabetes insipidus can be managed with amiloride, 5–10 mg administered twice a day (20). Hydrochlorthiazide, 25 mg twice a day, may have an additive effect.

2. *Metabolic Disturbances and Lead Nephropathy*

The interstitial disease caused by urates is characterized by the presence of uric acid crystals within the tubules and interstitium of the renal pyramids, accompanied by mononuclear and giant cell infiltration and fibrosis. Tophi are occasionally found in the interstitium. This form of kidney disease is rare now that allopurinol is frequently prescribed for hyperuricemic patients, with or without clinical gout. Moreover, because most patients with gout are also hypertensive, it is not clear to what extent the latter contributes to the renal insufficiency. Recently, some authors have proposed that the kidney damage apparent in gouty patients might represent lead rather than uric acid toxicity (21,22). An occupational history including the possible use of moonshine is helpful. Histologically, the so-called gouty and lead nephropathies share the same characteristics—tubulointerstitial scarring and nephrosclerosis—making it difficult to differentiate between them. When in doubt, lead excretion should be measured 24–72 hr after parenteral administration of 1–2 g of EDTA. More than 600 mg/24 hr of urinary lead is considered a positive test (23).

We have used allopurinol in hyperuricemic patients with gout and renal insufficiency and a negative EDTA test; however, in our limited experience, this approach has not prevented further progression of the kidney disease. Experience with the chronic use of EDTA as a chelating agent to treat lead nephropathy is limited (24), but should probably be tried. Other therapeutic modalities such as BAL, D-penicillanine, and 2,3-dimercaptosuccinic acid have also been tried with some success (25). It has been suggested that long-term low-level lead exposure could accelerate the age-related loss of renal function (26).

Oxalate nephropathy should be suspected in any elderly with an history of chronic inflammatory bowel disease or following intestinal bypass surgery for massive obesity (27). Hyperoxaluria (>40 mg/24 hr) is present in virtually every patient. Renal biopsy findings are nonspecific (unless oxalate crystals are seen) and consist of periglomerular and interstitial fibrosis as well as tubular atrophy and hyalinization of glomeruli. The presence of granular deposits of immunoglobulins and C_3 in the glomeruli of some patients suggests a possible immune pathogenesis. The possible beneficial effect of control of the hyperoxaluria or the underlying bowel disease (including the dismantling of the bypass) on the natural history of the disease has not been demonstrated but, in our opinion, should be tried.

5-Aminosalicylic acid, used to treat patients with moderately active inflammatory bowel disease, has also been associated with the development of chronic tubulointerstitial disease and renal insufficiency (27a). Other treatment modalities should be applied in these patients. Discontinuing the drug, however, is not generally associated with improvement in kidney function.

3. *Radiation Nephritis*

Chronic radiation nephritis is characterized clinically by proteinuria, hypertension, and renal insufficiency. The time elapsing between exposure (usually following an excess of 2500 rad to both kidneys) and development of renal disease is 1–14 years (28). With the newer techniques of radiation administration, this form of kidney disease is seen less frequency. Our own experience is limited to only one elderly patient who developed progressive renal insufficiency following treatment for lymphoma compressing the spinal cord. Treatment is supportive and directed mainly at controlling hypertension, which is usually present.

Sarcoidosis (see Chapter 7). Granulomas are commonly found in the renal interstitium of autopsied patients with sarcoidosis. Renal insufficiency, proteinuria (usually less than 1500 mg/24 hr), and tubular dysfunction are relatively rare complications (29–31). On histological evaluation, noncaseating granulomas with giant cells are seen in the interstitium. Tubular atrophy and interstitial fibrosis are found with more advanced disease. Apart from the presence of mild mesangial expansion, the glomeruli are unremarkable. Dramatic improvement in kidney function may be seen following steroid administration (40–60 mg of prednisone daily).

4. *Idiopathic Interstitial Nephritis*

Occasionally, interstitial nephritis is found in elderly patients on kidney biopsy performed to evaluate renal insufficiency and proteinuria for which no cause can be found. In the absence of advanced interstitial fibrosis and extensive glomerular obsolescence, a short course (4–6 weeks) of prednisone (40–60 mg daily) is worth trying, as long as no contraindications to its use exist. We have occasionally seen a dramatic response, suggesting that the patient had a prolonged active interstitial nephritis of unknown origin.

B. Hereditary Nephropathies

1. *Adult Polycystic Kidney Disease*

Adult Polycystic Kidney Disease (APKD) is an autosomal dominant disorder caused by a mutation in at least one of three genes. In most patients the causative gene is linked to the short arm of chromosome 16 ($APKD_1$) (32). There is a small fraction of patients (10–15%) in whom a second locus on the long arm of chromosome 4 may be responsible for the disease ($APKD_2$) (33). The third locus has not yet been identified. Only 3–4% of patients with APKD are 60 years or older at the time of initial diagnosis (34,35). In 30 elderly patients seen during the past 12 years, the diagnosis of APKD was established by sonographic examination during investigation for hypertension and renal insufficiency, which are seen at presentation more often in the elderly than in younger patients with this disease. The incidence of other symptoms, such as back pain, renal colic, hematuria, and urinary tract infection, is similar to that in younger patients (36,37). The renal insufficiency in APKD is progressive. The rate of progression, however, varies from patient to patient and, as recently shown, depends on (a) the patient's genetic makeup—in those with $APKD_2$, renal insufficiency occurs at a later age and tends to progress more slowly than $APKD_1$ (38,39); (b) blood pressure—extensive arterio- and arteriolar nephrosclerosis are common histological findings in APKD patients with advanced renal failure (37); (c) left ventricular mass (40); (d) gender—males do worse than females (40,41); and (e) renal volume (40). APKD patients also have a higher incidence of intracranial saccular aneurysms, various cardiac valvular abnormalities (mitral valve prolapse or aortic or tricuspid insufficiency), and inguinal hernia (42). The incidence of these associated abnormalities in the elderly with APKD is not known.

The cause and mechanism of cyst formation in patients with APKD is not clear. Renal tubular epithelial cells taken from patients with APKD synthesize an abnormal basement membrane in tissue culture (43), lending support to the hypothesis that the cysts result from collapse or atrophy of tubules with a primary defect in the basement membrane (44). Also, epithelial cells within the cyst wall with an altered basement membrane could dedifferentiate and exhibit increased proliferation. Cysts with either proximal or distal tubular characteristics have been found in APKD patients (45). The solute content of proximal cyst fluid is similar to that of serum taken from the patient, whereas distal cysts contain fluid that has a lower sodium and chloride and a higher potassium, creatinine, and urea concentration than the serum. Fluid accumulates in the cysts by chloride-driven transepithial secretion which can be inhibited in vitro by either bumetamide or furosemide (46). Polycystin, a newly identified protein produced by APKD, appears to be a result rather than the cause of the cysts (47).

The management of hypertension, nephrolithiasis, and urinary tract infection in the elderly with APKD is similar to that described for these conditions in other elderly patients. Infection, however, may be present in the absence of pyuria or bacteriuria when it is confined to the cyst cavity (pyocyst). Clues to the diagnosis include the development of a new discrete area of palpable tenderness in the involved kidney, particularly if blood cultures are positive (48,49). Also, thickening and irregularity of the cyst wall or an increase in the attenuation value of the cyst content on CT scan, although not pathognomonic for infection, are suggestive (50). Follow-up scans should be repeated in these patients because the findings are similar in the presence of renal cell carcinoma, which can occur in APKD patients, although at a higher frequency in younger compared to older patients (51,52). Trimethoprim, norfloxacin, ciproflaxin, or clindamycin, at the usual doses, can be used. Patients who have abdominal pain or gross hematuria are best managed with bed rest, liberal fluid intake, and analgesics. Symptoms usually resolve within 48–72 hr We have never needed to resort to surgical reduction of a cyst for pain control in our elderly APKD patients (53).

V. NATURAL HISTORY OF CRF

In the elderly, as in younger patients, CRF tends to progress to ESRD, long after the initial injurious event has subsided. Several factors appear to be responsible for this phenomenon (53a):

1. The host. The decline in renal function in patients with presumed hypertensive nephrosclerosis is greater in men and blacks (54,55).
2. The disease. Some disease entities are associated with more rapid decline than others (56). Patients with APKD, as a group, progress faster than patients with other causes of CRF (57).
3. The degree of proteinuria. A strong positive correlation has been found by some investigators between the 24-hr urine protein excretion and the progression of CRF, regardless of the cause of the renal disease (58–60). There is evidence that filtered proteins associated with clinical proteinuria, either directly or through the release of various enzymes, exert a toxic effect on the glomeruli and tubules (61). In addition, ammonia produced from the metabolism of those proteins can initiate an inflammatory reaction which result in tubulointerstitial damage (62).
4. Hypertension (discussed in the following section).
5. Calcium deposition in the kidney. As discussed below, abnormalities in Ca/P metabolism are universally found in patients with advanced CRF. Because the calcium content of kidney tissue from patients with renal disease of varying severity correlates significantly with the serum creatinine and phosphorus (63,64), it has been postulated that renal calcium phosphate deposition may play a secondary pathogenetic role, accelerating the progression of the renal failure. Dietary phosphate restriction has been shown to preserve kidney function in experimental renal disease in rats (65). Unfortunately, similar data are not available for humans (66).
6. Hyperlipidemia. There is some experimental as well as clinical evidence (at least in diabetics) to suggest that abnormal lipid metabolism, a relatively common finding in patients with CRF (67), may be an independent risk factor in the pathogenesis and/or progression of renal disease (68–70 and Ref. 70a in Chapter 7). Presumably, changes in glomerular permeability increase the filtration of lipoproteins. Their accumulation in the mesangial cells could stimulate them to proliferate and produce excess basement membrane material (71,72). Hyperlipidemia may also increase platelet aggregation with subsequent release of a platelet growth factor. The latter could bind to receptors on the mesangial cells and induce cellular proliferation (71).

7. Perhaps most important are the intraglomerular adaptive changes, such as glomerular hyperfiltration and hypertension and/or glomerular hypertrophy, which follow experimental renal injury or a reduction in renal mass. Control of these adaptive changes by blood pressure reduction or protein restriction appear to slow the progression of the renal disease in these animals (73–75). Finally, various circulating and locally produced growth factors have been shown to play a role in glomerular hypertrophy and sclerosis (76). Their role in the progression of CRF in humans remains to be determined.

In recent years the rate of decline in kidney function in patients with CRF has been mapped by plotting the reciprocal of the serum creatinine (1/serum creatinine) against time, which usually is represented by a straight line, unique for each patient (77). This approach is clinically useful in that changes in the slope of the line can be used to assess the result of a therapeutic intervention or to determine the effects of a new acute process on kidney function. The use in the latter situation is particularly helpful to recognize potentially reversible events such as volume contraction, congestive heart failure, or urinary tract obstruction. There are certain drawbacks to this method, however. Spontaneous changes, not readily attributable to a complication or therapy, can occur (78). Also, it has been shown recently that there is a poor overall correlation between the decline in GFR and the 1/creatinine slope, particularly in the presence of a change in protein intake and/or antihypertensive drugs (79–81), although the correlation is closer when the serum creatinine is greater than 2.5 mg/dl. Despite these shortcomings, this method of assessing the progression of CRF is still quite useful.

VI. PROBLEMS RELATED TO CRF AND THEIR MANAGEMENT

A. Hypertension

Hypertension per se is not only the primary cause of renal insufficiency in a large number of elderly patients (particularly blacks) but also is usually present in all forms of CRF; the incidence varies with the type of disease, being most common in patients with glomerular and polycystic kidney disease. Ninety-five percent of elderly patients entering our ESRD program have, or had, a history of hypertension. The incidence of hypertension in patients with CRF before starting dialysis is approximately 85% in all age groups (82). In general, hypertension in patients with underlying renal disease is salt sensitive, suggesting that volume expansion is important in the pathogenesis (83). Once initiated, hypertension may be maintained because the vasculature is unable to accommodate the increased volume owing to a loss of balance between circulating vasoconstrictors and vasodilators normally produced by the kidneys (84). Since there is a significant positive correlation between mean arterial pressure (MAP) and the rate of decline in kidney function, hypertension in the presence of kidney disease should be managed aggressively (85–87). The ideal target level for blood pressure control has not been determined; a recent study in patients of varying ages with CRF due to nephrosclerosis showed that lowering the MAP to 98 mmHg did not improve the GFR slope compared to a similar group of patients with a MAP of 104 mmHg (60). Similar observations were made for patients with APKD, where a MAP of ≤113 mmHg was compared to a MAP of ≤95 mHg (57). However, in patients with proteinuria, especially blacks, the MAP should be brought to or less than 98 mmHg (88,88a). Patients should be monitored closely in anticipation of side effects related to decreased organ perfusion, particularly patients with coronary artery disease (89). In our experience, the elderly are able to tolerate this level of pressure as long as it is achieved slowly and precipitous drops in blood pressure are avoided.

The usual level of blood pressure control has been shown to slow the progression of CRF in a large variety of renal diseases (90–96). Based on a variety of experimental evidence, it has been postulated that hypertension contributes to glomerular damage because there is enhanced transmission of the systemic pressure to the adapted glomeruli in the setting of reduced renal mass (97). The converting-enzyme inhibitors or calcium channel blockers, by reversing these effects on the glomerulus, have been shown in animals to offer superior renal protection compared to other agents. Similar benefits in humans have been demonstrated for the converting-enzyme inhibitors (98–102).

Since the hypertension of CRF is associated with expansion of the plasma volume, patients should be placed on a low-sodium diet (2–3 g/day). In those who do not adhere to the salt restriction, a diuretic (furosemide, bumetanide, or torsemide) should be used either daily or intermittently, depending on the degree of weight loss. Kidney function and weight should be monitored carefully during the first 2–3 weeks of therapy, since there is a risk of superimposed acute renal failure secondary to volume contraction. The dose of furosemide is 40–320 mg/day and that of bumetanide is 0.5–5 mg/day, with the range for torsemide 20–200 mg/day.

The dosage schedule of antihypertensive drugs in the elderly with renal disease is identical to that outlined in Table 3 in Chapter 12. In general, the starting dose of a converting-enzyme inhibitor should be the lowest available, with upward tritration accomplished more slowly than in patients with normal kidney function. The maximum dosage is otherwise the same except for ramipril. The recommended maximum dosage for that drug is 5 mg if the GFR is less than 30 ml/min. No dosage change is necessary with the calcium channel blockers (103,104). With the availability of potent antihypertensive drugs, it is possible to control the blood pressure in patients with CRF without a diuretic, although some degree of salt restriction is usually necessary.

B. Phosphate Retention

Despite the changes in serum phosphate, parathyroid hormone (PTH), and 1,25(OH)2D_3 that occur with age (see Chapter 5), neither hyperphosphatemia nor renal osteodystrophy differs in severity in older compared to younger patients with CRF. No correlation was found between plasma 1,25$(OH)_2D_3$ and age in patients with CRF (105). Mean PTH and mean plasma phosphate levels in a group of 50 patients below the age of 60 were similar to those of 50 elderly patients evaluated by us who had a creatinine clearance of less than 10 ml/min. None were on phosphate binders when studied. The degree of hypocalcemia was also similar in the two groups. The hyperphosphatemia of CRF results mainly from a decrease in renal phosphate excretion because of a lower GFR. Serum levels of 1,25$(OH)_2D_3$ decrease because of decreased synthesis by the damaged proximal renal tubular cells (106). In addition to hypocalcemia, hyperphosphatemia and a low 1,25$(OH)_2D_3$ independently stimulate the parathyroid gland, resulting in hyperparathyroidism (107). The hypocalcemia is a consequence of decreased intestinal calcium absorption as well as skeletal resistance to the calcemic action of PTH and an altered feedback relationship between ionized calcium and PTH secretion (108–110). The first step in controlling hyperphosphatemia is dietary (see later section on dietary management of renal failure). This approach, unfortunately, is rarely successful by itself, necessitating the addition of phosphate binders. In recent years we have reserved the use of aluminum hydroxide for the occasional patient who has a very high serum phosphorous level (>10 mg/dl). Once the serum phosphorous has decreased to less than 6 mg/dl, we switch to calcium carbonate or calcium acetate administered with meals (111–113). If the serum phosphorus concentration is less than 6 mg/dl to start, we avoid aluminum hydroxide altogether and initiate therapy with calcium carbonate or acetate. The average daily dose required in our elderly population has been approximately 2000 mg of elemental calcium. Patients who have difficulty with the tablets can be switched to calcium glubionate syrup (neocalglucon). Each tablespoonful (15 ml) contains 345 mg of calcium. Sixty-five percent of our patients, despite achieving normophosphatemia, remain hypocalcemic (serum Ca < 8.5 mg/dl). In these patients, we add 1,25$(OH)_2D_3$ (calcitrol), starting at a dose of 0.125 μg/day and gradually increasing the dose until the serum calcium reaches 10.5–11.5 mg/dl. Serum PTH levels gradually decrease within a few months after this therapy is initiated. We have not routinely performed a bone biopsy prior to and after therapy in our patients, but in studies in which patients over the age of 65 were included, a significant improvement in hyperparathyroid bone disease has been observed when this approach has been used (114,115). The average patient requires between 0.25 and 0.50 μg/day of calcitrol. Like others (116), we have not seen any deleterious effect of this drug on kidney function, and calcitrol does not increase the risk of aluminum bone disease.

C. Metabolic Acidosis

Despite lower plasma aldosterone levels and a lower urinary ammonium excretion in the elderly compared to younger patients when subjected to an acid load, the acidosis as assessed by arterial pH and bicarbonate (see Chapter 7) seen in elderly patients with a given level of renal insufficiency is no more severe than that seen in younger patients. The urine pH is usually 5.5 or less, except when the renal disease is associated with a "voltage-dependent" renal tubular acidosis (see Chapter 3), in which case the acidosis is usually more pronounced and urine pH is greater than 6.

Initially, the metabolic acidosis is of the hyperchloremic type (non-anion gap acidosis). As the GFR falls below 20 ml/min, organic anions such as sulfate, phosphate, and others, which are not completely oxidized, are retained, giving way to an anion gap acidosis (117). The inability of the surviving nephrons to produce sufficient amounts of ammonia to meet the requirement for excretion of the daily metabolic acid production is a major factor in the pathogenesis of the acidosis associated with renal insufficiency. Also, some derangement in the intrarenal handling of filtered bicarbonate probably plays a role (118). Elderly patients with severe acidosis (serum bicarbonate < 20 mEq/L) require therapy. We use sodium bicarbonate, starting with 0.5 mEq/kg/day in divided doses, with slow upward titration to maintain the serum pH above 7.35 or total CO_2 above 19 mEq/L. Patients who cannot tolerate sodium bicarbonate can be given sodium citrate (bicitra). Each milliliter of bicitra is equivalent to 1 mEq of bicarbonate. Potassium citrate (polycitra K, containing 2 mEq K and the equivalent of 2 mEq bicarbonate/ml) is available for patients who cannot handle the amount of sodium required with sodium bicarbonate or citrate. Since citrate increases intestinal aluminum absorption, these two compounds should never be used together (119). The goal is to keep the plasma bicarbonate as close as possible to normal, as acidosis per se increases protein catabolism through the ubiquitin-proteasome pathway (120).

D. Anemia

Anemia is present in most elderly patients with CRF. In general, the lower the GFR, the more severe is the anemia. Significant variations do occur among individual patients (121), however, so it is necessary to rule out other causes such as gastrointestinal blood loss, or other chronic diseases such as rheumatoid arthritis or a malignancy before attributing the anemia to the renal disease. The most common malignancy found in our elderly population with anemia and renal failure is multiple myeloma. Since the erythrocyte sedimentation rate is frequently elevated in the elderly with CRF, reaching values over 100, particularly in those with diabetic nephropathy (122,123), the possibility of multiple myeloma is frequently an issue.

The anemia associated with CRF is, for the most part, secondary to a decrease in erythropoetin production by the peritubular interstitial cells (endothelial?) (124,125). Factors related to the uremic milieu per se are also of pathogenetic importance, since the endogenous amount of erythropoietin required to maintain the same level of erythropoiesis following renal transplantation is far less than the relatively large doses of exogenous erythropoietin needed in patients with uremia (126).

The anemia is relatively well tolerated in most patients; however, in a small number the presence of concomitant conditions such as recurring angina pectoris, congestive heart failure, marked fatigue, or malignancy makes it necessary to transfuse or administer erythropoietin periodically. We usually start our elderly patients with either 5000 or 10,000 units (depending on the severity of the anemia) of erythropoietin administered subcutaneously once a week. Hematocrit is monitored weekly for the first month and twice monthly thereafter until the therapeutic goal (generally a hematocrit >30%) is achieved (usually within 6–8 weeks). Serum iron, total iron-binding capacity, and ferritin levels should be determined on a regular basis. Oral iron supplementation in the usual dosage is required in most patients. Once the therapeutic goal is achieved, a maintenance bimonthly or monthly dose is prescribed. The drug is well tolerated and associated with an increase in exercise tolerance as well as an overall sense of well-being. Hypertensive patients may require additional antihypertensive therapy, since the drug can raise the blood pressure by enhancing the response of the vasculature to norepinephrine, endothelin, and vasoconstrictor prostanoids (127,128). Like others (129), we have not seen any acute worsening in kidney function with the use of erythropoietin. At the present time the drug is quite expensive, a factor that limits its use to those who can afford the expense or who have drug insurance coverage.

VII. DIETARY MANAGEMENT OF THE ELDERLY WITH CRF

Several studies have been carried out to evaluate whether lowering dietary protein can slow the progression of kidney failure through its effect on glomerular hyperfiltration, urinary concentrating ability, ammoniagenesis, and possibly other actions as well (130,131). A recent meta-analysis of previously published studies has revealed that dietary protein restriction effectively slows the progression of both diabetic and nondiabetic renal diseases (132).

The estimated rate of body protein synthesis in the elderly is approximately 3 g/kg/day, and the dietary protein requirement is 0.60–0.75 g/kg/day (133). Presently, the recommended approach is to reduce protein intake to approximately 0.8 g/kg/day in patients who are ingesting more, as determined from a 24-hr urine collection using the following formulas: estimated protein intake (g/day) = urea nitrogen intake (g/day) × 6.25; urea nitrogen intake (g/day) = urine urea nitrogen (g/day) + (0.031 × kg body weight) (134). Since the average protein intake in our elderly population with CRF is 1.04 ± 0.40 g/kg, it is evident that most people require some form of restriction. Compliance, however, is difficult to achieve. We strongly suggest that the patient be followed carefully by a dietitian, since a reduction in dietary caloric intake is often associated with protein restriction, which potentially could lead to malnutrition (135), particularly in patients with a very low GFR (136).

VIII. CONCURRENT MEDICAL PROBLEMS AND THEIR MANAGEMENT

The majority of elderly with CRF have other co-morbid conditions such as heart disease and heart failure, peripheral vascular disease, and organic brain syndrome that predispose them to frequent hospitalizations and put them at increased risk of further deterioration of renal function. Acute renal failure superimposed on CRF is the most common complication encountered in the hospitalized elderly. Volume contraction due to vigorous diuresis during the management of heart failure and continuance of a diuretic and a low-sodium diet in the hospitalized hypertensive elderly patient with poor oral intake are the most common causes for acute worsening of kidney function in these patients. The usual evidence of volume contraction, such as poor skin turgor or an orthostatic drop in blood pressure, may not be present. Weight loss, a low urine sodium (less than 20 mEq/L, not always present when prerenal azotemia is superimposed on CRF or if a diuretic has been continued), and an unchanged urinary sediment are helpful signs. Management is straight forward, but the patient must be monitored carefully to prevent fluid overload. Prognosis for recovery is excellent.

The use of nephrotoxic antibiotics, NSAIDs, contrast-media administration, and acute tubular necrosis due to sepsis or cardiogenic shock are the other major causes of worsening of kidney function in the elderly with CRF. In these patients the history and physical findings are most helpful, and examination of the urine may not provide any useful information. Although the acute renal failure may be reversible, in some patients dialysis may be necessary. Furthermore, particularly in patients with underlying diabetic nephropathy, kidney function may not return to premorbid levels, and the patient may require maintenance dialysis.

Obstruction, mainly in males and especially those receiving sedatives, must be ruled out. In addition, acute interstitial nephritis (AIN) secondary to drugs (or infection) should be kept in mind. AIN, particularly when secondary to NSAIDs, may occur in the absence of the usual clinical picture of fever, rash, eosinophilia, or eosinophiluria. Renal artery occlusion, particularly in patients with an abdominal aortic aneurysm or direct evidence of renal vascular disease (abdominal bruit, discrepancy in kidney size) or vascular disease elsewhere, will cause acute worsening of renal function, which can be detected by a renal scan and/or angiography. Finally, although rare, the possibility of acute glomerulonephritis should always be kept in mind and adequately ruled out by careful examination of the urine and urinary sediment (red cell casts, proteinuria).

IX. SURGERY IN THE ELDERLY WITH CRF

Preoperative, perioperative, and postoperative management of the elderly with CRF is similar to that in patients with normal kidney function. Even patients with advanced disease (serum creatinine of 3.5 mg/dl or greater or a creatinine clearance of 15–20 ml/min or less) do not necessarily require prophylactic dialysis; however, attention should be paid to fluid balance, blood pressure control, acid–base status, and serum potassium during the preoperative period. Patients with anemia should be transfused to achieve a hematocrit of 30%, particularly if there is clinical evidence of coronary artery disease. When potentially nephrotoxic drugs are needed, the dose should be adjusted and blood levels monitored carefully. For patients with a diastolic blood pressure greater than 110 mmHg who cannot take oral medication, blood pressure control should be achieved with any of the parenteral drugs discussed in Chapter 12. Despite careful monitoring of all these factors, the incidence of worsening kidney function is increased in these patients.

X. ELDERLY WITH END-STAGE RENAL DISEASE

As already mentioned, the number of elderly patients entering the ESRD program has been increasing in the United States, with similar trends also reported from Europe and Canada. Age per se should not play any role when considering renal replacement therapy in the elderly. Rather, attention should be paid to the presence of poor functional capacity and multiple co-morbid medical conditions with poor outcome, for whom therapy should probably not be offered (3,137–139). Those patients who are candidates for dialysis should have an angioaccess inserted once the creatinine clearance is below 10 ml/min, and even earlier in diabetics.

XI. INDICATIONS FOR INITIATING DIALYSIS IN THE ELDERLY

The indications for starting maintenance dialysis in the elderly are identical to those in younger patients. Uremic encephalopathy, pericarditis, gastritis, colitis, and neuropathy are absolute indications for immediate dialysis. These complications are seen less frequently in recent years because increasingly more elderly patients with CRF are diagnosed prior to reaching end stage, and dialysis is usually started prior to the onset of the complications noted above. Table 3 summarizes the symptoms and signs present at the time of their first dialysis in 118 elderly patients seen by us.

Table 3 Symptoms and Signs Present in 118 Elderly Patients Prior to Starting Maintenance Dialysis

	Number of patients (%)
Nonspecific	
Generalized weakness	68 (58)
Anorexia, weight loss, decreasing serum albumin	72 (61)
Nervous system	
Encephalopathy (dementia)	58 (49)
Peripheral neuropathy (symptomatic)	8 (7)
Gastrointestinal	
Nausea, vomiting	48 (41)
Bleeding	12 (10)
Cardiovascular	
Difficulty with volume homeostasis (fluid overload, CHF)	19 (16)
Pleuropericarditis	2 (2)
Other	
Markedly elevated serum creatinine (>10 mg/dl)	19 (16)

XII. HEMODIALYSIS (HD), CHRONIC PERITONEAL DIALYSIS (CPD), RENAL TRANSPLANTATION (RT)

The same treatment options available to younger patients with ESRD are available to the elderly. In 1993, in the United States, 59% of all patients with ESRD were on HD, 14% were on CPD, and 27% had a functioning RT. In the elderly, 83% were on HD, 12% were on CPD, and 5% had a functioning RT (140). In Germany and Portugal, only 5% of the elderly with ESRD are on CPD, compared to 50% in the United Kingdom (141). The choice of HD over CPD depends on several factors: patient's choice and/or ability, presence of an absolute contraindication to insertion of a peritoneal catheter, physician's expertise, and available resources. In general, there is no difference in mortality rate between the elderly on HD or CPD, except perhaps in diabetics, who have a higher mortality rate with CPD (3,142–145), although in one recent study a better survival rate was found in patients on CPD for the first 2 years when compared with HD (145a).

XIII. HEMODIALYSIS IN THE ELDERLY

In general, hemodialysis is as well tolerated in the elderly as in younger patients (3,146,147). An attempt should always be made to place a Brescia-Cimino AV-fistula as a route for angioaccess, since the overall complication rate is lower in patients with a fistula than with a graft. If a radiocephalic fistula cannot be constructed, an attempt should be made to use the brachial artery (148).

Presently, 14% of elderly undergoing hemodialysis in the United States have an AV-fistula, compared to 19% in younger patients. The percentages with a polytetrafluoroethylene (PTFE) graft are 50% and 44%, respectively (149). An AV-fistula has been possible in only 20% of our elderly patients, primarily because of venous disease. An attempt is always made to insert a PTFE graft in the remaining patients, as central venous catheters are used either as temporary access or for patients in whom the other two alternatives are no longer feasible. Less than 10% of our elderly patients belong to this category. Our 1-year patency rate for fistula is 40%, considerably better than that reported by others (150). Our 1-year graft patency rate is approximately 70%, similar to the 69% found by the same investigators (150). The most common problem associated with angioaccess in the elderly is clotting, which is usually amenable to either surgical or medical declotting, with a success rate of 88% (140). Clotting may be recurrent in patients with intradialytic hypotension from whatever cause and in those with systemic infection. Also, it is imperative to do an angiogram in those patients who clot to rule out stenosis of the graft venous anastomotic site, which usually can be corrected surgically. Steal syndrome is seen more frequently in diabetic patients and in those with severe peripheral vascular disease. Patients with access infection (usually a graft) should be hospitalized and started on antibiotics such as vancomycin or a penicillinase-resistant penicillin, since *Staphylococcus* is almost always the offending agent (99% of our cases). In the remaining 1%, *Enterococcus* or *Pseudomonas* was isolated. We have not had any success with medical therapy alone, and in every instance the graft required removal. The new access is usually placed 8–10 days later, after all the signs of infection have subsided. In the interim, HD is continued through endovascular catheterization.

Adequacy of HD in the elderly is assessed in the same way as in younger patients, using the sense of well-being, nerve conduction velocity, and regular monthly estimation of the urea index (urea index = Kt/V, where K = urea clearance through the dialyzer, t = treatment time, and V = the volume of distribution of urea). The clinician should aim for a urea index of 1.3–1.5 or a minimum urea reduction ratio target of 70% (urea reduction ratio = $1 - C_t/C_0$, where C_0 is predialysis BUN and C_t the BUN 5 min after dialysis (151–151a). Other methods of estimating Kt/V have been described (152). The incidence of intradialytic hypotension and erytropoietin requirements are similar in older and younger patients (149,153,154).

Symptomatic aluminum toxicity is quite rare in our experience. Routinely measured serum aluminum levels in our elderly patients have been low. Aluminum toxicity is manifest primarily by CNS involvement, including speech disturbances, dementia, convulsions, and extrapyramidal signs (155). Patients with osteomalacia may complain of generalized bone pain or proximal muscle weakness. These patients have a tendency to develop hypercalcemia when given calcitrol and usually have an elevated serum alkaline phosphatase (156). The serum aluminum level is often elevated but not necessarily so. A more than 20% rise in the serum aluminum level 5 hr after starting deferoxamine (28.5 mg/kg) has been found to correlate better than the serum aluminum level with the presence of stainable bone aluminum (157). The infusion is administered during dialysis, the rate not exceeding 15 mg/kg/hr. The definitive diagnosis of aluminum bone disease is made histologically (158), however. Deferoxamine, 20–80 mg/kg/week in single or divided doses administered either intravenously, intramuscularly, or intraperitoneally, is the agent of choice for the management of these patients (159). A high incidence of mucormycosis infection has been reported in patients treated with this drug (160).

The other forms of bone diseases associated with chronic renal insufficiency, adynamic and hyperparathyroid (osteitis fibrosa cystica), occur with the same frequency in the elderly as in younger patients. A definite diagnosis requires histological confirmation (161). In the past, patients with hyperparathyroid bone disease were routinely referred for parathyroidectomy (162). Since $1,25(OH)_2D_3$ administered intravenously or orally can directly inhibit PTH secretion (163) and ameliorate the biochemical and histological picture of osteitis fibrosa cystica in patients on maintenance hemodialysis (164,165), it is now the treatment of choice, with surgery reserved only for refractory cases. The results in elderly patients with this form of therapy are as good as in younger patients. The recommended starting dose is 1.0 μg administered either into the venous line or orally during the last few minutes of each dialysis treatment (3 times weekly), with monthly or bimonthly increments of 0.5 μg up to a maximum of 4.0 μg, as long as the serum calcium remains less than 11.5 mg/dl. The goal is to keep the serum PTH at 120–250 pg/ml (165a). Hypercalcemia is the major side effect. The use of $MgCO_3$ in conjunction with a 0.6 mg/dl dialysate Mg or a decreased dose of $CaCO_3$ should be tried in persistently hypercalcemic patients (166).

Pruritis is more common in the elderly than in younger uremic patients. This may be related, in part, to the skin changes which take place with aging. Pruritis, which can be either localized or generalized, tends to be worse during dialysis. The pathogenesis of uremic pruritis is probably multifactorial, including increased divalent ion skin content (167), lower skin water content, increased sensitivity to pruritogens, ischemic neuropathy, and an abnormal pattern of cutaneous innervation (168). Therapy is generally unsatisfactory. We usually start with maneuvers that contribute to keeping the skin moist, such as use of an oatmeal soap and baby oil applications. These simple maneuvers may provide some relief in a significant number of patients. Lidocaine infusion during dialysis, oral charcoal, and antihistamines have generally been unsuccessful. Ultraviolet irradiation within the sunburn spectrum, either through a real effect on skin or through a placebo effect, has been helpful (169,170).

Elderly on hemodialysis spend an average of 14–30 days a year in the hospital (142,171–173), somewhat more than the 11–12 days average for younger adults with ESRD (139). Approximately 30% of hospital time is for fluid overload or complications related directly to dialysis, such as angioaccess clotting and infection. The remaining causes for hospitalization include cardiovascular complications such as ischemic heart disease (three times as common in the elderly as in younger patients), congestive heart failure, cardiac arrhythmia (atrial fibrillation), or vascular insufficiency (particularly in diabetics), which account for over 30% of the time spent in the hospital. Gastrointestinal bleeding accounts for another 10%. The remainder is for a variety of other problems, including cancer.

Bleeding gastritis in elderly patients on dialysis is due mainly to uremia or the use of NSAIDs. Blood loss is usually minimal, since the bleeding tends to stop within 24 hr when dialysis time is increased or therapy is given with any of the H_2-blockers or misoprostol (for those on NSAIDs), 200 μg with meals and at bedtime. More severe bleeding occurs in patients with angiodysplasia, which is the second most common cause of gastrointestinal bleeding in the elderly with ESRD in our experience. The lesions can occur anywhere along the gastrointestinal tract and are usually multiple (174). The outcome is variable. In some patients, bleeding stops spontaneously. In others, a single bleeding site may be located by endoscopy and managed with laser photocoagulation or electrocautery (175). In still others, surgery may be necessary, particularly if the site of bleeding is localized (which is not always possible). The indications for surgery in these patients should be the same as for other patients with gastrointestinal bleeding. We usually continue HD under tight heparinization (or no heparin), as long as blood pressure is well maintained. Otherwise, we switch to peritoneal dialysis. Patients with a prolonged bleeding time can be given dDAVP, 0.3 mg/kg intravenously in one dose, or 0.6 mg/kg of conjugated estrogen 4 to 5 times, at 24-hr intervals (176,177). Patients with recurrent bleeding may be managed with long-term norethynodrel-mestranol therapy in dose ratios varying from 2.5 to 5 μg of norethynodrel per 0.075 to 0.1 mg of mestranol (178). Patients should be watched carefully for side effects related to the use of estrogens. We tend to discontinue the drug in patients who continue to bleed after 2–3 months of therapy or in those who have not bled for the same length of time. This latter approach is used by the authors and is not based on any controlled study.

Patients on maintenance HD can tolerate major surgery quite well. Dialysis is scheduled the day before for the patient undergoing elective surgery. Post-surgery HD can be safely performed as long as the amount of heparin used is kept to a minimum (179). Elderly males who require a prostatectomy are given dDAVP or estrogens prophylactically, as described previously, since they tend to bleed profusely after the procedure, unless the laser technique is used.

ESRD is associated with decreased life expectancy. The projected expected remaining years of life for patients below the age of 50 on dialysis is about one-fourth to one-sixth that for the general population. The ratio is about one-third for older patients (180). The expected 1-year survival for 65-year-olds is 98%, compared to 71% if the individual has ESRD; the 5-year survival is 93% and 22%, respectively. At the age of 80, it is 94% versus 55% for 1-year survival and 54% versus 7% for 5-year survival (139). In general, the mortality rate is higher for diabetics compared to patients with other forms of kidney diseases, for males compared to females, and for whites compared to blacks and other ethnic groups in the United States (180).

The three major causes of death in the elderly are cardiac (42%), infectious (13%), and cerebrovascular diseases (5%), similar to that in younger patients (181). Withdrawal from dialysis is responsible for a significant percentage of deaths in adults (181). It has been estimated that one of every six patients over the age of 60 on dialysis dies from withdrawal, 2.5–6 times the rate in younger patients (181,182). Whites are twice as likely to withdraw as blacks (181). The most common reason for withdrawing were failure to thrive and multiple medical problems already present in a great majority of elderly at the time of initiation of dialysis (183,184).

Age per se is not a risk factor for malnutrition in the elderly on HD, so the same attention to adequate protein (1 g/kg/day) and caloric intake (≥35k cal/kg/day) applies to them and should be pursued aggressively.

XIV. CPD IN THE ELDERLY

CPD (CAPD or CCPD) is generally well accepted by the elderly, with about 69% remaining on CPD at 3 years, 46% at 5 years, similar to that seen in younger patients (3). The number of elderly patients switching to HD because of infectious complications (50%), personal preference (18%), inadequate clearance (7%), or other reasons (25%) is similar to and for the same reasons for change seen in the overall CPD population. The adequate dose of peritoneal dialysis in the elderly is the same as for other adults, a minimum weekly *Kt/V* of 2.0 and/or a minimum weekly creatinine clearance of 60 L/1.73 m^2 (184a). Hospitalization in the elderly on CPD has been reported to be anywhere from 19 to 58 days per patient per year, apparently somewhat higher than for younger patients (185). Infections (peritonitis, exit-site, or tunnel infection) and cardiovascular problems account for the vast majority of case admissions (3,142,144). As noted earlier, mortality in the elderly on CPD is similar to that seen with HD with the exception of diabetics and perhaps during the first 2 years, as noted above. Cardiovascular complication (49–54%) and infections (12–22%) account for most of the deaths (122,124,158,159). A higher incidence of inguinal hernia, fluid leaks, and vascular ischemia of the lower extremities has been found in older patients on CAPD compared with younger patients (186). The clinical manifestations, bacteriology, and management of peritonitis in the elderly are similar to that of the general CPD population. Abdominal pain associated with a cloudy effluent containing >100 white blood cells/ml were present in

Table 4 Dosage of Antibiotics Currently Used in the Treatment of Peritonitis in CAPD Patients

Drug	Initial dose (mg per 2-L bag)	Maintenance dose (mg per 2-L bag)
Vancomycin	1000	30
Cefazolin	500–1000	250–500
Cefuroxime	1500	500
Ceftazidime	1000	100–250
Mezlocillin	500	500
Tobramycin, Gentamicin	120	8–12
Amikacin	350	12–15
Ciprofloxacin	750 orally	50
Imipenem	500–1000	100–200
Amphotericin B	None	2–8

all our patients. *Staphylococcus epidermis*, *Staphylococcus aureus*, and *Pseudomonas aeruginosa* are the most commonly encountered organisms. Antibiotic treatment is initiated intraperitoneally and continued until 3–5 days following either a negative peritoneal fluid culture or an effluent WBC count less than 100 cells/ml (187). In those patients who fail to respond after 96 hr of an appropriate antibiotic regimen and in those with fungal or tunnel infections, the catheter should be removed (188,189). Serious intraabdominal or gynecological pathology should also be ruled out in these patients. Persistent exit-site infections despite 2–3 weeks of antibiotic therapy is another indication for removing the catheter. A list of the currently used antibiotics for treating peritonitis and their dosage is shown in Table 4.

The optimal time period between catheter removal for peritonitis and reinsertion of a new one is usually given as 2–3 weeks. However, the two procedures have been carried out successfully at the same sitting (190). Additional data are needed, however, before recommending this approach in the elderly on CPD.

In the diabetic patient the extra glucose load associated with CPD may necessitate an increase in insulin dose. The insulin can be administered either subcutaneously or intraperitoneally. The latter route, however, has been found to be associated with a higher incidence of peritonitis in one recent study (191). As in younger patients, attention should be paid to nutritional status (185). Because of protein losses through the PD fluid, protein intake should be higher in patients on CPD than in those on HD (1.2–1.5 g/kg/day).

XV. RENAL TRANSPLANTATION IN THE ELDERLY

Age per se should not be considered a contraindication to renal transplantation (192–196), except for the very old (>75 years), even though only 5% of dialysis patients 56 years of age or older receive a kidney transplant, compared to 27% in the total dialysis population (140,197).

The problem of transplantation in the elderly is complicated by the fact that the two most common causes of ESRD in this age group are vascular (nephrosclerosis, ischemic nephropathy) and diabetes mellitus. Both entities are associated with a higher mortality rate in the elderly with ESRD compared to other renal diagnosis such as glomerulonephritis or APKD (180,198). Furthermore, the overall patient survival following the first cadaveric graft is significantly less in the elderly compared to younger patients. Also, graft survival is less for a cadaveric transplant recipient in whom the primary renal diagnosis is either diabetic or vascular, compared to other diseases (198).

Despite these problems, the superiority of dialysis over transplantation in the elderly is still not proven. Comparing survival rates between these two modalities cannot be done accurately because of patient selection. The mortality risk in dialysis patients on a waiting list for transplantation is only half the mortality risk in those not wait listed (199). In addition, results of studies addressing the quality of life with either dialysis or transplantation in the elderly have been conflicting (200).

Although these data do not paint a pretty picture, it may be possible to optimize the long-term success rate of transplantation in the elderly by careful preoperative evaluation. Since graft loss is due primarily to patient mortality from cardiovascular causes, the cardiac status prior to transplant should be evaluated, including a cardiac stress test, even in asymptomatic patients. If the latter is positive or the patient has symptoms suggestive of coronary artery disease, cardiac catherization should be performed. Evidence of peripheral vascular disease should be looked for, particularly in the carotid arteries. Gallbladder sonogram in every patient, mammogram in females, rectal examination and prostatic specific antigen level in males, and barium enema in patients with APKD are also recommended as part of the preoperative evaluation (200). Patient selection should then depend on the result of these evaluations and subsequent correction of problems, when possible.

The higher incidence of complications and poorer outcome reported in the elderly in earlier years were also related to overly aggressive immunosuppression (201). The first-year allograft survival for cadaveric recipients is similar in the elderly compared with younger patients in most of the recent series reported from the United states, Canada, Japan, Europe, and Australia (198,202–205). Five-year graft survival for all ages in Canada is 67% compared with 55% for the elderly, in Japan it is 60% for all ages and 49% for the elderly, in Australia it is 64% for all ages and 59% for the elderly. Transplant survival from living related donors is 91% at 1 year and 66% at 5 years in the elderly (203).

Given the known changes in immune function associated with aging, the principles of immunosuppresion in the elderly should be altered accordingly (206).

Initially the dose of cyclosporine should be 6–8 mg/kg/day. Either low-dose maintenance corticosteroid (0.5 mg/kg/day) and azathioprine added to cyclosporine or monotherapy with cyclosporine can be used (206). Cyclosporine-associated nephrotoxicity during the first year following transplantation occurs more commonly in the elderly than does graft rejection (207,208).

As mentioned earlier, death due to cardiovascular disease is the most common cause of graft loss in the elderly, with rejection accounting for only 13–28% (200). Infection accounts for the majority of the remaining deaths (200).

Although age is not an absolute contraindication for donation of a kidney, the 1-year survival rate for a kidney harvested from an elderly donor is lower than for a kidney originating from a younger donor (209). The outcome may be improved if a routine kidney biopsy is performed in donors over the age of 55, those who died from nontraumatic cerebrovascular accidents (210), or by keeping cold ischemic time to a minimum. Glomerulosclerosis greater than 20% in a donor kidney increases the risk of delayed graft function and poorer long-term outcome.

REFERENCES

1. McInnes EG, et al. Renal failure in the elderly. Q J Med 1987; 243:583–588.
2. Llera FG, Gregorio PG. Incidence of renal diseases in a geriatric unit. In: Macia Nuñez JF, Cameron JS, eds. Renal Function and Disease in the Elderly. London: Butterworths, 1987:208–236.
3. Ismail N, et al. Renal replacement therapies in the elderly. Am J Kidney Dis 1993;22:759–782.
4. Valderrabeno F, Jones EHP, Malick NP. Report on management of renal failure in Europe. Nephrol Dial Transplant 1995;10(suppl 5):1–25.
5. United States Renal Data System 1996 annual data report. II. Incidence and prevalence of ESRD. Am J Kidney Dis 1996;28(suppl 2):S34–S47.
6. Burkart J, et al. Major causes of ESRD in geriatric patients in northwest North Carolina (abstr 48). 22nd Annual Meeting of the American Society of Nephrologists. Washington, DC, Dec 1989.
7. Appel RG, et al. Renovascular disease in older patients beginning renal replacement therapy. Kidney Int 1995;48:171–176.
8. Sandler DP, et al. Analgesic use and chronic renal disease. N Engl J Med 1989;320: 1238–1243.
9. Adams DH, et al. Non-steroidal anti-inflammatory drugs and renal failure. Lancet 1986;1:57–59.
10. Murray TG, et al. Epidemiologic study of regular analgesic use and end-stage renal disease. Arch Intern Med 1983;143:1687–1693.
11. Buckalew VM Jr, Schey HM. Renal disease from habitual antipyretic analgesic consumption: an assessment of the epidemiologic evidence. Medicine 1986;11:291–303.
12. Sabatini S. Analgesic-induced papillary necrosis. Sem Nephrol 1988;8:41–54.
13. Bennett WM, DeBroe ME. Analgesic nephropathy. A preventable renal disease. N Engl J Med 1989;320:1269–1271.

14. Linton AL. Renal disease due to analgesics. Can Med Assoc J 1972;107:749–751.
15. Henrich WL. Analgesic nephropathy. Am J Med Sci 1988;295:561–568.
16. McCredie M, et al. Phenacetin and papillary necrosis: independent risk factor for renal pelvic cancer. Kidney Int 1985;30:81–84.
17. Hestbech J, et al. Chronic renal lesions following long-term treatment with lithium. Kidney Int 1977;12:205–213.
18. Boton R, Gaviria M, Battle DC. Prevalence, pathogenesis and treatment of renal dysfunction associated with chronic lithium therapy. Am J Kidney Dis 1987;10: 329–345.
19. Walker RG, Davies BM, Holwill BJ. A chronic pathological study of lithium nephrotoxicity. J Chron Dis 1982;35:685–695.
20. Battle DC, et al. Amelioration of polyuria by amiloride in patients receiving long term lithium therapy. N Engl J Med 1985;312:409–414.
21. Batuman V, et al. The role of lead in gouty nephropathy. N Engl J Med 1981;304: 520–523.
22. Colleoni N, D'Amato G. Chronic lead accumulation as a possible cause of renal failure in gouty patients. Nephron 1986;44:32–35.
23. Wedeen RP. Use of $CaNa_2$ EDTA Pb-mobilization test to detect occult lead nephropathy. Uremia Invest 1985;9:127–130.
24. Wedeen RP, Mallich DK, Batuman V. Detection and treatment of occupational lead nephropathy. Arch Intern Med 1979;139:53–57.
25. Bennett WM. Lead nephropathy. Kidney Int 1985;28:212–220.
26. Kim R, et al. A longitudinal study of low level lead exposure and impairment of renal function. JAMA 1996;275:1177–1181.
27. Drenick EJ, et al. Renal damage with intestinal bypass. Ann Intern Med 1978;89: 594–599.
27a. Elseviers MM. DeBroe ME. Epidemiology of toxic nephropathies. Adv Nephrol 1997;27:241–262.
28. Luxton RW. Radiation nephritis. A long term study of 54 patients. Lancet 1961;2: 1221–1224.
29. Bolton WK, et al. Reversible renal failure from isolated granulomatous renal sarcoidosis. Clin Nephrol 1976;5:88–92.
30. Muther RS, McCarron DA, Bennett WM. Granulomatous sarcoid nephritis: a cause of multiple renal tubular abnormalities. Clin Nephrol 1980;14:190–197.
31. Farge D, et al. Granulomatous nephritis and chronic renal failure in sarcoidosis. Am J Nephrol 1986;6:21–27.
32. Reeders ST, Grimino GG. The molecular genetics of autosomal dominant polycystic kidney disease. Sem Nephrol 1989;9:122–134.
33. Romeo G, et al. A second genetic locus for autosomal dominant polycystic kidney disease. Lancet 1988;2:8–11.
34. Gabow PA, Iklé DW, Holmes JH. Polycystic kidney disease: prospective analysis of nonazotemic patients and family members. Ann Intern Med 1984;101:238–247.
35. Delaney VB, et al. Autosomal dominant polycystic kidney disease. Presentation, complications and prognosis. Am J Kidney Dis 1985;5:104–111.
36. Milutinovic J, et al. Clinical manifestations of autosomal dominant polycystic kidney disease in patients older than 50 years. Am J Kidney Dis 1990;15:237–243.

37. Zeier M, et al. Adult dominant polycystic kidney disease. Clinical problems. Nephron 1988;49:177–183.
38. Parfrey PS, et al. The prognosis of autosomal dominant polycystic kidney disease: PKD 1 vs PKD 2. Kidney Int 1990;37:251A.
39. Torra R, et al. Linkage, clinical features, and prognosis of autosomal dominant polycystic kidney disease types 1 and 2. J Am Soc Nephrol 1996;7:2142–2151.
40. Johnson AM, Gabow PA. Identification of patients with autosomal dominant polycystic kidney disease at highest risk for end-stage renal disease. J Am Soc Nephrol 1997;8:1560–1567.
41. Choukroun G, et al. Factors influencing progression of renal failure in autosomal dominant polycystic kidney disease. J Am Soc Nephrol 1995;6:1634–1642.
42. Gabow PA, Schrier RW. Pathophysiology of adult polycystic kidney disease. Adv Nephrol 1989;18:19–32.
43. Wilson PD, et al. A new method for studying human polycystic kidney disease epithelia in culture. Kidney Int 1986;30:371–378.
44. Carone FA. Functional changes in polycystic kidney disease are tubulointerstitial in origin. Sem Nephrol 1988;8:89–92.
45. Huseman R, et al. Macropuncture study of polycystic kidney disease in adult human kidneys. Kidney Int 1980;18:375–385.
46. Wallace DP, Grantham JJ, Sullivan LP. Chloride and fluid secretion by cultured human polycystic kidney cells. Kidney Int 1996;50:1327–1336.
47. Geng L, et al. Identification and localization of polycystin, the PKD 1 gene product. J Clin Invest 1996;98:2674–2682.
48. Schwab SJ, Bander SJ. Cyst infection in autosomal dominant polycystic kidney disease. Am J Med 1987;82:714–718.
49. Sklar AH, et al. Renal infections in autosomal dominant polycystic kidney disease. Am J Kidney Dis 1987;10:81–88.
50. Levine E, Grantham JJ. The role of computed tomography in the evaluation of adult polycystic kidney disease. Am J Kidney Dis 1981;1:99–105.
51. Ng RCK, Suki WN. Renal cell carcinoma occuring in a polycystic kidney of a transplant recipient. J Urol 1980;124:710–712.
52. Keith DS, et al. Renal cell carcinoma in autosomal dominant polycystic kidney disease. J Am Soc Nephrol 1994;4:1661–1669.
53. Bennett WM, et al. Reduction of cyst volume for symptomatic management of autosomal dominant polycystic kidney disease. J Urol 1988;137:620–622.
53a. El Nahas AM: Progression of renal scarring: a balancing act. Adv Nephrol 1997;27: 67–84.
54. Shulman NB, et al. Prognostic value of serum creatinine and effect of treatment of hypertension on renal function. Hypertension 1989;13(suppl 1):80–93.
55. Rostand SG, et al. Renal insufficiency in treated essential hypertension. N Engl J Med 1989;320:684–688.
56. Brahm M, et al. Prognosis in glomerulonephritis. Acta Med Scand 1985;217:117–125.
57. Klahr S, et al. Dietary protein restriction, blood pressure control, and the progression of polycystic kidney disease. J Am Soc Nephrol 1995;5:2037–2047.
58. Williams PS, Fass G, Bone JM. Renal pathology and proteinuria determine progression in untreated mild/moderate chronic renal failure. Q J Med 1988;252:343–354.

59. Stenvinkel P, Alvestrand A, Bergström J. Factors influencing progression in patients with chronic renal failure. J Intern Med 1989;226:183–188.
60. Toto RD, et al. Strict blood pressure control and progression of renal disease in hypertensive nephrosclerosis. Kidney Int 1995;48:851–859.
61. Burton C, Harris KPG. The role of proteinuria in the progression of chronic renal failure. Am J Kidney Dis 1995;27:765–775.
62. Peruzzi L, et al. Tubulointerstitial responses in the progression of glomerular diseases. Kidney Int 1996;50:1310–1320.
63. Giminez LF, Solez K, Walker GW. Relation between renal calcium content and renal impairment in 246 human renal biopsies. Kidney Int 1987;31:93–99.
64. Ibels L, et al. Calcification in end stage kidneys. Am J Med 1980;71:33–37.
65. Ibels L, et al. Preservation of function in experimental renal disease by dietary restriction of phosphate. N Engl J Med 1978;298:122–126.
66. Alfrey AC. Effect of dietary phosphate restriction on renal function and deterioration. Am J Clin Nutr 1988;47:153–156.
67. Grützmacher P, et al. Lipoproteins and apolipoproteins during the progression of chronic renal disease. Nephron 1988;50:103–111.
68. Keane WF, Kasiske BL, O'Donnell MP. Hyperlipidemia and the progression of renal disease. Am J Clin Nutr 1988;47:157–160.
69. Harris PG, et al. Lovastatin ameliorates the development of glomerulosclerosis and uremia in experimental nephrotic syndrome. Am J Kidney Dis 1990;15:16–23.
70. Massy ZA, et al. Lipids, 3-hydroxy-3-methylglutaryl coenzyme A reductase inhibitors, and progression of renal failure. Adv Nephrol 1997;27:39–56.
71. Moorhead JF, et al. Lipid nephrotoxicity in chronic progressive glomerular and tubulo-interstitial disease. Lancet 1982;2:1309–1311.
72. Moorhead JF, et al. Injury to rat mesangial cells in culture by low density lipoproteins. Kidney Int 1989;35:433A.
73. Klahr S, Schreiner G, Ichikawa I. The progression of renal disease. N Engl J Med 1988;318:1657–1666.
74. Anderson S, Brenner BM. Progressive renal disease: a disorder of adaptation. Q J Med 1989;70:185–189.
75. Miller PL, et al. Glomerular hypertrophy aggravates epithelial cell injury in nephrotic rats. J Clin Invest 1990;85:1119–1126.
76. Fogo A, Ichikawa I. Glomerular growth promoter: the common channel to glomerulosclerosis. Contemp Issues Nephrol 1992;26:23–54.
77. Mitch WE, et al. A simple method for estimating progression of chronic renal failure. Lancet 1976;2:1326–1328.
78. Kirschbaum BB. Analysis of reciprocal creatinine plots in renal failure. Am J Med Sc 1986;291:404–407.
79. Walser M, Drew HH, LaFrance ND. Reciprocal creatinine slopes often give erroneous estimates of progression of chronic renal failure. Kidney Int 1989; 36(suppl 27):S81–S89.
80. MDRD Study Group. Creatinine filtration, secretion and excretion during progressive renal disease. Kidney Int 1989; 36(suppl 27):S73–S80.

81. Levey AS, et al. Effects of diet and antihypertensive therapy on creatinine clearance and serum creatinine concentration in the modification of diet in renal disease study. J Am Soc Nephrol 1996;7:556–565.
82. Blythe WB. Natural history of hypertension in renal parenchymal disease. Am J Kidney Dis 1985;5:A50–A56.
83. Koomans HA, et al. Sodium balance in renal failure: a comparison of patients with normal subjects under extremes of sodium intake. Hypertension 1985;7:714–721.
84. Ritz E, et al. Pathogenesis of hypertension in glomerular disease. Am J Nephrol 1989;9(suppl 1):85–90.
85. Maschio G, Oldrizzil, Rugiu C. Role of hypertension on the progression of renal disease in man. Blood Purific 1988;6:250–257.
86. Klahr S. The modification of diet in renal disease study. N Engl J Med 1989;320: 864–866.
87. Acone D, et al. Blood pressure and progression of renal failure in the elderly. Kidney Int 1996;49(suppl 55):S75–S77.
88. Peterson JC, et al. Blood pressure control, proteinuria, and the progression of renal disease. Ann Intern Med 1995;123:754–762.
88a. Lazarus JM, et al. Achievement and safety of a low blood pressure goal in chronic renal disease. The modification of diet in renal disease study group. Hypertension 1997;29:641–650.
89. Cruickshank JM. Coronary flow reserve and the J curve: relation between diastolic blood pressure and myocardial infarction. Br Med J 1988;297:1227–1230.
90. Pettinger WA, et al. Long term improvement in renal function after short term strict blood pressure control in hypertensive nephrosclerosis. Hypertension 1989;13: 766–772.
91. Brazy PC, Stead WW, Fitzwilliam JF. Progression of renal insufficiency: role of blood pressure. Kidney Int 1989;35:670–674.
92. Bergström J, et al. Stockholm clinical study on progression of chronic renal failure. An interim report. Kidney Int 1989;36(suppl 27):S110–S114.
93. Rosman JB, et al. Protein-restricted diets in chronic renal failure: a four year follow-up shows limited indications. Kidney Int 1989;36(suppl 27):S96–S102.
94. Mogensen CE. Long term antihypertensive treatment inhibiting progression of diabetic nephropathy. Br Med J 1982;285:685–688.
95. Parving HH, et al. Early aggressive antihypertension treatment reduces rate of decline in kidney function in diabetic nephropathy. Lancet 1983;1:1175–1177.
96. Kes P, Ratkovic-Gusic I. The role of arterial hypertension in progression of renal failure. Kidney Int 1996;49(suppl 55):S72–S74.
97. Baldwin DS, Neugarten J. Treatment of hypertension in renal disease. Am J Kidney Dis 1985;5:57–70.
98. Keane WF, et al. Angiotensin converting enzyme inhibitors and progressive renal insufficiency. Ann Intern Med 1989;111:503–516.
99. Abrahan PA, et al. Efficacy and renal effects of enalapril therapy for hypertensive patients with chronic renal insufficiency. Arch Intern Med 1988;148:2358–2362.
100. Ruilope LM, et al. Converting enzyme inhibition in chronic renal failure. Am J Kidney Dis 1989;13:120–126.

101. Brazy PC, Fitzwilliam JF. Progressive renal disease: role of race and antihypertensive medications. Kidney Int 1990;37:1113–1119.
102. Maschio G, et al. Effect of the angiotensin-converting enzyme inhibitor benazepril on the progression of chronic renal insufficiency. N Engl J Med 1996;334:939–945.
103. Faubert PF, Porush JG. Managing hypertension in chronic renal disease. Geriatrics 1987;42:49–59.
104. Heyka RJ, Vidt DG. Control of hypertension in patients with chronic renal failure. Clev Clin J Med 1989;56:65–76.
105. Pitts TO, et al. Hyperparathyroidism and 1,25 dihydroxyvitamin D deficiency in mild, moderate and severe renal failure. J Clin Endocrinol Metab 1988;67:876–881.
106. Francis RM, Peacock M, Barkworth SA. Renal impairment and its effects on calcium metabolism in elderly women. Age and Ageing 1984;13:14–20.
107. Lopez-Hilker S, et al. On the mechanism by which phosphate restriction reverses secondary hyperparathyroidism in advanced renal insufficiency. Clin Res 1989;37: 582A.
108. Coburn JW, et al. Study of intestinal absorption of calcium in patients with renal failure. Kidney Int 1973;3:264–272.
109. LLach F, et al. Skeletal resistance of endogenous parathyroid hormone in patients with early renal failure: a possible cause for secondary hyperparathyroidism. J Clin Endocrinol Metab 1975;41:339–345.
110. Lloyd HM, et al. The parathyroid glands in chronic renal failure: a study of their growth and other properties made on the basis of findings in patients with hypercalcemia. J Lab Clin Med 1989;114:358–367.
111. Schiller LR, et al. Effect of the time administration of calcium acetate on phosphorus binding. N Engl J Med 1989;320:1110–1113.
112. Malberti F, et al. Efficacy and safety of long term treatment with calcium carbonate as a phosphate binder. Am J Kidney Dis 1988;12:487–491.
113. Moriniere P, et al. A control of predialytic hyperphosphatemia by oral calcium acetate and calcium carbonate. Nephron 1992;60:6–11.
114. Nordal KP, Dahl E. Low dose calcitrol versus placebo in patients with predialysis chronic renal failure. J Clin Endocrinol Metab 1988;67:929–936.
115. Coen G, et al. Bone aluminum content in predialysis chronic renal failure and its relation to secondary hyperparathyroidism and $1,25(OH)_2$ D_3 treatment. Miner Electrol Metab 1989;15:295–302.
116. Baker LRI, et al. $1,25(OH)_2$ D_3 administration in moderate renal failure: a prospective double-blind trial. Kidney Int 1989;35:661–669.
117. Widmer B, et al. Serum electrolyte and acid base composition: the influence of graded degrees of chronic renal failure. Arch Intern Med 1979;139:1099–1102.
118. Warnock DG. Uremic acidosis. Kidney Int 1988;34:278–287.
119. Molitoris BA, et al. Citrate: a major factor in the toxicity of orally administered aluminum compounds. Kidney Int 1989;36:949–953.
120. Mitch WE, Goldberg AL. Mechanisms of muscle wasting. The role of the ubiquitin-proteasome pathway. N Engl J Med 1996;335:1897–1905.
121. Howard AD, et al. Analysis of the quantitative relationship between anemia and chronic renal failure. Am J Med SC 1989;297:309–313.

122. Tinetti ME, Schmidt A, Baum J. Use of ESR in chronically ill, elderly patients with a decline in health status. Am J Med 1986;80:844–848.
123. Schusterman N, et al. Factors influencing erythrocyte sedimentation in patients with chronic renal failure. Arch Intern Med 1985;145:1796–1799.
124. Lacombe C, et al. Peritubular cells are the site of erythropoietin synthesis in the murine hypoxic kidney. J Clin Invest 1988;81:620–623.
125. Eckardt KU, et al. Erythropoietin in polycystic kidneys. J Clin Invest 1989;84: 1160–1166.
126. Sun CH, et al. Serum erythropoietin levels after renal transplantation. N Engl J Med 1989;321:151–157.
127. Hand MF, et al. Erythropoietin enhances vascular responsiveness to norepinephrine in renal failure. Kidney Int 1995;48:806–813.
128. Bode-B;auoger SM, et al. Recombinant human erythopoietin enhances vasoconstrictor tone via endothelin and constrictor prostanoid. Kidney Int 1996;50:1255–1261.
129. Eschbach JW, et al. Treatment of the anemia of progressive renal failure with recombinant human erythropoietin. N Engl J Med 1989;321:158–163.
130. Bankir L, Bouby N, Tringh-Trang-Tan MM. Possible involvement of vasopressin and urine concentrating process in the progression of chronic renal failure. Kidney Int 1989; 36(suppl 27):S32–S37.
131. Nath K, Hostetter MK, Hostetter TH. Ammonia-complement interaction in the pathogenesis of progressive renal injury. Kidney Int 1989; 36(suppl 27):S52–S54.
132. Pedrini MT, et al. The effect of dietary protein restriction on the progression of diabetic and non-diabetic renal diseases: a meta analysis. Ann Intern Med 1996;124: 627–632.
133. Mitch WE. Uremia and the control of protein metabolism. Nephron 1988;49:89–93.
134. Goodship THJ, Mitch WE. Nutritional approaches to preserving renal function. Adv Intern Med 1988;33:337–357.
135. Cianciaruso B, et al. Dietary compliance to a low protein and phosphate diet in patients with chronic renal failure. Kidney Int 1989;36(suppl 27):S173–S176.
136. MDRD Study Group. Nutritional status of patients with different levels of chronic renal insufficiency. Kidney Int 1989;36(suppl 27):S184–S194.
137. Rotellar E, et al. Must patients over 65 be hemodialyzed? Nephron 1985;41:152–156.
138. Ponticelli C. Renal replacement therapy in the elderly. Q J Med 1989;268:667–668.
139. Latos DL. Chronic dialysis in patients over age 65. J Am Soc Nephrol 1996;7:637–646.
140. United States Renal Data System. III. Treatment modalities for ESRD patients. Am J Kidney Dis 1996;28(suppl 2):S48–S57.
141. Grapsa I, Oreopoulos DG. Practical ethical issues of dialysis in the elderly. Sem Nephrol 1996;16:339–352.
142. Mion C, et al. Maintenance dialysis in the elderly. A review of 15 years experience in Languedoc-Roussillon. Proc EDTA-ERA 1984;21:490–509.
143. Panarello G, et al. Dialysis for the elderly: survival and risk factors. Adv Peritoneal Dialysis 1989;5:49–51.

144. Williams AJ, et al. Continuous ambulatory peritoneal dialysis and haemodialysis in the elderly. Q J Med 1990;274:215–223.
145. Husebye DJ, et al. Psychological, social and somatic prognostic indicators in old patients undergoing long-term dialysis. Arch Intern Med 1987;147:1921–1924.
145a. Fenton SSA et al. Hemodialysis versus peritoneal dialysis: a comparison of adjusted mortality rates. Am J Kidney Dis 1997;30:334–342.
146. Cohen SL, Comty CM, Shapiro FL. The effect of age on the results of regular haemodialysis treatment. Proc Eur Dial Transplant Assoc 1970;7:254–258.
147. Ghaptous WN, et al. Long-term hemodialysis in the elderly. Trans Am Soc Artif Intern Organs 1971;17:125–128.
148. Feldman HI, Kabrin S, Wasserstein A. Hemodialysis vascular access morbidity. J Am Soc Nephrol 1996;7:523–535.
149. United States Renal Data System. IV. The USRDS dialysis morbidity and mortality study (Wave 1). Am J Kidney Dis 1996;28(suppl 2):S58–S78.
150. Hinsdale JG, Lipkowitz GS, Hoover EL. Vascular access for hemodialysis in the elderly: results and perspectives in a geriatric population. Dialysis and Transplant 1985;14:560–565.
151. Jindal KK, Goldstein MB. Urea kinetic modelling in chronic hemodialysis: benefits, problems and practical solutions. Sem Dialysis 1988;1:82–85.
151a. NKF-DOQI: II Hemodialysis dose. Am J Kidney Dis 1997;30(suppl 2):532–537.
152. Basila C, Casino F, Lopez T. Percent reduction in blood urea concentration during dialysis estimates *kt/V* in a simple and accurate way. Am J Kidney Dis 1990;15: 40–45.
153. Jacobs C, et al. Maintenance haemodialysis treatment in patients over 60 years. Demographic profile, clinical aspects and outcome. Proc EDTA-ERA 1984;21: 477–489.
154. Faubert PF, Porush, JG. Unpublished observations, 1989.
155. Arieff AI. Aluminum and the pathogenesis of dialysis encephalopathy. Am J Kidney Dis 1985;6:317–321.
156. Norris KC, et al. Clinical and laboratory features of aluminum-related bone disease: differences between sporadic and "epidemic" forms of the syndrome. Am J Kidney Dis 1985;6L:342–347.
157. Malluche HH, Faugere MC. Aluminum: toxin or innocent bystander in renal osteodystrophy. Am J Kidney Dis 1985;5:336–341.
158. Goodman WG. Bone disease and aluminum: pathogenic considerations. Am J Kidney Dis 1985;5:330–335.
159. Swartz RD. Deferoxamine and aluminum removal. Am J Kidney Dis 1985;5: 358–364.
160. Boelaert JR, et al. The role of deferoxamine in dialysis associated mucormycosis: report of three cases and review of the literature. Clin Nephrol 1988;29:261–266.
161. Torres A, et al. Bone disease in predialysis, hemodialysis, and CAPD patients: evidence of a better bone response to PTH. Kidney Int 1995;47:1434–1442.
162. Kaye M. Parathyroidectomy in endstage renal disease. J Lab Clin Med 1989;114: 334–335.
163. Dunlay R, et al. Direct inhibitory effect of calcitriol on parathyroid function (sigmoid curve) in dialysis. Kidney Int 1989;36:1093–1098.

164. Andress DL, et al. Intravenous calcitriol in the treatment of refractory osteitis fibrosa of chronic renal failure. N Engl J Med 1989;321:274–279.
165. Levine BS, Song M. Pharmacokinetics and efficacy of pulse oral versus intravenous calcitriol in hemodialysis patients. J Am Soc Nephrol 1996;7:488–496.
165a. Fournier A, et al. The clinical significance of adynamic bone disease in uremia. Adv Nephrol 1997;27:131–166.
166. Delmez JA, et al. Magnesium carbonate as a phosphorus binder: a prospective, controlled, crossover study. Kidney Int 1996;49:163–167.
167. Blackely JD, et al. Uremic pruritus skin divalent ion content and response to ultraviolet therapy. Am J Kidney Dis 1985;5:237–241.
168. Stähle-Vackdahl M. Uremic pruritus. Clinical and experimental studies. Acta Derm Venerol 1989;1(suppl 145):38.
169. Taylor R, et al. A placebo-controlled trial of UV-A phototherapy for the treatment of uraemic pruritus. Nephron 1983;33:14–16.
170. Gilchrist BA, et al. Relief of uremic pruritus with ultraviolet phototherapy. N Engl J Med 1977;297:136–138.
171. Schaefer K, et al. Optimum dialysis treatment for patients over 60 years with primary renal disease. Survival data and clinical results from 242 patients treated either by hemodialysis or hemofiltration. Proc EDTA-ERA 1984;21:510–523.
172. Westlie J, et al. Mortality, morbidity and life satisfaction in the very old dialysis patient. Trans Am Soc Artif Intern Organs 1984;30:21–30.
173. Carlson DM, et al. Hospitalization in dialysis patients. Mayo Clin Proc 1984;59:769–775.
174. Zuckerman GR, et al. Upper gastrointestinal bleeding in patients with chronic renal failure. Ann Intern Med 1985;102:588–592.
175. Almond MK. Laser therapy for lesions of the bronchial tree and gastrointestinal tract in the elderly. IM 1987;8:53–58.
176. Remuzzi G. Bleeding in renal failure. Lancet 1988;1:1205–1208.
177. Vigano G, et al. Dose-effect and pharmacokinetics of estrogens given to correct bleeding time in uremia. Kidney Int 1988;34:853–858.
178. Bronner MK, et al. Estrogen-progesterone therapy for bleeding gastrointestinal telangiectasias in chronic renal failure. An uncontrolled trial. Ann Intern Med 1986;105:371–374.
179. Camana RJ, et al. Heparin free dialysis: comparative data and results in high risk patients. Kidney Int 1987;31:1351–1355.
180. United States Renal Data System. V. Patient mortality and survival. Am J Kidney Dis 1996;28(suppl 2):S79–S92.
181. United States Renal Data System. VI. Causes of death. Am J Kidney Dis 1996; 28(suppl 2):S93–S102.
182. Neu S, Kjellstrand CM. Stopping long-term dialysis. An empirical study of withdrawal of life-supporting treatment. N Engl J Med 1986;314:14–20.
183. McKevitt PM, Jones JF, Marion RR. The elderly on dialysis: physical and psychosocial functioning. Dialysis and Transplant 1986;15:130–137.
184. O'Kràfe Schultz K, Powers MJ. Adjustment of older patients to hemodialysis. Dialysis and Transplant 1987;16:234–241.

184a. NKF-DOQI. V. Adequate dose of peritoneal dialysis. Am J Kidney Dis 1997; 30(suppl 2):586–592.
185. Churchill DN, Taylor DW, Keshaviah PR. Adequacy of dialysis and nutrition in continuous peritoneal dialysis: association with clinical outcomes. J Am Soc Nephrol 1996;7:198–207.
186. Nichols AJ, et al. Impact of continuous ambulatory peritoneal dialysis on treatment of renal failure in patients aged over 60 years. Br Med J 1984;288:18–19.
187. Gokal R, et al. Peritonitis in continuous ambulatory peritoneal dialysis. Lancet 1982;2:1388–1391.
188. Keene WF, et al. CAPD related peritonitis management and antibiotic therapy recommendations. Peritoneal Dialysis Bull 1987;7:55–68.
189. Nolph KD, Lindblad AS, Novak JW. Continuous ambulatory peritoneal dialysis. N Engl J Med 1988;318:1595–1600.
190. Paterson AD, et al. Removal and replacement of Tenckhoff catheter at a single operation: successful treatment of resistant peritonitis in continuous ambulatory peritoneal dialysis. Lancet 1986;2:1245–1247.
191. Selgas R, et al. Comparative study of two different routes for insulin administration in CAPD diabetic patients. A multicenter study. Adv Peritoneal Dialysis 1989;5: 182–190.
192. Delmonico F, Cosimi BA, Russell PS. Renal transplantation in the older age groups. Arch Surg 1975;110:1107–1109.
193. Ost L, et al. Cadaveric renal transplantation in patients of 60 years and above. Transplantation 1980;30:339–340.
194. Taube DH, et al. Successful treatment of middle aged and elderly patients with end stage renal disease. Br Med J 1983;286:2018–2020.
195. Schulak JA, et al. Kidney transplantation in patients of 60 years and above. Transplantation 1980;30:339–340.
196. Vivas CA, et al. Renal transplantation in patients 65 years old or older. J Urol 1992;147:990–993.
197. Kjellstrand CM. Age, sex and race inequality in renal transplantation. Arch Intern Med 1988;148:1305–1308.
198. Fenton S, et al. Renal replacement therapy in Canada: a report from the Canadian organ replacement register. Am J Kidney Dis 1995;25:134–150.
199. United States Renal Data System. VII. Renal transplantation. Am J Kidney Dis 1996;28(suppl 2):S103–S113.
200. Ismail N, Hakim RM, Helderman JH. Renal replacement therapies in the elderly: part II. Renal transplantation. Am J Kidney Dis 1994;23:1–15.
201. Jordon ML, et al. Renal transplantation in the older recipient. J Urol 1985;134: 243–246.
202. Sommer BG, et al. Renal transplantation in the middle aged and elderly uremic patient. The recent United States experience and results from a single institution. In: Oreopoulous D, ed. Geriatric Nephrology. Boston: Martinus Nijhoff Publ, 1986: 157–168.
203. Teraoka S, et al. Current status of renal replacement therapy in Japan. Am J Kidney Dis 1995;25:151–164.

204. Disney APS. Demography and survival of patients receiving treatment for chronic renal failure in Australia and New Zealand: report on dialysis and renal transplantation treatment from the Australia and New Zealand Dialysis and Transplant Registry. Am J Kidney Dis 1995;25:165–175.
205. Mallick NP, Jones E, Selwood N. The European (European Dialysis and Transplantation Association-European Renal Association) registry. Am J Kidney Dis 1995; 25:176–187.
206. Becker BN, et al. Renal transplantation in the older end stage renal disease patient. Sem Nephrol 1996;16:353–362.
207. Myers BD, et al. Cyclosporine-associated chronic nephropathy. N Engl J Med 1984;311:699–705.
208. Pirsch JD, et al. Cadaveric renal transplantation with cyclosporin in patients more than 60 years of age. Transplantation 1989;47:259–261.
209. Foster MC, et al. Use of older patients as cadaveric kidney donors. Br J Surg 1988;75:767–769.
210. Gaber LW. Glomerulosclerosis as a determinant of post-transplant function of older donor renal allografts. Transplantation 1995;60:334–339.

12

Hypertension in the Elderly

I. AGE AND BLOOD PRESSURE

From 60 to 80 years of age, systolic blood pressure increases an average of 4–7 mmHg per decade in the male and 6–9 mmHg in the female. After the age of 80, a drop in systolic pressure of 2–3 mmHg per decade is seen in both males and females. On the other hand, after the age of 50, the diastolic blood pressure decreases 1–3 mmHg per decade in both males and females (1–5). Thus, both pulse pressure and mean arterial pressure (MAP) increase with aging (Fig. 1). In general, systolic blood pressure in the elderly black male and female tends to be 4–6 mmHg higher than in their white counterparts, whereas diastolic blood pressure tends to be similar.

The rise in systolic pressure seen with age is a reflection of an increase in arterial stiffness resulting from degeneration of wall elastin and calcium deposition (6–8). As a result, the pulse waves reflected from peripheral vascular sites return earlier during ventricular ejection, causing a prolonged increase in intraventricular systolic pressure, the end point being a boost in the systolic and a decrease in the diastolic pressure. The rise in MAP is a reflection of an increase in total peripheral vascular resistance since cardiac output, the other variable component of the blood pressure, either decreases slightly or remains unchanged with age (9–12).

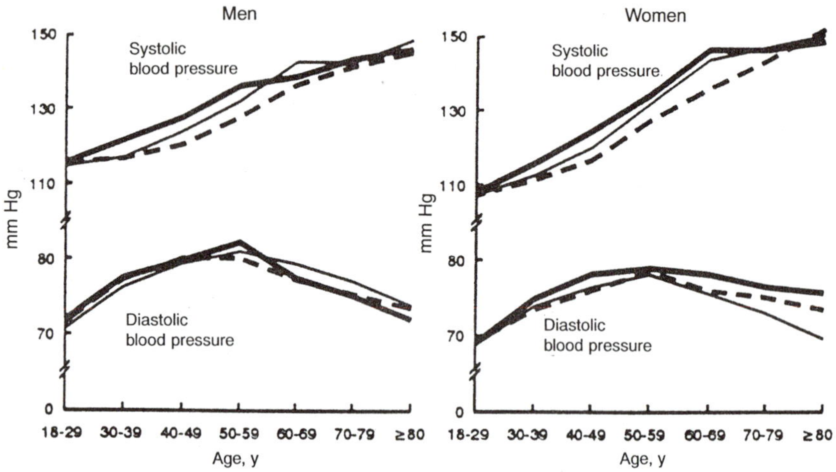

Figure 1 Mean systolic and diastolic blood pressures by age and race/ethnicity for men and women. U.S. population 18 years of age and older. (From Burt VL, et al. Trends in the prevalence, awareness, treatment, and control of hypertension in the adult US population. Hypertension 1995; 25:305–313.)

Besides the structural changes in the vasculature noted above, an alteration in muscular tone also contributes to the increase in peripheral vascular resistance seen with aging. Plasma norepinephrine levels increase with age (13), probably as a result of an increase in sympathetic activity mediated by an age-related change in baroreflex sensitivity (14,15). Alpha-adrenergic vasoconstrictor function remains intact with age, while dopamine- and beta-adrenergic-induced vasodilation is attenuated (16–18). This imbalance could lead to a state of relative vasoconstriction. It should be added, however, that in most recent studies, the β_2-adrenergic response in the elderly has been found to be identical to that of younger subjects (19). Aging is also associated with a decrease in erythrocyte sodium–potassium ATPase activity (20). If a similar defect is present in vascular smooth muscle cells, sodium transport out of these cells will decrease. Since the cellular concentration of calcium is linked to the sodium gradient across the cell membrane through a calcium–sodium exchanger, a small increase in cytoplasmic sodium may result in enough of an increase in intracellular calcium to produce an increase in smooth muscle tone.

Other vasoconstrictive agents such as vasopressin (see Chapter 1) and endothelin-1 (21) increase with age; however, their contribution to the age-related rise in blood pressure has not yet been adequately studied. Similarly, the increase in insulin resistance (22,23) and the progressive blunting of endothelium-derived vasodilation reported with aging (24,25) have not been clearly associated with the increase in blood pressure, although exogenous infusion of insulin in the normal elderly is associated with vasoconstriction of the forearm blood vessels compared to vasodilation in younger subjects (25a).

As discussed in Chapter 1, GFR tends to decrease with age, which probably contributes to renal sodium retention and expansion of the extracellular fluid volume, leading to an increase in blood pressure. It should be cautioned that this paradigm is only theoretical and is not based on direct studies (26). However, the importance of salt balance is suggested by the absence of an age-related increase in blood pressure in populations on a low salt intake (27). The higher blood pressure found in elderly blacks compared to whites might, in part, reflect their greater sensitivity to salt (28), a trait most likely genetically transmitted (29).

II. DEFINITIONS AND MEASUREMENT

Hypertension in the elderly is defined as a systolic blood pressure (SBP) >140 mmHg and/or a diastolic blood pressure (DBP) >90 mmHg, determined by averaging the blood pressures taken on three consecutive visits. The systolic pressure should be recorded at the first Korotkoff sound and the diastolic at the fifth phase, when the sound disappears, using a cuff width of 40–50% of the upper arm circumference and with the patient seated quietly for 3–5 min. The cuff should be deflated at a rate of 2–3 mmHg/sec (30). According to JNC V (30a), hypertension is classified as follows: stage 1 (mild), SBP 140–159 and DBP 90–99 mmHg; stage 2 (moderate), SBP 160–179 and DBP 100–109 mmHg; stage 3 (severe), SBP 180–209 and DBP 110–119 mmHg; stage 4 (very severe), SBP ≥210 and DBP >120 mmHg. Patients with a SBP >140 and DBP <90 mmHg are considered to have isolated systolic hypertension (ISH).

III. PREVALENCE

Figure 2 depicts the prevalence of essential hypertension in various age groups in a civilian, noninstitutionalized U.S. population (31). Data from National Health and Nutrition Examination Surveys (NAHNES) from 1960 to 1991 are shown in Fig. 3. Between NHANES I, II, and III, the prevalence of hypertension (BP >140/90 mmHg) was 64.7 among white males versus 81.7% among black males, 56.8% among white males versus 67.0% among black males, and 51% among white males versus 71.2% among black males, respectively. The values were 72.1% for white females versus 82.9% for black females in NHANES I, 61.3% versus 80.8% in NHANES II, and 05.0% versus 73.9% in NHANES III. Thus, there is a tendency for a decline in the prevalence of hypertension in elderly white males, white females, and black females between NHANES I and III, whereas an increase from 67% to 71.2% was noted in black males between NHANES II and

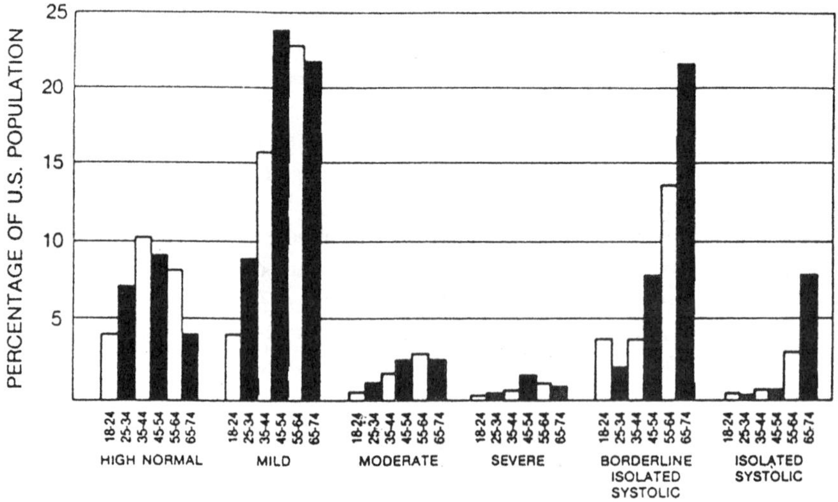

Figure 2 Percentage of the civilian noninstitutionalized population aged 18–74 years with hypertension, categorized by blood pressure (regardless of medication status) and by age, 1976–1980. (From Final report of the Subcommittee on Definition and Prevalence of Hypertension. 1984 Joint National Committee. Hypertension 1985; 7:457–468.)

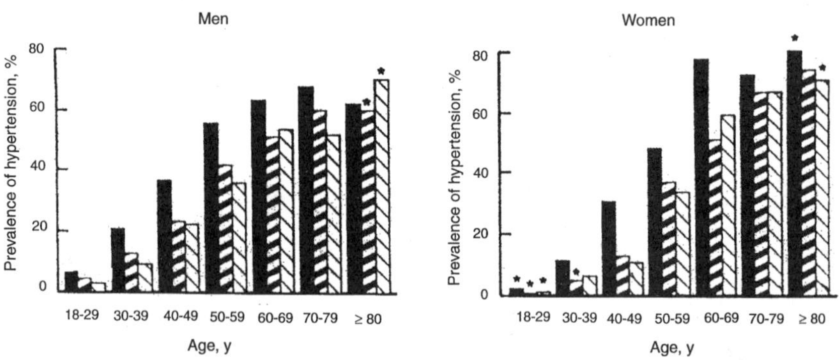

Figure 3 Prevalence of high blood presure by race and race/ecthnity for men and women, U.S. population 18 years of age and older. *Estimate based on sample size not meeting minimum requirements of the National Health and Nutrition Examination Survey III design or relative SEM greater than 30%. (From Burt VL, et al. Trends in prevalence, awareness, treatment, and control of hypertension in the adult US population. Hypertension 1995; 25:305–313.)

Table 1 Prevalence of Isolated Systolic Hypertension in the Elderly

Age (yr)	Prevalence (%)	Reference
60–69	6.8 (white males 5.3; black males 6.4; white females 7.4; black females 8.3)	(36)
65–90	14.4 (males)	
	22.8 (females)	(37)
65–74	7.3	(38)
60–64	3.3	(39)
60–64	12.7	(40)
80+	29.4	(40)
65–75	10–12	(41)
60–69	5.0	(33)
70–79	12.6	(33)
80+	23.6	(33)

III. As seen in Fig. 2, the incidence of mild, moderate, and severe hypertension is similar in the 45–54, 55–64, and 65–74 age groups, while isolated systolic hypertension is uncommon before the age of 55 and increases with age.

Table 1 summarizes the prevalence of ISH as reported in different studies. The wide spread in prevalence noted among these studies most likely reflects differences in methods used to diagnose ISH (33). In general, ISH is more prevalent in white and black females compared to their male counterparts, with the highest prevalence found among black females (32–35).

IV. HEMODYNAMICS

The hemodynamic parameters of hypertension are quite different in the elderly compared to younger patients. As noted, the systolic pressure tends to be higher and the diastolic lower in the elderly. Since the cardiac output in older hypertensives is lower than in younger hypertensives, the elevated blood pressure is due to a disproportionately higher total peripheral resistance (42), which is a function of arteriolar tone and, to a lesser degree, blood viscosity.

A. Pathogenesis of Enhanced Arteriolar Tone in the Elderly Hypertensive

Potentially reversible as well as irreversible factors are involved in the maintenance of increased arteriolar tone in the elderly hypertensive. The irreversible factors include the structural changes which occur with aging, such as wall thickening and degeneration of elastin, noted earlier. Not all the structural changes accompanying hypertension are irreversible, however, since significant regression in the thickness of the arterial tunica media may take place following prolonged antihypertensive therapy (43). This phenomenon results from changes in vascular smooth muscle cells, identical to the changes in myocardial cells in treated hypertensives who manifest reversal of left ventricular hypertrophy (44). What is not yet evident is whether these arterial changes constitute the primary event leading to the increased vascular resistance or are the result of the hypertension per se. Evidence showing an increase in synthesis and release of growth factors by the arterial wall of the hypertensive animal, together with the fact that the abnormal vasculature persists despite effective antihypertensive treatment, tends to favor the former possibility (45–47). In addition to structural changes, other potentially reversible factors capable of raising the peripheral resistance in the elderly hypertensive include the sodium and water content of arterial walls, neurohumoral factors, and divalent cations.

1. Sodium and Water Content of Arterial Wall

The role played by an increase in vascular smooth muscle content in the pathogenesis of hypertension is still controversial (48). To date there are no data available comparing the sodium content of the arterial wall in elderly normotensive and hypertensive subjects.

2. Neurohumoral Factors

Several circulating vasoactive substances can modify vascular tone. Theoretically, an increase in the activity or sensitivity to a vasoconstrictor, not accompanied by a proportional increase in the activity or sensitivity to a vasodilator, will increase vascular tone and thereby peripheral vascular resistance. A decrease in the activity or sensitivity to a vasodilator without a similar decrease in the activity or sensitivity to a vasoconstrictor will have the same effect.

As discussed in Chapter 1, plasma renin activity (PRA) decreases with age. Moreover, the levels are lower in elderly hypertensives compared to normotensives. On the other hand, plasma aldosterone (PA) is similar in the normotensive and hypertensive elderly, which may be a reflection of an increased sensitivity of the adrenal gland to angiotensin II (AII) in the elderly hypertensive (49). A similar change in sensivity of the vasculature to AII does not seem to play a pathogenetic role in hypertension of the elderly, even though the plasma AII level is lower in the hypertensive compared to the normotensive elderly, since AII receptor density and affinity are the same in both groups (50). The sympathetic nervous system does not appear to be responsible for the increase in peripheral resistance associated with the hypertension of the elderly. Although circulating norepinephrine levels increase with age, there is either no difference between normotensive and hypertensive elderly (51) or the levels are high in normotensives (52,53). It should be emphasized, however, that the net effect of the autonomic nervous system on the vasculature is the result of the interaction between the vasoconstrictive effect of the

α_2 receptor and the vasodilatory effect of the β_2 receptor. Even though catecholamine levels may be lower in the elderly hypertensive, the impaired β_2-adrenergic-mediated vasodilation noted in this group could result in an unopposed effect of the constrictive effect of the α_2 receptor and subsequent increase in total peripheral resistance (54). This impaired β_2-adrenergic response has been attributed to an alteration in the interactions between the G protein and its receptor (55).

Because of its vasoconstrictive property, arginine vasopressin has been implicated in the pathogenesis of hypertension associated with chronic renal insufficiency in humans (56,57). Information is lacking concerning the contribution of vasopressin to hypertension seen in the elderly. Plasma vasopressin levels are similar in normotensive and hypertensive white elderly but significantly higher in hypertensive compared to normotensive black elderly (58). Insulin resistance, as mentioned earlier, increases with age and could potentially play a role in the pathogenesis of hypertension in the elderly by increasing sodium reabsorption and shifting the pressure–natriuresis curve in favor of a higher renal perfusion pressure, by stimulating the sympathetic nervous system and by increasing vascular smooth muscle tone through modification of cation (Mg/Ca) fluxes across cell membranes (23,59,60). Higher plasma insulin levels have been found in elderly hypertensives compared with normotensives (23). In a more recent study, however, the increase in insulin resistance seen with aging was more apparent in those elderly without hypertension. The higher level found in earlier studies could have been due to the concomitant use of various antihypertensive drugs, which can independently interfere with insulin sensitivity (61). It therefore appears that the role of insulin resistance in the pathogenesis of hypertension in the elderly is, if anything, minimal.

The concentration of vasodilator peptides such as vasoactive intestinal peptides (VIPs) and opioid peptides in the hypertensive animal and plasma substance P in human hypertensives may be reduced (62,63). The role played by these substances in the pathogenesis of hypertension remains to be elucidated, however. Although the concentration of kallikreins has been found to be higher in the urine of hypertensive patients compared to normal subjects over the age of 60 (64), a role of the kinins in the pathogenesis of hypertension remains to be elucidated (65). There are data suggesting that some patients with essential hypertension have reduced renal synthesis of prostaglandins (primarily PGE_2) (66). Similar observations have also been made in elderly hypertensives (67). Atrial natriuretic peptide (ANP), although closely linked to blood pressure regulating systems, does not appear to play a role in the pathogenesis of hypertension (68,69).

3. *Divalent Ions*

Both calcium and magnesium have been found to play a role in the pathogenesis of hypertension (70–72). Significant controversy still exists, however, and the issue is complicated by the fact that serum ionized calcium and magnesium levels vary with PRA in essential hypertensives (73,74). The higher the PRA, the lower is the serum magnesium level and the more magnesium loading lowers the blood pressure (75). Compared to normotensive subjects, the serum ionized calcium level is lower in low-renin hypertensives and higher in high-renin patients, suggesting a role for calcium deficit in the former group and calcium excess in the latter (76,77). Since the prevalence of low-renin hypertension is highest in the elderly (42,78), it is quite possible that alterations in calcium metabolism due to a basic defect in the plasma membrane contribute to the hypertension seen in this group (79,80). The hypotensive effect of oral calcium supplementation in the elderly is rather modest, however (81). Furthermore, the antihypertensive property of calcium supplementation might be related to its natriuretic property rather than to a direct effect of this cation on total peripheral resistance (82).

4. *Other Factors*

Endothelium-derived relaxing factor (EDRF) is a substance released by vascular endothelium which mediates relaxation induced by some vasodilators such as acetylcholine, bradykinin, and adenosine 5'-diphosphate (83). It stimulates soluble guanilate cyclase to increase cyclic GMP levels in vascular smooth muscle. GMP then mediates relaxation, probably through its actions on intracellular free calcium (84). As noted earlier, the endothelium-derived vasodilation is blunted in aging. Apart from the loss of the renal response to L-arginine infusion in elderly hypertensive (85), the possibility of an impairment in endothelium-dependant vascular relaxation in this group identical to that seen in younger hypertensives remains to be explored (86). Thus, direct evidence for a pathogenetic role of nitric oxide in elderly hypertensives is lacking.

Endothelin is a potent vasoconstrictor peptide released by endothelial cells in response to various chemical and physical stimuli (87), and binds specifically to human vascular smooth muscle cells (88). The plasma endothelin level does not differ significantly between normotensive and elderly hypertensives (89), but is higher in black compared to white hypertensives (89a). Endothelin I levels are higher in the cerebrospinal fluid of older hypertensives, with the levels correlating significantly with both systolic and diastolic blood pressures (90). Based on the evidence available, it appears that the contribution of endothelin to the pathogenesis of hypertension in the elderly remains to be clarified.

As noted earlier, total peripheral resistance is primarily a function of vascular smooth muscle tone and, to a lesser extent, blood viscosity, The latter has not been studied specifically in the elderly hypertensive, but in hypertensives in their fifth decade an increase in blood viscosity proportional to the severity of the hypertension has been found (91,92). The increase in blood viscosity might be secondary to the hypertension itself, however, since the blood viscosity does decrease in these patients following therapy with prazosin, a vasodilator (93).

The hemodynamics of ISH reflect an exaggeration of the hemodynamic changes which occur with aging. The cardiac index in the elderly with ISH is similar to the cardiac index in the normotensive elderly, whereas the total peripheral resistance is higher (94). The wide pulse pressure is due to a marked decrease in arterial compliance. In general, the greater the arterial stiffness, the higher is the systolic pressure and the lower is the diastolic pressure (8).

Finally, the presence of the angiotensin gene $M^{235} \rightarrow T$ polymorphism (the methionine or threonine at residue 235) has been reported to be a marker in the elderly which may predispose them to both isolated systolic and diastolic hypertension (94a).

V. CLINICAL MANIFESTATIONS AND DIAGNOSIS

As in younger patients, hypertension in the elderly is usually diagnosed during routine physical examination or during evaluation for other, unrelated conditions. Occasionally, patients will present with headache or vertigo or, rarely, with accelerated hypertension manifested by encephalopathy, cardiac, and/or renal failure. The presence of a bruit (particularly in diastole) in the abdomen, flank, or costovertebral angle, suggesting the presence of renovascular disease, should always be looked for on physical examination. Baseline laboratory evaluation of the hypertensive elderly is similar to that of younger patients and includes a CBC, BUN, creatinine, electrolytes, glucose, lipid profile, urinalysis, and electrocardiogram (95). An increase in cardiovascular mortality has been found by some, but not by others, in the elderly hypertensive with microalbuminumuria (30–200 μg/min) (95a,96). A renal sonogram and a 24-hr urine for protein excretion and creatinine clearance are obtained if proteinuria and/or renal insufficiency is present. Patients with any suggestion of heart disease are sent for an echocardiogram in order to rule out the syndrome of hypertensive hypertrophic cardiomyopathy, so that therapy may be tailored adequately (97,98).

Ambulatory blood pressure measurement (ABPM) is a noninvasive way of constantly monitoring blood pressure through the use of a portable automatic device. ABPM in the elderly hypertensive has consistently shown a daytime systolic blood pressure (SBP) on the average 20 mmHg lower than clinic measurements. The difference between diastolic blood pressures (DBP) is smaller or not observed (99–106a). Three ABPM patterns at night can be seen: (a) the SBP either rises or remains unchanged (nondipper); (b) a 10–20% drop in SBP is observed (dipper); (c) the drop in SBP is greater than 20% (extreme dipper). The latter pattern tends to occur with a greater frequency in elderly with ISH (103). In the early morning hours, patients either experience a steep increase in SBP upon waking and rising, or the SBP starts to rise gradually during sleep and reaches its peak upon rising (107).

The evidence that hypertension is a powerful predictor of cardiovascular morbidity and mortality is based mainly on clinic measurements. ABPM adds to the diagnostic precision of clinic blood pressure measurements and should be helpful in the diagnosis of "white coat" hypertension (108,109) and in the evaluation of the severity of the hypertension, since it correlates more closely with indices of end-organ damage. For instance, cardiac and cerebrovascular involvement are more prevalent in nondippers and in those patients with a steep rise in blood pressure when waking and rising (100–103). Silent cebrovascular damage as assessed by MRI has also been found to correlate with nocturnal SBP (103a) and with a higher frequency in extreme dippers (103).

VI. INDICATIONS FOR THERAPY

It is the authors' opinion that some form of therapeutic intervention (nonpharmacological and/or pharmacological) is indicated in every elderly person with a blood pressure greater than 160 SBP or 90 mmHg DBP. This approach is supported by those studies which demonstrate an increase in total mortality as well as in mortality from stroke and cardiovascular disease in the elderly (age 60–79) with elevated blood pressure, whether systolic and/or diastolic (110–117a). Furthermore, the results from several studies with therapeutic interventions recently summarized by Applegate, Thijis et al., and Lever and Ramsey (118–120) (Table 2) have shown that therapy reduces cardiovascular mortality by 10–32% (or 1.4–2.2% of patients each year). The decrease in cardiovascular mortality is due to a significant reduction (9–50%) in cerebrovascular mortality as well as in coronary mortality (9–40%). Noncardiovascular mortality, however, does not appear to be significantly affected. The benefits of therapy have been shown to outweigh the risks (121).

Results from the Systolic Hypertension in the Elderly Program (SHEP) have demonstrated that therapy might prevent cardiovascular complications in 1.1% of patients each year (122). The rate reduction of strokes was 36%. The rate reduction of heart failure among patients with prior myocardial infarction was 80% (122a). Moreover, the SHEP study and preliminary data from SYST-Euro and other studies have shown that these patients tolerate antihypertensive drugs well (122–131). The goal of therapy, as recommended by the Working Group on Hypertension in the Elderly (131) and others (132–134), is to reduce the SBP to the range of 140–160 mmHg and the DBP to below 90 mmHg. Some caution should be exercised, since a higher incidence of myocardial infarction and/or mortality has been observed by some in elderly patients in whom the DBP was decreased below 85 mmHg (115,135–139a). This phenomenon (the J curve) might be related to the presence of widespread atherosclerosis and, more specifically, severe coronary disease (>85% stenosis) in many of these patients (139b). Since coronary flow reserve virtually disappears with this degree of stenosis, a fall in DBP below 85 mmHg would be accompanied by an equivalent fall in coronary flow (140–142).

In the controlled study reported by the European Working Party on High Blood Pressure in the Elderly (EWPHE) (143), an increase in mortality was noted in patients with the lowest blood pressure, whether they were on medicine or on placebo. In both groups, patients with the lowest blood pressures were characterized by lower body weight and hemoglobin levels, suggesting that a deterioration of general health was the cause of their higher mortality rather than the drug-induced drop in blood pressure (144). Furthermore, in the SHEP study a reduction in cardiovascular events in the treated patients was noted despite a fall in DBP from a mean of 77 to 68 mmHG (122). Thus, there is significant controversy with regard to the concept of the J curve in the treatment of hypertension and coronary artery disease (145,146).

Controversy also exists concerning the results of treating either systolic or diastolic hypertension in elderly over 75 years of age. In one study involving both male and female Finnish patients over 85, a significantly higher 5-year survival rate was found in the hypertensive (59%) compared to normotensive (28%) subjects (147). Similar observations have been made by Lauger et al. (148,149) in American men but not in women 75 years and over. They concluded that a 5-mmHg fall in diastolic blood pressure is associated with a poor survival in men, more so if they are on antihypertensive drugs. In the EWPHE study, patients in this older age group did not benefit significantly from therapy, but the number treated was relatively small (150). In a study reported by Heikinheimo et al. (151) in patients aged 84 to 88 years, following the first year of follow-up the lowest mortality rate was found in subjects with a SBP between 140 and 169 mmHg and a DBP between 70 and 99 mmHg. Values outside those ranges, either above or below, were associated with an increase in mortality, particularly of cardiac origin. Guzik et al. (152) found that hypertension (BP >140/90) is a modestly important risk factor in the development of cardiovascular disease in the 75–85 years range. In the SHEP study (122), a statistically significant benefit of treatment was noted in patients 80 years and older (21 events in the active treatment group compared to 38 events in the placebo group).

Based on these data, our approach to therapy in patients over the age of 75 varies according to the functional status of the patient and is similar to that followed by others (153). In those patients who are active and otherwise well, we start with a single drug at a low dose followed by a slow titration process in order to bring the pressure to approximately 160/90 mmHg. The occurrence of any significant side effect is an indication to either stop at the best-tolerated dose (even if the blood pressure goal is not achieved) or discontinue therapy altogether. Frail and severely debilitated elderly with multiple other problems and free from signs of cardiovascular disease (154) are probably better left untreated.

Table 2 Design and Outcome of Randomized Trials of the Treatment of Hypertension in the Elderly

Study	Type	Age	Pressure (mmHg)	Blood pressure medication	Outcome
VA (1970)	Randomized, double blind, placebo controlled	60–69	90–114 (DBP)	HCTZ and reserpine	Decrease (32%) in cardiovascular morbidity, did not reach significance.
HDFP (1979)	Randomized, special care vs. referred care	60–69	90–115 (DBP)	CTLD and reserpine or alpha-methyldopa	Statistically significant, 16.4% reduction in total mortality for special care group.
Austr (1980)	Randomized, double blind, placebo controlled	60–69	95–109 (DBP)	CTZ and various second-step agents	Reduction (39%) in trial end points for the treatment subgroup; did not reach statistical significance.
Kuramoto (1981)	Randomized, double blind, placebo controlled	60–90+	90–110 (DBP) 160–200 (SBP)	TCTZ-alpha-methyldopa hydralazine	Decrease (12%) in cardiovascular complications; did not reach significance.
EWPHE (1985)	Randomized, double blind, placebo controlled	60–97	90–119 (DBP) 160–239 (SBP)	HCTZ-triamterene and alpha-methyldopa	Significant (38%) reduction in cardiac mortality, (32%) reduction in cerebrovascular mortality was not quite significant.
Coope (1986)	Randomized, single blind, no placebo, no controls	60–79	$\geq$ 105 (DBP) $\geq$ 170 (SBP)	Beta-blocker and BNFZD	Significant reduction (30%) in fatal strokes, no effect on myocardial infarction.

STOP (1991)	Randomized, double blind, placebo controlled	70–84+	90–120 (DBP) 170–280 (SBP)	HCTZ-amiloride and/or beta-blocker	Significant reduction (27%) in total mortality Reduction (36%) in cardiovascular, morbidity and mortality. Reduction (24%) in stroke morbidity and mortality.
SHEP (1991)	Randomized, double blind, placebo controlled	60+	<90 (DBP) 160–219 (SBP)	CLTD and/or atenolol	Significant reduction (36%) in stroke reduction and major cardiovascular events.
MRC (1992)	Single blind, randomized, placebo controlled	65–74	<115 (DBP) 160–209 (SBP)	HCTZ-amiloride or atenolol	Significant reduction (25%) in stroke and (17%) in all cardiovascular events.
STONE (1996)	Single blind, placebo controlled	60–79	≥96 (DBP) ≥160 (SBP)	Nifedipine captopril-DHCT	Significant reduction (58%) in stroke and severe arythmia.
Syst-Eur (1997)	Randomized, placebo controlled	60+	160–219 (SBP) <95 (DBP)	Nifedipine with added enalapril and/or hydrochlorothiazide, if necessary	Significant reduction (42%) in stroke and (26%) in cardiac end points (congestive heart failure or myocardial infarction).

ABBREVIATIONS: VA, Veterans Administration Cooperative Study; HDFP, Hypertension Detection and Follow-up Program; Autr, Australian Trial on Mild Hypertension; EWPHE, European Working Party on Hypertension in the Elderly; STOP, Swedish Trial in Old Patients with Hypertension; SHEP, Systolic Hypertension in the Elderly Program; MRC, Medical Research Council trial; STONE, Shanghai trial of nifedipine in the elderly; Syst-Eur, systolic hypertension in Europe; DBP, diastolic blood pressure; SBP, systolic blood pressure; HCTZ, hydrochlorothiazide; CTZ, chlorothiazide; BNFZD, benfluorothiazide; CTLD, chlorthalidone; TCTZ, trichlormethiazide; DHCT, dihydrochlorothiazide.

Sources: Applegate WB. Hypertension in elderly patients. Ann Intern Med 1989; 110:901–915.

Thijis L, et al. A meta analysis of outcome trials in elderly hypertensives. J Hypertens 1992; 10:1103–1109.

Lever AF, et al. Treatment of hypertension in the elderly. J Hypertens 1995; 13:571–579.

Gong L, et al. Shanghai trial of nifedipine in the elderly (STONE). J Hypertens 1996; 14:1237–1245.

Presented at the European Society of Hypertension, June 1997 (Syst-Eur).

A. Pseudo-hypertension

SBP and DBP, as measured by the cuff, are respectively 5 mmHg lower and 5–10 mmHg higher than intraarterial pressures. Pseudo-hypertension is defined as a cuff-to-intraarterial SBP difference greater than 10 mmHg and to a cuff-to-intraarterial DBP difference greater than 15 mmHg (155). Since intraarterial pressure is not measured routinely, pseudo-hypertension can be clinically detected by inflating the blood pressure cuff above the SBP and carefully palpating either the radial or brachial artery (Osler's maneuver). If either of these vessels remains palpable, the test is considered positive for pseudo-hypertension (156). The automatic infrasonic recorder (IR), which detects the subaudible oscillations in the arterial wall under an occluding cuff, might also help in diagnosing pseudo-hypertension in the elderly (157). The incidence of this phenomenon in the elderly hypertensive has been variably reported as 0–5%, a reflection of selection bias (158–163). Pseudo-hypertension is probably not very common in an unselected elderly population (164). Pseudo-hypertension should be ruled out in any treated elderly who experience symptoms suggestive of a low pressure, such as fainting spells, chronic fatigue, etc., at a time when cuff blood pressure readings are still in the hypertensive or even normotensive range.

B. "White Coat" Hypertension

"White coat" hypertension is defined as an elevated blood pressure in the clinic or physician's office but normal at other times (usually at home or by ABPM). Since the clinic SBP readings are higher than the readings with ABPM, as discussed previously, it is not surprising that a significant number of elderly (8%) with ISH will have SBP in the normal range on ABPM (108,108a,110). Studies comparing the long-term effects of pharmacological intervention compared with placebo in these patients are lacking. In a small group of elderly patients with "white coat" hypertension treated with doxazosin, an alpha-blocker, a lower blood pressure was achieved in the clinic without affecting the ambulatory blood pressure (165). Some enrollees in the ongoing Syst-Eur study are undergoing clinic readings as well as ABPM, which may provide additional data related to this problem (104). We usually treat these patients, particularly if other risk factors for cardiovascular diseases such as cigarette smoking, lipid disorders, left ventricular hypertrophy, and/or sedentary lifestyle are present.

VII. THERAPY FOR HYPERTENSION IN THE ELDERLY

Once the decision to treat is made, the following factors should be considered.

1. Postural hypotension. This condition, defined as a greater than 10% drop in supine MAP, is present in 10–20% of elderly hypertensives and is more common in women (166–168a). Several mechanisms have been

proposed and include an age-related impairment in the homeostatic mechanisms of blood pressure regulation and/or blunted sympathetic nerve activity (168). In general, the higher the SBP, the more prevalent is orthostatic hypertension. Attempts should be made to identify these patients prior to initiating therapy, as it will significantly influence which drugs to use (168). Also, a drop in SBP of greater than 20 mmHg is present in 24–36% of elderly patients within 75 min of eating a meal (169–174). In 11% of these patients, the SBP may drop below 100 mmHg (172). In general, greater drops are found in patients on vasodilators and/or other cardiovascular drugs, with some becoming symptomatic (172–174). Those patients who develop orthostatic hypotension have a higher insulin response to a glucose load and a blunted increase in cardiac output when compared with controls. It is postulated that the vasodilatory effect of insulin superimposed on impairment in the sympathetic nervous system response to insulin are responsible for this phenomenon (175).

2. Drug interactions. Up to 40% of elderly hypertensives have a concomitant medical problem which requires some form of therapy. In one study of 102 elderly hypertensives, the average number of medications per patient was 3.6 (176). The possibility of drug–drug interaction is significant in these patients. Among the most common offenders are the nonsteroidal antiinflammatory drugs (NSAIDs) (176a) (with the exception, perhaps, of sulindac), which could interfere with the antihypertensive action of beta-blockers, the angiotensin-converting enzyme inhibitors (ACEIs), and diuretics (177–182). Tricyclic antidepression agents will interfere with the antihypertensive effect of reserpine and clonidine. ACEIs may lead to dangerous hyperkalemia in a patient on supplemental potassium (particularly if the patient is also taking an NSAID).
3. Cost. Most elderly patients live on rather limited budgets and often do not have adequate insurance to cover the cost of drugs. The thiazide diuretics are among the cheapest drugs available, followed by central adrenergic agonists and vasodilators. The beta-blockers are intermediate in price and the alpha-adrenergic blockers, calcium channel blockers, and ACEIs are the most expensive (118,183,184).

A. Nonpharmacological Therapy

1. Diet

We usually recommend mild salt restriction (2–3 g Na diet) to our elderly patients with hypertension, based on the results of the recent meta-analysis of previously published trials (185). Even though the decreases in blood pressure after salt restriction were larger in older hypertensive individuals, the response varies from patient to patient (186–190). Fish oil (8 g/day) has been found to have an additive hypotensive effect to a low-sodium diet in a small group of elderly subjects (191). Supplemental potassium (60–65 mEq/day) has been associated with a reduction in both clinic and ABPM, but caution should be exercised in the elderly with superimposed renal insufficiency or taking an ACEI and/or an NSAID. Also, the benefits obtained from potassium supplementation are minimal (192), particularly in a patient on a low-sodium diet (193–197). Calcium supplementation (1 g elemental Ca) has been shown to result in a modest decrease in MAP in a small number of elderly hypertensives (198,199). Obese patients are encouraged to lose weight, since a positive correlation has been found between blood pressure and weight in all age groups (5,200,201), and weight reduction in the obese leads to a fall in blood pressure (202,203). When feasible, the patient should be referred for nutritional counseling, since merely instructing the patient to lose weight is not sufficient in most instances (204). Finally, alcohol consumption should be curtailed in patients who take more than a 1 oz of ethanol per day (2 drinks of spirits or its equivalent in wine or beer) (205–208).

2. *Exercise*

Exercise in the elderly hypertensive is as well tolerated as in the elderly normotensive (209). Furthermore, low-intensity exercise, such as walking for 1 hr thrice weekly, has been shown to be associated with a decrease in both systolic and diastolic pressure in the elderly (210). The hypotensive effects of exercise are probably multifactorial and include changes in cardiac output, total peripheral vascular resistance, and, possibly, blood viscosity (211).

B. Drug Therapy

The drugs that control blood pressure in elderly patients are the same as those used in the treatment of hypertension in other age groups. It should be kept in mind, however, that pharmacokinetics and pharmacodynamics change with age, and that other co-morbid states are frequently present in the elderly which require a more considered approach than is used in the usual stepped-care regimens. Dose titration should be slower than in younger patients (211a), and attention should be paid to factors which could improve compliance. In one recent study (211b), good compliance was associated with the use of calcium channel blockers and angiotensin-converting enzyme inhibitors. The presence of co-morbid cardiac disease, multiple drug use, and multiple physician visits were generally associated with poor compliance.

1. *Diuretics*

The thiazide diuretics and their equivalent are both safe and effective for treating either isolated systolic or systolic and diastolic hypertension in the elderly (150,212–215a). It is recommended that therapy be started at the lowest dose, with graded increases (Table 3). The use of more than 25 mg/day of hydrochlorothiazide or its equivalent is probably not warranted, as side effects increase without a significant further drop in blood pressure (216–219). Initiation of thiazide therapy is associated with a decrease in intravascular volume and an upward shift in the pressure–natriuresis relationship which are, in part, responsible for the antihypertensive effect (220,221). The decrease in blood pressure, however, is maintained primarily through a decrease in total peripheral vascular resistance, probably by activating vasodepressor substances such as prostacyclin (222,223). Thiazides should not be used in the presence of serum creatinine of 2.5 mg/dl or greater. One exception, however, is metolazone, which can be added to a loop diuretic (furosemide, bumetanide, or torsemide) to manage elderly hypertensives with chronic renal insufficiency. The most common side effects associated with the thiazides in the elderly are hypokalemia, cardiac arrhythmias, hyponatremia (mainly in females), and hypomagnesemia (224). When a loop diuretic is used, careful attention should be paid to volume status in order to prevent excessive volume contraction. Indapamide is an indolines diuretic which has been used successfully in treating the elderly. As with the thiazides, normotension is maintained through its effect on total peripheral resistance (225,226).

2. *Alpha$_2$-Adrenergic Receptor Agonists*

The α_2-adrenergic receptor agonists include methyldopa, clonidine, guanadrel sulfate, guanabenz acetate, and guanfacine HCl. They lower blood pressure through either a central or peripheral stimulation of the α_2-adrenergic receptor. As a consequence, norepinephrine release is decreased and sympathetic tone reduced (227). Methyldopa can be used in the elderly with mild to moderate hypertension. We usually start with a dose of 125 mg twice a day with slow upright titration, since the drug can decrease cardiac output in the elderly (228) and induce severe orthostatic hypotension, especially when used in combination with a diuretic (229,230). Other common side effects include sleep disturbances and drowsiness (231). The starting dose for clonidine is 0.05 mg every 12 hr, with slow titration up to 0.6 mg daily (232). Clonidine has also been used successfully in combination with a thiazide diuretic (233). Common side effects are dryness of the mouth and orthostasis. Rebound (overshoot) hypertension and the clonidine withdrawal syndrome (headache, nausea, palpitations, tremor) have been reported within 12 to 48 hr after abrupt discontinuation of the drug. This problem, although uncommon, is important for the forgetful elderly patient. Therefore, a prudent approach is not to use the drug in these patients (234). A transdermal patch of the drug is available as TTS-1, TTS-2, TTS-3 and programmed to deliver 0.1 mg, 0.2 mg, and 0.3 mg, respectively, of clonidine per day for 7 days. This preparation offers certain advantages for the elderly, including a weekly interval between doses, which facilitates compliance. Blood concentrations are stable, and the incidence of side effects is significantly reduced (235,236). The drug is, in our experience,

Table 3 Drugs Used in the Elderly Hypertensive Patient

Class and drug	Starting dosage	Maintenance dosage	Frequency	Reference
Diuretics				
Hydrochlorothiazide (Hydrodiuril, Esidrix)	25 mg	25–50 mg	Once a day	(150,212–219,263)
Methylclothiazide (Enduron)	2.5 mg	2.5–5.0 mg	Once a day	
Chlorthalidone (Hygroton)	12.5 mg	12.5–25 mg	Once a day	
Metolazone (Zaroxolyn, Diulo)	1.25 mg	1.25–10 mg	Once a day	
Indapamide (Lozol)	2.5 mg	2.5 mg	Once a day	(225,226)
Furosemide (Lasix)	40 mg	40–240 mg	Once a day	
Bumetanide (Bumex)	1 mg	1–6 mg	Once a day	
Torsemide (Demadex)	5 mg	5–200 mg	Once a day	
α_2-Adrenergic agonists				
Methyldopa (Aldomet)	250 mg	250–1000 mg	Once a day	(228–231)
Clonidine (Catapres)	0.1 mg	0.1–0.3 mg	Q 8–12 hr	(232,233)
Clonidine patch (Clonidine TTS)	TTS-1	TTS-1–3	Weekly	(235,236)
Guanadrel Sulfate (Hylorel)	5 mg	5–30 mg	Once a day	(237)
Guanabenz Acetate (Wytensin)	4 mg	4–32 mg	Once a day	
Guanfacine Hcl (Tenex)	0.5 mg	0.5–1 mg	Once a day	
α_1-Adrenergic antagonists				
Doxazosin (Cardura)	1 mg	1–16 mg	Once a day	(241)
Prazosin (Minipress)	2 mg	2–20 mg	Q 8–12 hr	(238,239)
Terazosin (Hytrin)	1 mg	1–40 mg	Once a day	(242)
Beta-Adrenergic antagonists				
Propanolol (Inderal)	20 mg	20–100 mg	Q 8–12 hr	
Propanolol LA (Inderal LA)	40 mg	40–400 mg	Once a day	(243)
Timolol (Blocadren)	10 mg	10–60 mg	Q 12 hr	(261)
Nadolol (Corgard)	10 mg	10–120 mg	Once a day	(262)
Metoprolol (Lopressor)	25 mg	25–300 mg	Once a day	(263,264,415)
Metoprolol extended release (Toprol)	50 mg	50–400 mg	Once a day	
Atenolol (Tenormin)	25 mg	25–100 mg	Once a day	(262,265)
Pindolol (Visken)	5 mg	5–20 mg	Q 12 hr	(266,267)
Acebutolol (Sectral)	200 mg	200–800 mg	Once a day	
Labetalol (Normodyne, Trandate)	100 mg	100–400 mg	Q 12 hr	(256,257,268,269)
Carteolol (Cartrol)	2.5 mg	2.5–10 mg	Once a day	
Betaxolol (Kerlone)	10 mg	10–20 mg	Once a day	

Penbutolol (Levatol)	10 mg	10–20 mg	Once a day	
Bisoprolol (Zebeta)	2.5 mg	2.5–20 mg	Once a day	
Carvedilol (Coreg)	12.5 mg	12.5–50 mg	Once a day	
Vasodilators				
Hydralazine (Apresoline)	25 mg	25–50 mg	Q 6 hr	
Minoxidil (Loniten)	2.5 mg	2.5–40 mg	Once a day	(208)
Angiotensin II-converting enzyme inhibitors				
Captopril (Capoten)	12.5 mg	12.5–50 mg	Q 8–12 hr	(215–220)
Enalapril (Vasotec)	2.5 mg	2.5–20 mg	Q 12 hr	(178,221,222)
Lisinopril (Zestril, Prinivil)	20 mg	20–40 mg	Once a day	(223,224)
Benazepril (Lotensin)	10 mg	10–40 mg	Q 12–24 hr	
Quinapril (Accupril)	10 mg	10–80 mg	Q 12–24 hr	
Ramipril (Altace)	2.5 mg	2.5–20 mg	Q 12–24 hr	
Fosinopril (Monopril)	10 mg	10–40 mg	Once a day	
Moexipril (Univasc)	7.5 mg	7.5–30 mg	Q 12–24 hr	
Trandolapril (Mavik)	1 mg	1–8 mg	Q 12–24 hr	
Calcium channel antagonists				
Dihydropyridines				
Nifedipine (Procardia, Adalat)	30 mg	30–80 mg		(302,303)
Amlodipine (Norvasc)	5 mg	5–10 mg	Once a day	(311,315)
Nicardipine (Cardene SR)	10 mg	10–30 mg	Q 12 hr	(307–310)
Isradipine (Dyna Circ)	1.25 mg	1.25–10 mg	Q 12 hr	(290,313,314)
Nisoldipine (Sular)	10 mg	10–40 mg	Once a day	
Felodipine (Plendil)	5 mg	5–20 mg	Once a day	(300,312)
Nondihydropyridines: phenylakylamines				
Verapamil (Calan SR, Covera-HS, Verelan, Isoptin SR)	120 mg	160–360 mg	Q 12–24 hr	(303–305)
Nondihydropyridines: benzothiazepines				
Diltiazem (Cardizem CD, Cardizem SR, Dilacor XR, Tiazac)	60 mg	60–120 mg	Once a day	(306)
Others				
Bepridil (Vascor)	200 mg	200–400 mg	Once a day	
Mibefradil (Posicor)	50 mg	50–100 mg	Once a day	
Angiotensin II-receptor antagonists				
Losartan (Cozar)	25 mg	25–100 mg	Once a day	(292)
Valsartan (Diovan)	80 mg	80–320 mg	Once a day	(416)
Irbesartan (Avapro)	75 mg	75–300 mg	Once a day	

efficient in elderly with mild hypertension; however, in a significant number of our patients we had to discontinue it because of the development of a bothersome contact dermatitis. The other α_2-agonists, guanadrel sulfate, guanabenz acetate, and guanfacine HCl, are long acting and can be used once a day in elderly with mild to moderate hypertension (237). Their side effects are identical to those of clonidine.

3. *Alpha$_1$-Adrenergic Receptor Antagonists*

Doxazoxin, prazosin, and terazosin lower blood pressure by blocking the vasoconstrictive effects of the α_1-receptor, thereby decreasing total peripheral resistance. These drugs are, in general, well tolerated by elderly with mild hypertension. Dizziness is the most common side effect (238,239). It is recommended that the first dose, usually 1 mg, be given prior to bedtime in order to minimize the risk of severe postural hypotension, which occurs occasionally (so-called first-dose response). Uptitration should be undertaken slowly, to a maximum of 10 mg twice a day for prazosin, 16 mg daily for doxazosin, and 40 mg per day for terazosin. Those drugs are advantageous to the hypertensive elderly male with symptomatic prostatic hypertrophy, as they can decrease the frequency of urination in these patients (240–242). They may be particularly useful in patients who refuse prostatic surgery or who are considered poor surgical risks.

4. *Beta-Adrenergic Receptor Antagonists*

Several beta-antagonists are available in the United States, including nonselective β_1- and β_2-antagonists (propanolol, timolol, nadolol, penbutolol); selective β_1-antagonists (metoprolol, atenolol, betaxolol, bisoprolol); nonselective β_1- and β_2- and a selective alpha$_1$ α_1-adrenergic antagonist (labetolol, carvedilol); beta-blockers with intrinsic sympathomimetic activity (pindolol, acebutolol, carteolol). Beta-blockers are well tolerated by the elderly hypertensive, with an incidence of side effects similar to younger patients (243–245). Mental performance does not appear to be adversely affected (246–248).

The antihypertensive action of the beta-adrenergic antagonists depends on their ability to attenuate the effects of catecholamines at beta-adrenoreceptors localized in the heart, the brain, and presynaptic nerve endings of the heart and blood vessels (249). The net effect is diminished central sympathetic discharge and peripheral norepinephrine release. Acutely, the cardiac output decreases and the total peripheral vascular resistance increases or remains unchanged. With prolonged therapy, cardiac output returns toward the pretreatment level and total peripheral resistance decreases (250–252). The effect of the drug on the vasculature may be secondary to its ability to antagonize AII enhancement of sympathetic nerve stimulation by increasing prostaglandin levels in vascular tissue (253,254). The choice of beta-blockers should be based on the physician's familiarity with the drug, patient compliance, and co-morbid problems.

In general, the antihypertensive efficacy and side effects profile are the same among the various drug groups (255). They can be used alone or in combination with a diuretic in the elderly with diastolic hypertension as well as ISH (122,256,257). Kirkendall (258) and Lessem et al. (259) have discussed the theoretic advantages of using a beta-blocker with intrinsic sympathomimetic activity or with an α_1-adrenergic antagonist in the elderly, related to the lesser depression of cardiac function with these agents. Contraindications to the use of these drugs in the older hypertensives are similar to those for younger patients and include chronic obstructive disease, most patients with congestive heart failure, heart block, and peripheral vascular disease (260). The starting and maintenance doses for the various beta-blockers are outlined in Table 3.

5. *Vasodilators*

Hydralazine and minoxidil act directly on the vascular smooth muscle to lower total peripheral resistance through changes in potassium channels (270). Although these drugs are well tolerated in the elderly, they usually cannot be used as monotherapy because they cause tachycardia and salt retention. Minoxidil is usually reserved for the treatment of severe hypertension and requires the addition of a beta-blocker and a diuretic to block the reflex tachycardia and salt retention (271). Patients in whom a beta-blocker is contraindicated should receive clonidine to correct the tachycardia (272). Minoxidil can also be associated with hypertrichosis, a complication that is poorly tolerated by females. This problem usually remits within 2–3 weeks after the drug has been discontinued, but occasionally the hypertrichosis can persist for months. The starting and maintenance doses for these drugs are outlined in Table 3.

6. *Angiotensin II-Converting Enzyme Inhibitors*

ACEIs exert their antihypertensive effect by lowering total peripheral resistance. They do not have any effect on cardiac output (273). In addition to reducing angiotensin II activity, the ACEIs stimulate prostaglandin synthesis and potentiate the activity of bradykinin resulting from kinase inhibition (274). The use of a bradykinin inhibitor, aprotinin, or a prostaglandin inhibitor, indomethacin, can blunt the antihypertensive effects of ACEIs (275). These agents are usually well tolerated by the elderly; however, first-dose hypotension has been reported, accompanied by reversible renal, cardiac, or cerebral ischemia (276,277). Patients at risk for this effect are those taking diuretics as well as those who are hypovolemic, hyponatremic, or in congestive heart failure. Treatment should be initiated at a low dose and the patient monitored carefully. Acute renal failure can occur in patients with bilateral renal artery stenosis or renal artery stenosis to a solitary kidney (see Chapter 10). Since these drugs can induce hyperkalemia (particularly in patients with renal insufficiency), serum potassium should be measured on a regular basis. Other, less common side effects include skin rash, neutropenia, chronic cough with or without wheezing (more common in females), and angioedema (273). Captopril, as well as other agents (see Table 3), has been used successfully in elderly with mild to moderate hypertension, either as monotherapy or together with a diuretic (278–289). There is no evidence to suggest any difference in therapeutic efficacy of one agent over the other. These agents are also effective in treating elderly with ISH (290–291a). Starting and maintenance doses for the various agents are summarized in Table 3.

7. *Angiotensin II Receptor Antagonists*

Losartan, valsartan, and irbesartan are nonpeptide AII receptor antagonists that are highly selective and specific for the AT_1 receptor subtype. Since they block the vasoconstrictive effect of AII on the vasculature, their antihypertensive effect results from a decrease in total peripheral resistance. In contrast to ACEIs, these drugs do not interfere with bradykinin metabolism, therefore offering the potential advantage of a decreased incidence of the side effects associated with ACEIs. Dizziness is the most commonly reported side effect. The drug can be used alone or in combination with a diuretic (292). Their efficacy in patients with ISH remains to be determined.

8. *Calcium Channel Blockers*

Calcium channel blockers (CCBs) are very efficient in lowering blood pressure in the elderly (293), with treatment failure rates lower than with atenolol and enalapril (294). A positive correlation has been found between age and the magnitude of the arterial pressure reduction by CCBs (295) that might, in part, be due to the lower PRA seen with aging. Indeed, the blood pressure-lowering effect of these drugs is inversely related to pretreatment PRA (296). They lower total peripheral vascular resistance by interfering with calcium influx, which is mediated by binding of the neurotransmitter, norepinephrine, to its receptor on the vascular smooth muscle (297). Despite their similar effects on peripheral vascular resistance, these drugs have differing effects on cardiac function. They can all affect inotrophy and chronotrophy, with verapamil having the most negative effects, followed by diltiazem, and the dihydropyridine group having the least effect (293). Mibefradil, a member of a new class of selective T-type calcium channel blocker, decreases heart rate but does not appear to cause a negative inotropic effect (297a). Those differences should be kept in mind when considering CCBs in patients with heart failure and/or atrioventricular conduction defects. The recommended doses in the elderly are described in Table 3. The most common side effect in the elderly is constipation, which at times can be quite troublesome. Headaches and pedal edema are not as common (298). CCBs are effective for ISH, as well as for systolic/diastolic hypertension in the elderly (290). There is a possibility that CCBs provide additional cardiovascular protection independent of their BP control in the elderly (299,300), keeping in mind that short-acting CCBs, such as nifedipine, particularly at high doses, have been associated with an increased risk of myocardial infarction (300a,300b). It is hoped that some answer will be provided by the ongoing Shell study (301). Finally, an increased risk of cancer has been found in elderly on long-term CCBs (301a). As noted by these authors, the evidence provided "is not sufficient to recommend withdrawal of treatment from current users." Finally, in a recent meta-analysis of the currently available data, Stason et al. concluded that long-acting nifedipine was a safe drug in patients with hypertension (301b).

9. Antihypertensive Drugs and Lipids

Recently there has been a great deal of interest in the effects of various antihypertensive drugs on lipid metabolism. The subject has been reviewed extensively (316–320). To summarize, thiazide diuretics can increase triglycerides, total cholesterol, VLDL and LDL, at least short term and, possibly, long term (2 years or longer); HDL, however, is not changed. These effects are greater in blacks. In the elderly these alterations appear to be dose dependent, since significant hyperlipidemia did not develop at the dose used (25–50 mg/day of chlorthalidone) in the EWPHE study (150). Similar observations have also been made by others (321). The effects of beta-blockers on plasma lipids depend on the agent used. Nonselective and selective $beta_1$-antagonists increase triglycerides, total cholesterol, and LDL cholesterol, while decreasing HDL (5–19%). Pindolol decreases LDL while increasing HDL, whereas labetolol, atenolol, and carvedilol do not affect lipid levels at all (322,322a). The α_1-adrenoreceptor antagonists decrease triglycerides and total cholesterol in diabetics. ACEIs lower triglycerides and total cholesterol in diabetics. CCBs do not alter plasma lipids, apart from nifedipine, which increases HDL cholesterol. A prudent approach is to follow lipid levels in every patient treated with any of the agents known to affect lipid levels adversely, or to avoid these agents altogether in patients with significant elevations of total and LDL cholesterol (323).

10. Effect of Antihypertensive Drugs on Left Ventricular Hypertrophy

Left ventricular hypertrophy (LVH) is commonly found in the elderly at the time of initial diagnosis of hypertension: 13–29% by EKG and 55–83% by echocardiogram (324–327). Twenty-six percent of elderly patients with ISH have LVH on echocardiogram (327a). In one recent study, echocardiographic abnormalities were compared among normotensive elderly (NT), those with diastolic hypertension (DH), and those with ISH (327b). The findings were divided into concentric remodeling, concentric and eccentric left ventricular hypertrophy (LVH). Concentric remodeling was present in 56% of patients with DH, 43% of those with ISH, and 12% of those with NT. Concentric LVH was found in 7% with DH, 5% with ISH, and in none with NT. Eccentric LVH occurred in 2% of DH patients, 4% of ISH, and 2% of NT.

Over the past few years LVH has been identified as not being entirely pressure dependent and a major risk factor for sudden death, myocardial infarction, and congestive heart failure (327–330). Physical examination and the EKG, the two most commonly used means of detecting LVH, are relatively insensitive. The echocardiogram is more sensitive but relatively expensive (331). In general, its routine use is not warranted in elderly hypertensive for evaluating the presence of LVH when the EKG is normal, but should be obtained when this information is necessary for appropriate therapy, particularly if the diagnosis of hypertensive hypertrophic cardiomyopathy is being considered (97,98). Furthermore, the results of an ongoing prospective study carried out to determine whether reducing or reversing LVH in the elderly will improve its inherent ominous prognosis are not yet available (327). Finally, reduction of LVH parallels the reduction in arterial blood pressure with all classes of drugs discussed in Table 3, with the exception of vasodilators. The beta-blockers, CCBs, and ACEIs reduce left ventricular mass by reducing wall hypertrophy, whereas the diuretics act through a reduction in left ventricular diameter (332–333a). The effect on the left ventricular mass is more pronounced with ACEIs; whether these agents will prove to be superior to the others in reducing the risks associated with LVH remain to be determined (333).

C. Antihypertensive Therapy and Quality of Life

As discussed earlier, the treatment of hypertension in the elderly is effective in reducing cardiovascular mortality. However, a significant number of hypertensive elderly have age-related decreases in functional capacity as well as various chronic medical problems. Therefore, the clinician should direct his or her attention to the possibility that antihypertensive treatment per se might worsen the quality of life of their patients, keeping in mind that hypertension itself is generally symptomless. This issue has been addressed recently by several authors looking at the effects of various antihypertensive drugs (diuretics, beta-blockers, CCBs, and ACEIs) on the well-being of elderly patients, whether measured by cognitive functioning, physical or emotional well-being, or social terms. The overall conclusion is that elderly patients taking these antihypertensive drugs maintain cognitive function and quality of life (334–340a). In some patients, long term adequate blood pressure control might even reverse cognitive impairment associated with uncontrolled hypertension as long as the systolic blood pressure does not fall below 135 mmHg (341,341a).

D. Hypertensive Emergencies and Urgencies in the Elderly

Hypertensive emergencies refer to patients with a markedly elevated blood pressure (DBP usually ≥130 mmHg) associated with concomitant acute end-organ involvement such as grade IV Keith-Wagoner-Barker retinopathy, encephalopathy, left ventricular failure, acute renal failure, or dissecting aortic aneurysm. The blood pressure in these patients has to be lowered immediately. Patients presenting with similarly high blood pressures but without evidence of acute end organ damage are referred to as hypertensive urgencies, and require agressive blood pressure reduction but not by the use of intravenous drugs (342).

In 315 patients with hypertensive emergencies reported by Lip et al. (343), 38 (12%) were over the age of 65 (343a). In a more recent report from Italy (344), in 68% of patients with hypertensive emergencies the clinical manifestations were usually those of the target organ(s) involved. The CNS is the organ that is most commonly involved, with patients presenting with confusion and agitation. The presence of coma or focal neurological signs are suggestive of an intracerebral bleed. Pulmonary congestion or edema are the most common cardiac presentations, usually associated with LVH and occasionally, evidence of acute myocardial infarction. Patients with acute renal failure may be asymptomatic, with the diagnosis made only after blood chemistries become available. The urine may have red cells and proteinuria, but these are not invariably present. The pathological lesion characteristic of malignant hypertension is that of fibrinoid necrosis of the arteriolar wall with subsequent endothelial damage. In the kidneys, the glomeruli are relatively spared, apart from some tuft collapse or wrinkling of the glomerular basement membrane (345).

For patients with a hypertensive emergency, we usually initiate therapy with sodium nitroprusside infused at the rate of 0.5 mg/kg/min and titrate up to 10 mg/kg/min, as necessary. The mean dose required to control blood pressure (vide infra) is approximately 1 mg/kg/min. Labetolol, administered as a bolus of 20, 40, or 80 mg or as a continuous infusion of 1–3 mg/min, has been used successfully in the elderly (346). The blood pressure-lowering effect of this agent is not accompanied by reflex tachycardia, making it the drug of choice in the management of elderly with a dissecting aneurysm. Parenteral nicardipine can also be used with a starting dose of 5 mg/hr. The infusion rate may be increased by 2.5 mg/hr every 5 min up to a maximum of 15 mg/hr. Once the goal BP is achieved, the infusion rate is decreased to 3 mg/hr.

Other parenteral drugs are available and include diazoxide, enalaprilat, trimethaphan camsylate, and phentolamine. Diazoxide is given as a bolus of 50–100 mg, and repeated every 10–15 min until a maximum of 300 mg is administered. Enalaprilat is also administered as a bolus of 1.25 mg, which can be repeated every 6 hr. Trimethaphan camsylate is used as a continuous infusion of 1 mg/min and phentolamine at 0.1–0.5 mg/min. This latter drug is reserved for patients with pheochromocytoma. We generally try to avoid diazoxide in patients with heart failure and dissecting aneurysm, since tachycardia and salt retention are common side effects (347). Whenever possible, oral therapy should be started concomitant with parenteral therapy, preferably with short-acting agents to facilitate rapid changes.

It is not presently clear what is a safe target blood pressure in elderly with a hypertensive emergency. We aim for a MAP of 120 mmHg (approximately

160/100 mmHg), based on evidence recently reviewed by Ledingham (348). The mortality rate in patients who have experienced a hypertensive emergency is increased—as high as 45% in one study in which patients were followed for an average of 3 years (343a). The cause of death is usually renal failure, stroke, or myocardial infarction.

Once the blood pressure is brought under control, the prognosis for reversal of target-organ dysfunction is usually good. We routinely evaluate elderly patients with a hypertensive emergency for the presence of renovascular disease. The yield in our experience has been over 70%. Three of the 7 patients reported by Given et al. (349), and 1 of the 3 reported by Cressman et al. (346) had renovascular disease, a significantly higher percentage than is found in the general hypertensive population.

The goal in lowering the blood pressure in patients with a hypertensive urgency is the same as outlined above. Hypertensive urgencies are encountered more frequently in a geriatric practice than hypertensive emergencies (344). The majority of our patients have had severe hypertension in the pre- or postoperative period. In these patients, unless absolutely contraindicated (in which case parenteral therapy should be used), the oral route is the preferred method of controlling the blood pressure. Clonidine is the most commonly used drug (350). The starting dose is 0.1 or 0.2 mg, followed by 0.1 mg every hour, with a maximum dose of 0.7 mg (351,352). Short-acting nifedipine has been used extensively in the past (353–358), but is associated with serious adverse effects. Recent recommendation is for the drug not to be used in this clinical setting (358a). Other regimens have been recommended, including captopril, 25–50 mg every 4–6 hr (359), labetolol, 200–400 mg every 6–12 hr (360), a combination of minoxidil, 2.5–10 mg every 4–6 hr, with a beta-blocker and a diuretic (361). In contrast to patients with a hypertensive emergency, the overwhelming majority of elderly with hypertensive urgencies have essential hypertension, so a routine search for renovascular disease is not warranted.

VIII. SECONDARY HYPERTENSION

Renovascular hypertension and hypertension of renal insufficiency are the two most common forms of secondary hypertension in the elderly and are dealt with separate chapters. The other forms of secondary hypertension seen in the elderly include pheochromocytoma, primary hyperaldosteronism, and other adrenocortical diseases.

A. Pheochromocytoma

Pheochromocytoma is seen in 0.2–0.7% of patients with hypertension (362). Approximately 22% of reported patients were over the age of 60 (363–370). These tumors are located intraadrenally in 75% of cases and extraadrenally in the remainder. Common extraadrenal sites include abdominal, peripheral nerves, intrathoracic, and intravesical. In addition to hypertension, which is present in 92% of elderly patients with pheochromocytoma (sustained in 50% and paroxysmal in 42%), the patients may complain of headaches, diaphoresis, palpitations, and various gastrointestinal symptoms (367,369,371). Orthostatic hypotension is seen occasionally, and hyperglycemia is observed quite frequently. Because of the nonspecific nature of these findings, the diagnosis is often made only at autopsy (31% of the time) (366). It is not clear whether this number is applicable to the elderly. Hypercalcemia or evidence of pituitary dysfunction, suggestive of multiple endocrine neoplasia, are rare in the elderly. The presence of neurofibromatosis and hypertension should raise the suspicion of this entity.

The hypertension seen in pheochromocytoma, as in essential hypertension, is associated with an increase in total peripheral resistance. Since no strong correlation exists between blood pressure and the level of catecholamines in patients with pheochromocytoma, other modulating factors are probably at work (372,373). The state of the patient's circulating blood volume, which may be reduced because of the catecholamine-induced venoconstriction, is probably important (374). A generalized increase in sympathetic nervous system activity is also present, since clonidine, an inhibitor of central sympathetic outflow as well as presynaptic receptors, decreases blood pressure in patients with pheochromocytoma without changing plasma catecholamines (375). Vasodilators (dopamine, prostaglandins) secreted by the tumor may also modulate the blood pressure, since a negative correlation has been found between the ratio of dopamine to norepinephrine and blood pressure, suggesting that the blood pressure is determined by a balance of vasoconstrictor and vasodilator substances (376). Finally, the high level of circulating catecholamines is likely to be associated with a down-regulation of the vascular smooth muscle cell receptors, thereby decreasing their sensitivity to these agents (377). Furthermore, aging itself has been shown to induce a state of relative insensitivity to catecholamines (378).

The laboratory investigation of pheochromocytoma usually starts with a 24-hr urinary collection for metanephrine levels. The upper limit of normal in our elderly patients is similar to that reported in the essential hypertensive population at large, 1.8 mg/24 hr. This test is quite reliable (379), with the major drawback being the 24-hr urine collection, which may not be complete (particularly in the elderly), leading to errors. In these patients, plasma catecholamines should be determined. The patient should be in a fasting state and have a large-bore needle inserted into a vein at least 30 min prior to the test, with the patient kept supine in a quiet room. The plasma norepinephrine (NE) level for both normotensive and essential hypertensive elderly is less than 700 pg/ml, and plasma epinephrine (E) is less than 150 pg/ml (14,51,380). Values for plasma NE or E in our elderly patients with proven pheochromocytomas have been greater than 2000 pg/ml. Patients with values less than 2000 pg/ml but higher than normal with a high clinical suspicion for pheochromocytoma should be considered for the clonidine-suppression test. This consists of measuring NE and E prior to and 2–3 hr after the oral administration of 0.3 mg of clonidine. A fall in NE and E to a level below 500 pg/ml is evidence against the presence of a pheochromocytoma (379). Recently, the determination of plasma metanephrines has been found to be the most accurate of the tests for diagnosing pheochromocytoma. One major drawback, however, is its limited availability (381).

Once the diagnosis of a pheochromocytoma has been confirmed biochemically, an abdominal CT scan should be obtained. With tumors larger than 1.0 cm, this test has a localizing precision of 96% (382,383). Nuclear magnetic resonance imaging (MRI) is no more accurate or sensitive, but is much more expensive (384). Its advantage consists of the fact that neither contrast media nor ionizing radiation is involved. Patients with clinical and biochemical evidence of a pheochromocytoma and a negative CT scan or MRI should be referred for radioisotope imaging, using 131_I-metaiodobenzyl-guanidine (mIBG), which is a guanethidine analog possessing an affinity for chromaffin tissue. It is actively concentrated in pheochromocytoma cells, providing a functional means of tumor localization. Images are recorded 24, 48, and 72 hr after intravenous injection of 0.5–1.0 mCi. This test has a diagnostic sensitivity of about 85% and specificity of about 98% (385,386). Other diagnostic tests, such as measurement of platelet catecholamines, arteriography, and catecholamine venous sampling, can be tried. Their usefulness, however, is limited.

The management of pheochromocytoma in the elderly is surgical. One or two weeks prior to surgery, alpha-adrenergic blockade should be initiated to reduce operative morbidity and mortality (387). Phenoxybenzamine blocks both postsynaptic α_1- and presynaptic α_1- and α_2-receptors. The starting dose is 10 mg every 12 hr, which can be slowly increased every 48–72 hr until the blood pressure is controlled. The average daily dose varies from 40 to 100 mg in the elderly. Orthostatic hypotension is the most common side effect. Because the drug increases the rate as well as the contractile force of the heart, angina may be precipitated in patients with marginal coronary perfusion, a common finding in the elderly (369). In these patients, careful addition of a beta-blocker to control heart rate should be considered, but only after the pressor effect of the phenoxybenzamine has been established. Prazosin, a specific postsynaptic alpha$_1$-blocker, is an alternative to phenoxybenzamine. One major advantage is the lower incidence of tachycardia with this agent. The starting dose is 1 mg every 8 hr. The average daily dose varies between 8 and 12 mg. Labetolol, both alpha- and beta-blockers, CCBs, (388,389), and adenosine (100–500 ug/kg), an antagonist of the cardiovascular effects of catecholamines (390), have been advocated as alternatives to phenoxybenzamine and prazosin. Experience with these drugs in the elderly is rather limited at the present time.

Despite a higher incidence of symptomatic heart disease in older compared to younger patients, the perioperative mortality is similarly low, approximately 1%

(369,371). The surgical excision is curative in 65–70% of patients. In the remaining, hypertension persists despite a return of plasma catecholamines to normal. The frequency of neurological and/or cardiac disability in these patients has been high (369). Persistent elevation of catecholamines despite excisional surgery suggests either multiple primary lesions or metastases from a malignant pheochromocytoma. Clues to malignancy include large tumors, extensive areas of necrosis, and a predominance of small cells (391). The correct approach for these patients is a whole-body mIBG scan. Patients with metastatic disease should be referred to an oncologist for appropriate management (388). Elderly patients judged unfit for surgery can be managed with blocking agents long term, as outlined above.

A paroxysmal rise in blood pressure and symptoms suggesting pheochromocytoma could occur in pseudopheochromocytoma (392), baroreceptor failure (393), and ischemic nephropathy (Chapter 13). In pseudopheochromocytoma the symptoms are due to hyperactivity of both beta- and alpha-adrenergic receptor function. The Valsalva maneuver is associated with marked elevation in SBP (>50 mmHg), but plasma and urinary catecholamines are normal. In baroreflex failure, past history of damage to the brainstem might be present, and episodes of hypertension may alternate with hypotension. Plasma catecholamine concentrations are elevated only during the paroxysms of hypertension and decrease following the administration of clonidine (see clonidine-suppression test). In ischemic nephropathy the paroxysms of blood pressure elevation are usually associated with pulmonary edema and normal urinary and plasma catecholamines.

B. Primary Aldosteronism

Primary aldosteronism is a form of secondary hypertension that is seen in 0.3–0.4% of the general hypertensive population (362). Six percent of these patients are 60 years and older (394,395). Although the disease is rare, it should be considered in an elderly hypertensive presenting with significant hypokalemia (serum K <3.1 mEq/L), either unprovoked or following conventional diuretic therapy, an elevated serum bicarbonate level, and a high urinary K (>30 mEq/L). The hallmark of the diagnosis is an elevated plasma aldosterone associated with hyporeninemia. The autonomous secretion of aldosterone is, in the majority of cases, secondary to a unilateral adrenocortical adenoma; occasionally, bilateral adrenal hyperplasia or an adenocarcinoma is found (396,397).

The hypertension of primary aldosteronism is associated with a hyperkinetic circulatory state, including higher cardiac output, faster heart rate, and a larger intravascular volume, compared with patients of the same sex and age with essential hypertension (398). The hypokalemia resulting from urinary K losses and the increase in urinary hydrogen losses resulting in the alkalosis are due to the effects of aldosterone on the distal part of the nephron (see Chapter on K metabolism). Whereas increased aldosterone production in patients with a unilateral lesion is due to a primary increase in biosynthesis of aldosterone by the adenoma cells, in those with bilateral adrenal hyperplasia the increased secretion of a glycoprotein of probable pituitary origin may be the stimulus for the cells of the adrenal zona glomerulosa to overproduce aldosterone (399).

Since the therapy for an adenoma is surgery and that for a bilateral hyperplasia is pharmacological intervention, it is important that these two entities be differentiated, a task made easy by the use of a CT scan of the adrenal glands, taking very thin (5-mm) tomographic views (396,400). False negative results occur in about 10% of the patients. Therefore, in those patients in whom biochemical findings suggest the presence of an adenoma but in whom the CT scan results are not definitive, adrenal venous sampling from both veins during continuous ACTH infusion should be attempted. Specimens are assayed for mineralo- and glucocorticoids. Once collection is completed, venography is performed in order to confirm the location of the catheter tip (401). This procedure, if completed successfully, is very accurate. A major problem is the difficulty in cannulating the right adrenal vein. Adrenal scans using 131_{I}-iodocholesterol can be used. This test provides both anatomical and functional information, but the sensitivity is less than with a CT scan (72%). Furthermore, the isotope is expensive and not readily available (402).

Hypertension associated with hypokalemia, an increase in urinary K, and/or metabolic alkalosis can occur in patients ingesting compounds with mineralocorticoid-like activity, such as licorice, carbenexolone, or certain nasal sprays (403). In these patients the plasma aldosterone is either within normal limits or low in contrast to primary aldosteronism.

The treatment of an aldosterone-producing adenoma is surgical. Patients are usually prepared with spironolactone (100–800 mg/day) or amiloride (20–40 mg/day) to correct hypokalemia. Spironolactone may also control the hypertension. The prognosis following adrenalectomy is usually good, with 70–80% of patients achieving normotension (396,404). In the elderly the prognosis is probably not as good, but there is no definitive information available. Patients who are unable to tolerate surgery or those with idiopathic hyperaldosteronism can be managed with spironolactone, 100–400 mg/day, in three to four divided doses. Amiloride, 10–40 mg/day in a single dose, may also be used (405). Although this drug does control hypokalemia, additional agents are usually required to control the blood pressure. Triamterene, 100 mg twice a day, has also been used successfully along with a thiazide diuretic (406,407). Nifedipine and enalapril have been tried in a small number of patients (408,409).

IX. CUSHING'S SYNDROME

Cushing's syndrome is present in 0.1–0.3% of the hypertensive population (362). This entity as a cause of hypertension in the elderly is very rare (410,411). As in younger patients, the presence of a cushingoid appearance (moon face, truncal obesity, proximal muscle weakness, increase in facial hair) in a hypertensive elderly should raise the possibility of this syndrome, particularly if the patient is also diabetic. The diagnosis can be confirmed by measurement of the plasma cortisol, ACTH, daily urine free cortisol excretion and a low-dose (2 mg) dexamethasone suppression test, together with radiological evaluation (MRI for patients suspected of having a pituitary lesion, or CT scan if looking for an adrenal tumor). If an ectopic production of ACTH by a tumor is suspected, petrosal sinus sample for ACTH might have to be done (412). The pathogenesis of hypertension in this syndrome is most likely multifactorial, with an imbalance between the activity of various vasoconstrictive and vasodilatory agents, as well as abnormalities in the renin-angiotensin axis (413). The treatment is usually surgical. Metyrapone, 750 mg every 4 hr, may be tried in patients considered to be poor surgical risks (411).

Hypertension associated with the therapeutic use of glucocorticoid is not uncommon in the elderly. Risk factors include a lower than normal total serum calcium and/or a positive family history of hypertension (414).

REFERENCES

1. Boe J, Humerfelt S, Wedervang F. The blood pressure in a population. Blood pressure readings and height and weight determinations in the adult population of the city of Bergen. Acta Med Scand 1957;321(suppl):1–336.
2. Dyer AR, et al. Hypertension in the elderly. Med Clin NA 1977;61:513–529.
3. Avolio AP, et al. Effects of aging on changing arterial compliance and left ventricular load in a Northern Chinese urban community. Circulation 1983;68:50–58.
4. Kotchen JM, McKean HE, Kotchen TA. Blood pressure trends with aging. Hypertension 1984;4(suppl III):128–134.
5. Phillips SJ, O'Fallon WM, Whisnant JP. A population-based model for predicting blood pressure. Mayo Clin Proc 1988;63:700–706.
6. Gozna ER, et al. Age related changes in the mechanics of the aorta and pulmonary artery of man. J Appl Physiol 1974;36:407–411.
7. O'Roarke M. Arterial stiffness, systolic blood pressure and logical treatment of arterial hypertension. Hypertension 1990;15:339–347.
8. Meaney E, et al. Vascular dynamics in isolated systolic arterial hypertension. Clin Cardiol 1995;12:721–725.
9. Amery A, et al. Hypertension in the elderly. Acta Med Scand 1981;210:221–229.
10. Gordon JM, et al. Echocardiographic measurements in normal subjects: evaluation of an adult population without clinically apparent heart disease. JCU 1979;7: 439–447.
11. Rodeleffer RJ, et al. Exercise cardiac output is maintained with advancing age in healthy human subjects: cardiac dilatation and increased stroke volume compensate for a diminished heart rate. Circulation 1984;69:203–215.
12. Walsh RA. Cardiovascular effects of the aging process. Am J Med 1987;82(suppl 1B):34–40.

13. Sowers JR, Rubenstein LZ, Stern N. Plasma norepinephrine responses to posture and isometric exercise increase with age in the absence of obesity. J Gerontol 1983;38: 315–317.
14. Pfiefer MA, et al. Differential changes of autonomic nervous system function with age in man. Am J Med 1983;75:249–258.
15. Shinada K, et al. Age-related changes of baroreflex function, plasma norepinephrine and blood pressure. Hypertension 1985;7:113–117.
16. Buehler FR, et al. Plasma catecholamines and cardiac, renal and peripheral vascular adrenoreceptor mediated rsponses in different age groups of normal and hypertensive subjects. Clin Exp Hypertens 1980;2:409–426.
17. Van Brummelen P, Buhler FR, Kiowski W. Age related decrease in cardiac and peripheral vascular responsiveness to isoprenaline: studies in normal subjects. Clin Sci 1981;60:571–577.
18. Kuchel OG, Kuchel GA. Peripheral dopamine in pathophysiology of hypertension. Interaction with aging and lifestyle. Hypertension 1991;18:709–721.
19. Klein C, et al. Age does not alter human vascular and nonvascular B_2-adrenergic responses to isoproterenol. Clin Pharm Ther 1988;44:573–578.
20. Gambert SR, Duthie EH. Effect of age on red-cell membrane sodium potassium dependant adenosine triphosphatase (Na^+-K^+ ATPase) activity in healthy man. Gerontology 1983;38:23–28.
21. Komatsumoto S, Mara M. Changes in the level of endothelin-1 with aging. Nippon Ronen Igakkai Zasshi 1995;32:664–669.
22. Stolk RP, et al. Insulin, hypertension and antihypertensive drugs in elderly patients: the Rotterdam Study. J Hypertens 1996;14:237–242.
23. Giugliano D, et al. Impaired glucose metabolism and reduced insulin clearance in elderly hypertensives. Am J Hypertens 1992;5:345–353.
24. Gerhard M, et al. Aging progressively impairs endothelium-dependent vasodilation in forearm resistance vessels of humans. Hypertension 1996;27:849–853.
25. Taddei S, et al. Mechanisms determining aging related impaired endothelial function in normotensive subjects. Am J Hypertens 1996;9:52A.
25a. Hausberg M. et al: Contrasting autonomic and hemodynamic effects of insulin in healthy elderly versus young subjects. Hypertension 1997;29:700–705.
26. Brenner BM, Garcia DL, Anderson S. Glomeruli and blood pressure. Less of one, more the other? Am J Hypertens 1988;1:335–347.
27. Corvalho JJM, et al. Blood pressure in four remote populations. Hypertension 1989; 14:238–246.
28. Bowers JR, et al. Salt sensitivty in blacks. Salt intake and natriuretic substances. Hypertension 1988;12:485–490.
29. Luft FC, et al. Differences in response to sodium administration in normotensive white and black subjects. J Lab Clin Med 1977;90:555–562.
30. Kirkendall WM, et al. Recommendations for human blood pressure determinations by sphygmomanometers. Subcommittee of the AHA Postgraduate Education Committee. Circulation 1980;62:1146A–1155A.
30a. Joint National Committee. Fifth report of the Joint National Committee on Detection, Evaluation, and Treatment of High Blood Pressure. Arch Intern Med 1993;153: 154–183.

31. Joint National Committee. Hypertension prevalence and the status of awareness, treatment and control in the United States. Hypertension 1985;7:457–468.
32. Burt VL, et al. Trends in the prevalence, awareness, treatment, and control of hypertension in the adult US population. Hypertension 1995;26:60–69.
33. Staessen J, Amery A, Fafard R. Isolated systolic hypertension in the elderly. J Hypertens 1990;8:393–405.
34. Cohen CE. Prevalence of hypertension among the elderly in an urban community. J Am Geriatr Soc 1975;23:165–168.
35. Curb DJ, et al. Determinants of isolated systolic hypertension. Am J Epidemiol 1985;121:371–376.
36. Hypertension detection and follow-up program (HDFP): isolated systolic hypertension in 14 communities. Am J Epidemiol 1985;121:362–370.
37. Wilking SVB, et al. Determinants of isolated systolic hypertension. JAMA 1988; 260:3451–3455.
38. Shekelle RB, Ostfeld AM, Klawans HL Jr. Hypertension and risk of stroke in an elderly population. Stroke 1974;5:71–75.
39. Garland C, Barrett-Connor E. Isolated systolic hypertension and mortality after age 60 years: a prospective population-based study. Am J Epidemiol 1983;118:365–376.
40. Smith WM, et al. Blood pressure characteristics of a population aged 60 to 90 years: SHEP. J Hypertens 1986;4(suppl 5):64A.
41. Harlan WR, et al. High blood pressure in older Americans. The first national health and nutrition examination survey. Hypertension 1984;6:802–809.
42. Messerli FH, et al. Essential hypertension in the elderly: hemodynamics, intravascular volume, plasma renin activity and circulating catecholamine levels. Lancet 1983;2:983–986.
43. Heagerty AM, Bund SJ, Aalkjaer C. Effects of drug treatment on human resistance arteriole morphology in essential hypertension: direct evidence of structural remodeling of resistance vessels. Lancet 1988;2:1209–1211.
44. Fouad-Tarazi FM, Liebson PR. Echocardiographic studies of regression of left ventricular hypertrophy in hypertension. Hypertension 1987;9(suppl II):65–68.
45. Sarzani R, Brecher P, Chobanian AV. Growth factor expression in aorta of normotensive and hypertensive rats. J Clin Invest 1989;83:1404–1408.
46. Naftilan AJ, Pratt RE, Dzau J. Induction of platelet-derived growth factor A-chain and C-myc gene expressions by angiotensin II in cultured rat vascular smooth muscle cells. J Clin Invest 1989;83:1419–1424.
47. Aalkjaer C, et al. Abnormal structure and function of isolated subcutaneous resistance vessels from essential hypertensive patients despite antihypertensive treatment. J Hypertens 1989;7:305–310.
48. Simon G. Is intracellular sodium increased in hypertension? Clin Sci 1989;76: 455–461.
49. Stern N, et al. Circadian rhythm of plasma renin activity in older normal and essential hypertensive man: relation with inactive renin, aldosterone, cortisol and REM sleep. J Hypertens 1986;4:643–550.
50. Druggan J, et al. Effects of aging and hypertension on plasma-angiotensin II and platelet angiotensin II receptor density. Am J Hypertens 1972;5:687–693.

51. Kawamoto A, et al. Cardiovascular regulatory functions in elderly patients with hypertension. Hypertension 1989;13:401–407.
52. Goldstein DS, et al. Age-dependance of the hypertensive-normotensive differences in plasma norepinephrine. Hypertension 1983;5:100–107.
53. Stern N, et al. Dissociation of 24-hour catecholamine levels from blood pressure in older men. Hypertension 1985;7:1023–1029.
54. Yamada Y, et al. Age-related changes in muscle sympathetic nerve activity in essential hypertension. Hypertension 1989;13:870–877.
55. Feldman RD, Tan CM, Chorazyczewski J. G-protein alterations in hypertension and aging. Hypertension 1996;26:725–732.
56. Crofton JT, et al. Importance of vasopressin in the development and maintenance of DOC-salt hypertension in the rat. Hypertension 1979;1:31–38.
57. Gavras J, et al. Effects of a specific inhibitor of the vascular action of vasopressin in humans. Hypertension 1984;6(suppl 1):156–160, 156–160.
58. Burztyn M, et al. Pressor hormones in elderly hypertensive persons. Racial differences. Hypertension 1990;15(suppl 1):88–92.
59. Byyny RL, et al. Cytosolic calcium and insulin resistance in elderly patients with essential hypertension. Am J Hypertens 1992;5:459–464.
60. Paolisso G, et al. Effects of magnesium and nifedipine infusions on insulin action, substrate oxidation, and blood pressure in aged hypertensive patients. Am J Hypertens 1993;6:920–926.
61. Stolk RP, et al. Insulin, hypertension and antihypertensive drugs in elderly patients: the Rotterdam Study. J Hypertens 1996;14:237–242.
62. Said Sami I. Vasoactive peptides. State of-the-art review. Hypertension 1983;5(suppl 1):17–26.
63. Faulhaber HD, et al. Evidence of decreased plasma P levels in human essential hypertension and influence of prazosin treatment. Biomed Biochem Acta 1983;42: 1019–1025.
64. Margolies HS. Kallikreins and kinins. Hypertension 1995;26:221–229.
65. Naka O, et al. The effect of aging on urinary kallikrein excretion in normotensive subjects and in patients with essential hypertension. J Clin Endocrinol Metab 1981; 52:1023–1026.
66. Tan SY, Bravo E, Mulrow PJ. Impaired renal prostaglandin E_2 biosynthesis in human hypertensive states. Post Med 1978;1:76–85.
67. Mackenzie T, et al. The importance of age on prostaglandin E_2 secretion in normal and hypertensive men. Nephron 1984;38:178–182.
68. Lang RE, Unger T, Genten D. Atrial natriuretic peptide: a new factor in blood pressure control. J Hypertens 1987;5:255–271.
69. Oparil S. The elusive role of atrial natriuretic peptide in hypertension. Mayo Clin Proc 1995;70:1015–1017.
70. Kesteloot H, Geboers J. Calcium and blood pressure. Lancet 1982;1:813–815.
71. McCarron DA. Low serum concentrations of ionized calcium in patients with hypertension. N Engl J Med 1982;307:226–228.
72. Altura BM, et al. Magnesium deficiency and hypertension: correlation between magnesium-deficiency diets and microcirculatory changes in situ. Science 1984;223: 1315–1317.

73. Resnick LM, et al. Divalent cations in essential hypertension. Relations between serum ionized calcium, magnesium and plasma renin activity. N Engl J Med 1983; 309:888–891.
74. Kesteloot H, Joossens JV. Relationship of dietary sodium, potassium, calcium and magnesium with blood pressure. Hypertension 1988;12:594–599.
75. Resnick LM, Gupta RK, Laragh JH. Intracellular free magnesium in erythrocytes of essential hypertension: relation to blood pressure and serum divalent cations. Proc Natl Acad Sci USA 1984;81:6511–6515.
76. Resnick LM, Muller FB, Laragh JH. Calcium-regulating hormones in essential hypertension: relation to plasma renin activity and sodium metabolism. Ann Intern Med 1986;105:649–654.
77. Resnick LM, et al. Dietary calcium modifies the pressor effects of dietary salt intake in essential hypertension. J Hypertens 1986;4(suppl 6):679–681.
78. Niarchos AP, Laragh JH. Renin dependency in isolated systolic hypertension. Am J Nephrol 1984;77:407–414.
79. Postnov YV, Orlov SN. Cell membrane alterations as a source of primary hypertension. J Hypertens 1984;2:1–6.
80. Bohr DF, Webb RO. Vascular smooth muscle membrane in hypertension. Ann Rev Pharmacol Toxicol 1988;28:389–409.
81. Tabuchi Y, et al. Hypotensive effect of a long-term oral calcium supplementation in elderly patients with essential hypertension. J Clin Hypertens 1986;2:254–256.
82. Lasaridis AN, et al. Increased natriuretic ability and hypotensive effect during short term high calcium intake in essential hypertension. Nephron 1989;51:517–523.
83. Gryglewski RJ, Botting RM, Vane Jr. Mediators produced by the endothelial cell. Hypertension 1988;12:530–548.
84. Griffith TM, et al. Endothelium-derived relaxing factor. J Am Coll Cardiol 1988;12: 797–806.
85. Campo C, et al. Aging abolishes the renal response to L-arginine infusion in essential hypertension. Kidney Int 1996;49(suppl 55):S126–S128.
86. Panza JA, et al. Effect of increased availability of endothelium-derived nitric oxide precursor on endothelium-dependant vascular relaxation in normal subjects and in patients with essential hypertension. Circulation 1993;87:1475–1481.
87. Yanagisawa M, et al. A novel potent vasoconstrictor peptide produced by vascular endothelial cells. Nature 1988;332:411–415.
88. Clozel M, Fischli W, Guilly C. Specific binding of endothelin on human vascular smooth muscle cells in culture. J Clin Invest 1989;83:1758–1761.
89. Fernandez-Cruz A, et al. Plasma endothelin is increased in young essential hypertensives but not in elderly essential or diabetic hypertensives. J Hypertens 1993; 11(suppl 5):S146–147.
89a. Ergul S, et al. Racial differences in plasma endothelin-1 concentrations in individuals with essential hypertension. Hypertension 1996;28:652–655.
90. Nakajima M, et al. Endothelin 1 in cerebrospinal fluid in elderly patients with hypertension and dementia. Hypertension 1994;24:97–100.
91. Letcher RL, et al. Direct relationship between blood pressure and blood viscosity in normal and hypertensive subjects. Role of fibrinogen and concentration. Am J Med 1981;70:1195–1202.

92. Linde T, et al. Blood viscosity and peripheral vascular resistance in patients with untreated essential hypertension. J Hypertens 1993;11:731–736.
93. Letcher R, Chien S, Laragh J. Changes in blood viscosity accompanying the response to prazosin in patients with essential hypertension. J Cardiovasc Pharmacol 1979;1(suppl 6):S8–S20.
94. Galarza CR, et al. Diastolic pressure underestimates age-related hemodynamic impairment. Hypertension 1997;30:809–816.
94a. Johnson AG, et al. T polymorphism of the angiotensinogene gene predicts hypertension in the elderly. J Hypertens 1996;14:1061–1065.
95. Gifford RS Jr, et al. Office evaluation of hypertension. A statement for health professionals by a writing group of the Council for High Blood Pressure Research, American Heart Association. Hypertension 1989;13:283–293.
95a. Damsgaard EM, et al. Microalbuminuria as predictor of increased mortality in elderly people. Br Med J 1990;300:297–300.
96. Agewall S, et al. Does microalbuminuria predict cardiovascular events in nondiabetic men with treated hypertension? Am J Hypertens 1995;8:337–342.
97. Topol EJ, Traill TA, Fortrein NJ. Hypertensive hypertrophic cardiomyopathy of the elderly. N Engl J Med 1985;312:277–283.
98. Pearson AC, Gudipati CV, Labovitz AJ. Systolic and diastolic flow abnormalities in elderly patients with hypertensive hypertrophic cardiomyopathy. J Am Coll Cardiol 1988;12:989–995.
99. Kobrin J, et al. Diurnal variation of blood pressure in elderly patients with essential hypertension. J Am Geriatr Soc 1984;32:896–899.
100. Suzuki Y, et al. The cardiac functional reserve in elderly hypertensive patients with abnormal diurnal change in blood pressure. J Hypertens 1992;10:173–179.
101. Shimada K, et al. Diurnal blood pressure variations and silent cerebrovascular damage in elderly patients with hypertension. J Hypertens 1992;10:875–878.
102. Shimada K, et al. Silent cerebrovascular disease in the elderly. Hypertension 1990; 16:692–699.
103. Kario K, et al. Nocturnal fall of blood pressure and silent cerebrovascular damage in elderly hypertensive patients. Hypertension 1996;27:130–135.
103a. Kohara K, et al. Asymptomatic cerebrovascular damages in essential hypertension in the elderly. Am J Hypertens 1997;10:829–835.
104. Thijs L, et al. Ambulatory blood pressure monitoring in elderly patients with isolated systolic hypertension. J Hypertens 1992;10:693–699.
105. Cox J, et al. Relationship between measured blood pressure in the clinic and by ambulatory monitoring and left ventricular size as measured by electrocardiogram in elderly patients with isolated systolic hypertension. J Hypertens 1993;11:269–276.
106. Fotherby MD, Potter JF. Reproductibility of ambulatory and clinic blood pressure measurements in elderly hypertensive subjects. J Hypertens 1993;11:573–579.
106a. Sega R, et al. Ambulatory and home blood pressure normality in the elderly. Data from the Pamela population. Hypertens 1997;30(part 1):1–6.
107. Kuwajima I, et al. Cardiac implications of the morning surge in blood pressure in elderly hypertensive patients: relation to arising time. Am J Hypertens 1995;8: 29–33.

108. Silagy CA, McNeil JJ, McGrath BP. Isolated systolic hypertension: does it really exist on ambulatory blood pressure monitoring? Clin Experim Pharmacol Physiol 1990;17:203–206.
108a. Trenkwalder P, et al. White coat hypertension in the elderly. Am J Hypertens 1993; 6:132A, 1431.
109. Winberg N, et al. 24-H ambulatory blood pressure in 352 normal Danish subjects, related to age and gender. Am J Hypertens 1995;8:978–986.
110. Ruddy MC, et al. The relationship of plasma renin activity to clinic and ambulatory blood pressure in elderly people with isolated systolic hypertension. J Hypertens 1988;6(suppl 4):S412–S415.
111. Shekelle RB, Ostfeld AM, Klawans HL Jr. Hypertension and risk of stroke in an elderly population. Stroke 1974;5:71–74.
112. Kannel WB, Dawber TR, McGee DL. Perspective on systolic hypertension. The Framingham Study. Circulation 1980;61:1179–1182.
113. Borhani NO. Prevalence and prognostic significance of hypertension in the elderly. J Am Geriatr Soc 1986;34:112–114.
114. Landahl S, Lernfelt B, Sundh V. Blood pressure and mortality in old age. Eleven years' followup of a 70 year old population. J Hypertens 1987;5:745–748.
115. Coope J, Warrender TS, McPherson K. The prognostic significance of blood pressure in the elderly. J Hum Hypertens 1988;2:79–88.
116. Ueda K, et al. Prognosis and outcome of elderly hypertensives in a Japanese community: results from a long term prospective study. J Hypertens 1988;6:991–997.
117. Glynn RJ, et al. Evidence for a positive linear relation between blood pressure and mortality in elderly people. Lancet 1995;345:825–829.
117a. Weijenberg MP, Feskens EJM, Kromhout D. Blood pressure and isolated systolic hypertension and the risk of coronary heart disease and mortality in elderly men (the Zutphen Eldery Study). J Hypertens 1996;14:1159–1166.
118. Applegate WB. Hypertension in elderly patients. Ann Intern Med 1989;110: 901–915.
119. Thijs L, et al. A meta-analysis of outcome trials in elderly hypertensives. J Hypertens 1992;10:1103–1109.
120. Lever AF, Ramsey LE. Treatment of hypertension in the elderly. J Hypertens 1995; 13:571–579.
121. Fletcher A, et al. Risks and benefits in the trial of the European Working Party on high blood pressure in the elderly. J Hypertens 1991;9:225–230.
122. SHEP Copperative Research Group. Prevention of stroke by antihypertensive drug treatment in older persons with isolated systolic hypertension. Final results of the Systolic Hypertension in the Elderly (SHEP). JAMA 1991;265:3255–3264.
122a. Kostis JB, et al. Prevention of heart failure by antihypertensive drug treatment in older patients with isolated systolic hypertension. JAMA 1997;278:212–216.
123. Slovick DJ, et al. SYST-EUR multicentre trial on the treatment of isolated systolic hypertension in the elderly: first interim report. J Hum Hypertens 1993;7:201–203.
124. Gifford RW Jr. Isolated systolic hypertension in the elderly. Some controversial issues. JAMA 1982;247:781–785.
125. Seligman AW, Alderman MH, Davis TK. Systolic hypertension: occurence and treatment in a defined community. J Am Geriatr Soc 1979;27:135–138.

126. Vardan S, et al. Systolic hypertension in the elderly. Hemodynamic response to long term thiazide diuretic therapy and its side effects. JAMA 1983;250:2807–2813.
127. Garland BJ, et al. Effects of treatment for isolated systolic hypertension on cognitive status and depression in the elderly. J Am Geriatr Soc 1988;36:1015–1022.
128. Goldstein G, et al. Treatment of hypertension in the elderly: II cognitive and behavioral function. Results of a Department of Veterans Affairs cooperative study. Hypertension 1990;15:361–369.
129. Dustan HP. Isolated systolic hypertension: a long-neglected cause of cardiovascular complications. Am J Med 1989;86:368–369.
130. Breckenridge MB, Kostis JB. Isolated systolic hypertension in the elderly: results of a statewide survey of clinical practice in New Jersey. Am J Med 1989;86: 370–375.
131. The Working Group on Hypertension in the Elderly: statement on hypertension in the elderly. JAMA 1986;256:70–74.
132. Larochelle P, et al. Recommendation from the Consensus Conference on Hypertension in the Elderly. Can Med Assoc J 1986;135:741–745.
133. Davidson RA, Caranasos GJ. Should the elderly hypertensive be treated? Arch Intern Med 1987;147:1933–1937.
134. McFate Smith W. The case for treating hypertension in the elderly. Am J Hypertens 1988;1:173S–178S.
135. Applegate WB, et al. Control of systolic blood pressure in elderly black patients. J Am Geriatr Soc 1983;30:391–392.
136. Applegate WB, Dismuke Se, Runyan JW. Treatment of hypertension in the elderly: a time for caution? J Am Geriatr Soc 1984;321–323.
137. Cruickshank JM, Thorp JM, Zacharies FJ. Benefits and potential harm of lowering high blood pressure. Lancet 1987;1:581–584.
138. Alderman MH, et al. Treatment-induced blood pressure reduction and the risk of myocardial infarction. JAMA 1989;262:920–924.
139. Bulpitt CJ, et al. Relation between treated blood pressure and death from ischemic heart disease at different ages: a report from the Department of Health hypertension care computing project. J Hypertens 1992;10:1273–1278.
139a. Merlo J, et al. Incidence of myocardial infarction in elderly men being treated with antihypertensive drugs: population based cohort study. Br Med J 1996;313:457–461.
139b. Bots ML, et al. Low diastolic blood pressure and atherosclerosis in elderly subjects. Arch Intern Med 1996;156:843–848.
140. Cruickshank JM. Coronary flow reserve and the J curve relation between diastolic blood pressure and myocardial infarction. Br Med J 1988;297:1227–1230.
141. Strandgaard S, Hannso S. Why does antihypertensive treatment prevent stroke but not myocardial infarction? Lancet 1987;2:658–660.
142. Editorial: How far to lower blood pressure? Lancet 1987;2:251–252.
143. Staessen J, et al. Relation between mortality and treated blood pressure in elderly patients with hypertension: report of the European Working Party on High Blood Pressure in the Elderly. Br Med J 1989;298:1552–1556.
144. Cox JP, O'Brien E, O'Malley K. The J-shaped curve in elderly hypertensives. J Hypertens 1992;10(suppl 2):S17–S23.

145. MacMahon S, et al. Blood pressure, stroke and coronary heart disease. Part 1, prolonged differences in blood pressure: prospective observational studies corrected for the regression dilution bias. Lancet 1990;335:765–774.
146. Collins R, et al. Blood pressure, stroke and coronary heart disease. Part 2, short-term reductions in blood pressure: overview of randomised drug trials in their epidemiological context. Lancet 1990;335:827–838.
147. Mattilea K, et al. Blood pressure and five-year survival in the very old. Br Med J 1988;296:887–889.
148. Lauger RD, Ganiats TG, Barrett-Connor E. Paradoxical survival of elderly man with high blood pressure. Br Med J 1989;298:1356–1358.
149. Lauger RD, et al. Blood pressure change and survival after age 75. Hypertension 1993;22:551–559.
150. Amery A, et al. Mortality and morbidity results from the European Working Party on High Blood Pressure in the Elderly trial. Lancet 1985;2:1349–1354.
151. Heikinheimo RJ, et al. Blood pressure in the very old. J Hypertens 1990;8:361–367.
152. Guzik HJ, et al. Hypertension: Cardiovascular implications in a cohort of old old. J Am Geriatr Soc 1992;40:348–353.
153. Weber MA, Neutel JM, Cheung DG. Hypertension in the aged: a pathophysiologic basis for treatment. Am J Cardiol 1989;63:25H–32H.
154. Lernfelt B, et al. Overtreatment of hypertension in the elderly? J Hypertens 1990; 8:483–490.
155. Zweifler AJ, Shahab ST. Pseudohypertension: a new assessment. J Hypertens 1993; 11:1–6.
156. Messerli FH, Ventura HO, Amodes O. Osler's maneuver and pseudohypertension. N Engl J Med 1985;312:1548–1551.
157. Hla KM, Feussner JR. Screening for pseudohypertension. A qualitative non-invasive approach. Arch Intern Med 1988;148:673–676.
158. O'Callaghan WG, et al. Accuracy of indirect blood pressure measurement in the elderly. Br Med J 1983;286:1545–1546.
159. Hla KM, Vokaty KA, Feussner JR. Overestimation of diastolic blood pressure in the elderly: magnitude of the problem and a potential solution. J Am Geriatr Soc 1985; 33:659–663.
160. Pitlik SD, et al. Overestimation of blood pressure in the elderly. Isr J Med 1986; 22:435–437.
161. Prochazka AV, Martel R. Osler's maneuver in outpatient veterans. J Clin Hypertens 1987;3:554–558.
162. Spence JD, Sibbald WJ, Cape RD. Pseudohypertension in the elderly. Clin Sci Mol Med 1978;55:3995S–402S.
163. Varder S, et al. Systolic hypertension. Direct and indirect blood pressure measurements. Arch Intern Med 1983;143:935–938.
164. Kuwajima I, et al. Pseudohypertension in the elderly. J Hypertens 1990;8:429–432.
165. Pickering TG, Levenstein M, Walmsley P. Differential effects of Doxazosin on clinic and ambulatory pressure according to age, gender and presence of white coat hypertension. Am J Hypertens 1994;7:848–852.
166. Mader SL. Aging and postural hypotension. An update. J Am Geriatr Soc 1989;37: 129–137.

167. Applegate WB, et al. Prevalence of postural hypotension at baseline in the Systolic Hypertension in the Elderly Program (SHEP). Cohort. J Am Geriatr Soc 1991;39: 1057–1064.
168. Masuo K, et al. Changes in frequency of orthostatic hypotension in elderly hypertensive patients under medications. Am J Hypertens 1996;9:263–268.
168a. Vanhanen H, et al. Associations of orthostatic blood pressure in older patients with isolated systolic hypertension. J Hypertens 1996;14:943–949.
169. Lipsitz LA, et al. Postprandial reduction in blood pressure in the elderly. N Engl J Med 1983;309:81–83.
170. Lipsitz LA, Fullerton KJ. Postprandial blood pressure reduction in healthy elderly. J Am Geriatr Soc 1986;34:267–279.
171. Peitzman SJ, Berger SR. Postrandial blood pressure decrease in well elderly persons. Arch Intern Med 1989;149:286–288.
172. Vaitkevicius PV, et al. Frequency and importance of postprandial blood pressure reduction in elderly nursing-home patients. Ann Intern Med 1991;115:865–870.
173. Aronow WS, Ahn C. Postprandial hypotension in 499 elderly persons in a long-term health care facility. J Am Geriatr Soc 1994;42:930–932.
174. Jansen R WMM, Kelly-Gagnon MM, Lipsitz LA. Intraindividual reproducibility of postprandial and orthostatic blood pressure changes in older nursing home patients: relationship with chronic use of cardiovascular medications. J Am Geriatr Soc 1996;44:383–389.
175. Masuo K, et al. Mechanisms mediating postprandial blood pressure reduction in young and elderly subjects. Am J Hypertens 1996;9:536–544.
176. Anderson RJ, Reed G, Kirk LM. Therapeutic considerations for elderly hypertensives. Clin Ther 1982;5:25–38.
176a. Mulkerrin EC, Clark BA, Epstein FH. Increased salt retention and hypertension from non-steroidal anti-inflammatory agents in the elderly. Q J Med 1997;90: 411–415.
177. Swartz SL, et al. Captopril-induced changes in prostaglandin production: relationship to vascular responses in normal man. J Clin Invest 1980;65:1257–1264.
178. Webster J. Interactions of NSAIDs with diuretics and beta-blockers. Mechanisms and clinical implications. Drugs 1985;30:32–41.
179. Ebel DL, Rhymer AR, Stahl E. Effect of sulindac, piroxicam and placebo on the hypotensive effect of propranolol in patients with mild to moderate essential hypertension. Adv Ther 1985;2:131–142.
180. Wong DG, et al. Effect of non-steroidal anti-inflammatory drugs on control of hypertension by beta-blockers and diuretics. Lancet 1986;1:997–1001.
181. Oates JA. Antagonism of antihypertensive drug therapy by non-steroidal anti-inflammatory drugs. Hypertension 1988;11(suppl II):4–6.
182. Gurwitz JH, et al. The impact of ibuprofen on the efficacy of antihypertensive treatment with hydrochlorothiazide in elderly persons. J Gerontol A, Biol Sci Med Sci 1996;51:M74–M79.
183. Dustan HP. Calcium channel blockers. Potential medical benefits and side-effects. Hypertension 1989;13(suppl I):137–140.
184. Stason WB. Cost and quality trade-offs in the treatment of hypertension. Hypertension 1989;13(suppl I):145–148.

185. Midgley JP, et al. Effect of reduced dietary sodium on blood pressure, a meta-analysis of randomized controlled trials. JAMA 1996;275:1590–1597.
186. Richards AM, et al. Blood-pressure response to moderate sodium restriction and to potassium supplementation in mild essential hypertension. Lancet 1984;1:757–761.
187. Weinberger MH, et al. Dietary sodium restriction as adjunctive treatment of hypertension. JAMA 1988;259:2561–2565.
188. Luft FC, Weinberger MH. Review of salt restriction and the response to antihypertensive drugs. Hypertension 1988;11(suppl I):229–232.
189. Australian National Health and Medical Research Council Dietary Salt Study Management Committee. Fall in blood pressure with modest reduction in dietary salt intake in mild hypertension. Lancet 1989;1:399–402.
190. Fotherby MD, Potter JF. Effects of moderate sodium restriction on clinic and 24-hour ambulatory blood pressure in elderly hypertensive subjects. J Hypertens 1993;11:657–663.
191. Cobiac L, et al. A low-sodium diet supplemented with fish oil lowers blood pressure in the elderly. J Hypertens 1992;10:87–92.
192. Gelijnse JM, et al. Dietary electrolyte intake and blood pressure in older subjects: the Rotterdam Study. J Hypertens 1996;14:737–741.
193. MacGregor GA, et al. Moderate potassium supplementation in essential hypertension. Lancet 1982;2:567–570.
194. Kaplan NM, et al. Potassium supplementation in hypertensive patients with diuretic-induced hypokalemia. N Engl J Med 1985;312:746–749.
195. Krishna GG, Miller E, Kapoor S. Increased blood pressure by having potassium depletion in normotensive men. N Engl J Med 1989;320:1177–1182.
196. Grimm RH Jr, et al. The influence of oral potassium chloride on blood pressure in hypertensive men on a low-sodium diet. N Engl J Med 1990;322:569–574.
197. Fotherby MD, Potter JF. Potassium supplementation reduces clinic and ambulatory blood pressure in elderly hypertensive patients. J Hypertens 1992;10:1403–1408.
198. Morris CD, McCarron DA. Calcium supplementation reduces blood pressure in older systolic hypertensives. J Hypertens 1986;4(suppl 5):S562A.
199. Morris CD, McCarron DA. Effect of calcium supplementation in an older population with mildly increased blood pressure. Am J Hypertens 1992;5:230–237.
200. Berchtold P, et al. Obesity and hypertension: cardiovascular response to weight reduction. Hypertension 1982;4(suppl III):50–55.
201. Smith WCS, et al. Urinary electrolyte excretion, alcohol consumption and blood pressure in the Scottish Heart Health Study. Br Med J 1988;297:329–330.
202. Rouse IL, et al. Blood-pressure lowering effect of a vegetarian diet: controlled trial in normotensive subjects. Lancet 1983;1:5–9.
203. Editorial. Weight reduction in hypertension. Lancet 1985;1:1251–1252.
204. Ramsay LE, et al. Weight reduction in a blood pressure clinic. Br Med J 1978;2:244–245.
205. Saunders JB, Beevers DE, Paton A. Alcohol-induced hypertension. Lancet 1981;2:653–656.
206. Subcommittee on Nonpharmacological Therapy of the 1984 Joint Committee on Detection, Evaluation and Treatment od High Blood Pressure. Non-pharmacological approaches to the control of high blood pressure. Hypertension 1986;8:444–467.

207. Trevisan M, et al. Alcohol consumption, drinking pattern and blood pressure: analysis of data from the Italian National Research Council Study. Int J Epidemiol 1987; 16:520–527.
208. Palmer AJ, et al. Alcohol intake and cardiovascular mortality in hypertensive patients. Report from the Department of Health Hypertension Care Computing Project. J Hypertens 1995;12:957–964.
209. Mountain SJ, et al. Altered hemodynamics during exercise in older essential hypertensive subjects. Hypertension 1988;12:479–484.
210. Hagberg JM, et al. Effect of exercise training in 60 to 69 year-old persons with essential hypertension. Am J Cardiol 1989;64:348–353.
211. Arakawa K. Antihypertensive mechanism of exercise. J Hypertens 1993;11:223–229.
211a. National High Blood Pressure Education Program Working Group report on hypertension in the elderly. Hypertension 1994;23:275–285.
211b. Monane M, et al. The effects of initial drug choice and comorbidity on antihypertensive therapy compliance. Am J Hypertens 1997;10:697–704.
212. Myers MG. Hydrochlorothiazide with or without amiloride for hypertension in the elderly. Arch Intern Med 1987;147:1026–1030.
213. Freis ED. Age and antihypertensive drugs (hydrochlorothiazide, bendromethiazide, nadolol and captopril). Am J Cardiol 1988;61:117–121.
214. Leehay DJ, Hartman E. Comparison of diltiazem and hydrochlorothiazide for treatment of patients 60 years of age or older with systemic hypertension. Am J Cardiol 1988;62:1218–1223.
215. Vardan S, et al. Systolic hypertension in the elderly: hemodynamic response to long term diuretic therapy and its side effects. JAMA 1983;250:2807–2813.
215a. Curb JD, et al. Effect of diuretic-based antihypertensive treatment on cardiovascular disease risk in older diabetic patients with isolated systolic hypertension. JAMA 1996;276:1886–1892.
216. Gifford RW Jr. Management of isolated systolic hypertension in the elderly. J Am Geriatr Soc 1986;34:106–111.
217. Morledge JH, et al. Isolated systolic hypertension in the elderly. A placebo-controlled, dose response evaluation of chlorthalidone. J Am Geriatr Soc 1986;34: 199–206.
218. Medical Research Council's trials of treatment of mild hypertension: comparison of the antihhypertensive efficacy and adverse reactions to two doses of bendrofluazide and hydrochlorothiazide and the effect of potassium supplementation on the hypotensive action of bendrofluazide. J Clin Pharmacol 1987;27:271–277.
219. Materson BJ, et al. Treatment of hypertension in the elderly. I. Blood pressure and clinical changes. Results of a Department of Veteran's Affairs cooperative study. Hypertension 1990;15:348–360.
220. Freis ED, Reda DJ, Materson BJ. Volume (weight) loss and blood pressure response following thiazide diuretics. Hypertension 1988;12:244–250.
221. Saito F, Kimura G. Antihypertensive mechanisms of diuretics based on pressure-natriuresis relationship. Hypertension 1996;27:914–918.
222. Webster J, et al. Antihypertensive action of bendraflumethiazide: increased prostacyclin production? Clin Pharm Ther 1980;28:751–754.

223. O'Connor DT. Response of the renal kallikrein-kinin system, intravascular volume and renal hemodynamics to sodium restriction and diuretic treatment in essential hypertension. Hypertension 1982;4(suppl III):72–78.
224. MacLennan WJ. Diuretics in the elderly: how safe? Br Med J 1988;296:1550.
225. Plante GE, Dessurault DL. Hypertension in elderly patients. A comparative study between indapamide and hydrochlorothiazide. Am J Med 1988;84(suppl IB): 98–103.
226. Werning C, Weitz T, Ludwig B. Assessment of indapamide in elderly hypertensive patients with special emphasis on well-being. Am J Med 1988;84(suppl IB):104–108.
227. Langer SZ, Cavero I, Massingham R. Recent developments in noradrenergic neurotransmission and its relevance to the mechanism of action of certain antihypertensive agents. Hypertension 1980;2:372–382.
228. Messerli FH, et al. Antiadrenergic therapy: special aspects in hypertension in the elderly. Hypertension 1981;3(suppl II):226–229.
229. Jackson G, et al. Inappropriate antihypertensive therapy in the elderly. Lancet 1976;2:1317–1318.
230. Jansen PAF, et al. Contribution of inappropriate treatment for hypertension to pathogenesis of stroke in the elderly. Br Med J 1986;293:914–917.
231. Applegate WB, et al. Comparison of the use of reserpine versus alphamethyldopa for the second step treatment of hypertension in the elderly. J Am Geriatr Soc 1985;33:109–115.
232. Thananopavarn C, Golub MS, Sambhi MP. Clonidine in the elderly hypertensive. Monotherapy and therapy with a diuretic. Chest 1983;83:410–411.
233. Weber MA, Drayer JIM, Gray DR. Combined diuretic and sympatholytic therapy in elderly patients with predominant systolic hypertension. Chest 1983;83:416–418.
234. Whitsett TL, et al. Abrupt cessation of clonidine administration: a prospective study. Am J Cardiol 1978;41:1285–1290.
235. Klein C, et al. Transdermal clonidine therapy in elderly mild hypertensives: effects on blood pressure, plasma norepinephrine and plasma glucose. J Hypertens 1985; 3(suppl 4):81–84.
236. Schmidt GR, Schuna AA, Goodfriend TL. Transdermal clonidine compared with hydrochlorothiazide as monotherapy in elderly hypertensive males. J Clin Pharmacol 1989;29:133–139.
237. Owens SD, Dunn MI. Efficacy and safety of guanadrel in elderly hypertensive patients. Arch Intern Med 1988;148:1515–1518.
238. Cheung DG, et al. Mild hypertension in the elderly. A comparison of prazosin and enalapril. Am J Med 1989;86(suppl 1B):87–99.
239. Ram CVS, et al. Antihypertensive therapy in the elderly. Effects on blood pressure and cerebral blood blow. Am J Med 1987;82(suppl 1A):53–57.
240. Kirby RS, et al. Prazosin in the treatment of prostatic obstruction. A placebo-controlled study. Br J Urol 1987;60:136–142.
241. Guthrie RM. Doxazosin for the treatment of patients with hypertension and symptoms of benign prostatic hyperplasia. Am J Hypertens 1996;9:118A.
241a. Kaplan SA, Kaplan NM. Alpha-blockade: monotherapy for hypertension and benign prostatic hyperplasia. Urology 1996;48:541–550.

242. Dauer AD. Terazosin: an effective once-daily monotherapy for the treatment of hypertension. Am J Med 1986;80(suppl 5B):29–34.
243. Hamdy C, et al. Use of long-acting propranolol (Inderal LA) in the management of elderly hypertensive patients. Eur J Clin Pharmacol 1982;22:379–381.
244. Wikstrand J, Berglund G. Antihypertensive treatment with beta blockers in patients aged over 65. Br Med J 1982;285:850.
245. Forrest WA. The treatment of hypertension in older patients;a comparative study between a diuretic, a beta receptor antagonist and their fixed combination. Practitioner 1982;226:777–778.
246. Frohlich ED. Beta-blockers and mental performance. Arch Intern Med 1988;148: 888–778.
247. Gango FM, et al. The effect of beta-blockers on mental performance on older hypertensive patients. Arch Intern Med 1988;148:779–784.
248. Bird AS, Blizard RD, Mann AH. Treating hypertension in the older person: an evaluation of the association of blood pressure level and its reduction with cognitive performance. J Hypertens 1990;8:147–152.
249. Buhler FR, et al. Betablockers and calcium antagonists: cornerstone of antihypertensive therapy. Drugs 1983;25(suppl 2):50–57.
250. Frohlich ED, et al. The paradox of beta-adrenergic blockade in hypertension. Circulation 1968;37:417–421.
251. Wikstrand J, et al. Increased cardiac output and lowered peripheral resistance during metoprolol treatment. Acta Med Scand 1983;672(suppl):105–110.
252. Hartford M, et al. Cardiovascular and renal effects of long-term antihypertensive therapy. JAMA 1988;259:2553–2557.
253. Jackson EK, Campbell WB. A possible antihypertensive mechanism of propranolol: antagonism of angiotensin II enhancement of sympathetic nerve-transmission through prostaglandins. Hypertension 1981;3:23–33.
254. Beckmann ML, et al. Propranolol increases prostacyclin synthesis in patients with essential hypertension. Hypertension 1988;12:582–588.
255. Cressman MD, Gifford RW Jr, Vidt DG. Geriatric hypertension controversies: uses of newer agents. Geriatrics 1985;40:53–68.
256. Silberman J, et al. Isolated systolic hypertension (ISH) in the elderly: treatment with labetolol. Clin Pharmacol 1988;28:908–959, 55A.
257. DeQuattro V, et al. Labetol blunts morning pressor surge in systolic hypertension. Hypertension 1988;11(suppl 1):198–201.
258. Kirkendall WM. Treatment of hypertension in the elderly. Am J Cardiol 1986;57: 63C–68C.
259. Lessem JN, Weber MA. Antihypertensive treatment with a dual-acting beta-blocker in the elderly. J Hypertens 1993;11(suppl 4):S29–S36.
260. Roberts DH, et al. Placebo-controlled comparison of captopril, atenolol, labetalol and pindolol in hypertension complicated by intermittent claudication. Lancet 1987;2:650–653.
261. Hosie J, Vallé-Jones JC, Clifford PD. Long term usage of Prestim (Timolol/bendrofuazide) in the management of mild to moderate hypertension in general practice. Br J Clin Pract 1983;11/12:393–396.

262. O'Callaghan WG, et al. Antihypertensive and renal hemodynamic effects of atenolol and nadolol in elderly hypertensive patients. Br J Clin Pharmacol 1983;16:417–421.
263. Wikstrand J, et al. Antihypertensive treatment with metoprolol or hydrochlorothiazide in patients aged 60 to 75 years. JAMA 1986;255:1304–1310.
264. Wikstrand J. New concepts in the treatment of elderly hypertensive patients. Am Heart J 1988;116:296–304.
265. Andersen GS. Atenolol versus bendroflumethiazide in middle-aged and elderly hypertensives. Acta Med Scand 1985;218:165–172.
266. Perrson I. Treatment of hypertension in the elderly with pindolol and clopamide. J Am Geriatr Soc 1978;26:337–340.
267. Marks AD, et al. An office-based primary care trial of pindolol (Visken) in essential hypertension. Curr Med Res Opin 1986;10(S):297–307.
268. Eisalo A, Virta P. Treatment of hypertension with labetalol. Acta Med Scand 1982;665(suppl):129–133.
269. Abernathy DR, et al. Pharmacodynamics and disposition of labetalol in elderly hypertensive patients. J Clin Pharmacol 1985;25:468A.
270. Meisheri KD, Cipkus KLA, Taylor CA. Mechanism of action of minoxidil-sulfate induced vasodilation: a role for increased K permeability. J Pharmacol Exp Ther 1988;245:751–760.
271. Spitalewitz S, Porush JG, Reiser IW. Minoxidil, nadolol and a diuretic. Once-a-day therapy for resistant hypertension. Arch Intern Med 1986;146:822–886.
272. Velasco M, et al. Cardiovascular hemodynamic interactions between clonidine and minoxidil in hypertensive patients. Chest 1983;83(suppl 3):360–364.
273. Williams GH. Converting-enzyme inhibitors in the treatment of hypertension. N Engl J Med 1988;319:1517–1525.
274. Zusman RM. Renin and non-renin mediated antihypertensive actions of converting enzyme inhibitors. K Int 1984;25:969–983.
275. Mimran A, Targhetta R, Laroche B. The antihypertensive effect of captopril: evidence for an influence of kinins. Hypertension 1980;2:732–737.
276. Reid JL, et al. Angiotensin-converting enzyme inhibitors in the elderly. Am Heart J 1989;117:751–754.
277. Chobanian AV. The use of angiotensin-converting enzyme inhibitors in elderly patients with hypertension. J Am Geriatr Soc 1987;35:269–270.
278. Jenkins AC, Knill JR, Dreslinski GR. Captopril in the treatment of the elderly hypertensive patient. Arch Intern Med 1985;145:2029–2031.
279. Tuck ML, et al. Low-dose captopril in mild to moderate geriatric hypertension. J Am Geriatr Soc 1986;34:693–696.
280. Creisson C, Baulac L, Lenfant B. Captopril/hydrochlorothiazide combination in elderly patients with mild-moderate hypertension. A double-blind, randomized, placebo-controlled study. Postgrad Med J 1986;62(suppl 1):139–141.
281. Ambrosio GB, Zamboni S, Botta G. Captopril in elderly hypertensive patients. Results from a multicenter Italian trial. The Study Group on Captopril in the Elderly. Am J Med 1988;84(suppl 3A):152–154.
282. Cox JP, et al. A double blind evaluation of captopril in elderly hypertensives. J Hypertens 1989;7:299–303.

283. Woo J, et al. Singleblind randomized, cross-over study of angiotensin converting enzyme inhibitor and triamterene and hydrochlorothiazide in the treatment of mild to moderate hypertension in the elderly. Arch Intern Med 1987;1471:1386–1389.
284. Woo J, Woo KS, Valalance-Owen J. The use of the angiotensin-converting enzyme (ACE) inhibitor enalapril in the treatment of mild to moderate hypertension in the elderly. Br Clin Pract 1987;41:845–847.
285. Cooper WD, Glover DR, Kimber GR. The influence of age on the blood pressure response to enalapril. Gerontol 1987;33(suppl 1):48–54.
286. Laher MS, et al. Antihypertensive and renal effects of lisinopril in older patients with hypertension. Am J Med 1988;85(suppl 3B):38–43.
287. Gomez HJ, Smith SG, Moncloa F. Efficacy and safety of lisinopril in older patients with essential hypertension. Am J Med 1988;85(suppl 3B):35–37.
288. Mondal BK, et al. Enalapril in the long-term treatment of elderly hypertensives. Nephron 1990;55(suppl 1):96–97.
289. Hawkins DW, et al. A multicenter analysis of the use of enalapril and lisinopril in elderly hypertensive patients. J Am Geriatr Soc 1994;92:1273–1276.
290. Tomlinson B, et al. Sustained release isradipine compared with spirapril in the treatment of elderly patients with isolated systolic hypertension. Am J Hypertens 1994; 7:35S–39S.
291. Silagy C, McNeil JJ, McGrath BP. Treatment for isolated systolic hypertension: a comparison of atenolol, enalapril hydrochlorothiazide and isradipine. Am J Hypertens 1993;6:115A, 1071.
291a. Israili ZH, Hall WD. ACE inhibitors. Differential use in elderly patients with hypertension. Drugs Aging 1995;7:355–371.
292. Goldberg AI, Dunlay MC, Sweet CS. Safety and tolerability of losartan potassium, an angiotensin II receptor antagonist, compared with hydrochlorothiazide, atenolol, felodipine and angiotensin-converting enzyme inhibitors for the treatment of systemic hypertension. Am J Cardiol 1995;75:793–795.
293. Piepho RW, Sowers JR. Antihypertensive therapy in the geriatric patient I: a review of the role of calcium channel blockers. J Clin Pharmacol 1989;29:193–200.
294. Applegate WB, et al. A randomized controlled trial of the effects of three antihypertensive agents on blood pressure control and quality of life in older women. Arch Intern Med 1991;151:1817–1823.
295. Bolli P, et al. Using age and plasma renin to design antihypertensive therapy. Calcium channel blockers in hypertension. Epstein SE, ed. New York: USA Biomedical Information Corp, 1986.
296. Resnick LM, Nicholson JP, Laragh JH. Calcium metabolism and the renin-aldosterone system in essential hypertension. J Cardiovasc Pharmacol 1985;7(suppl 6): 187–193.
297. Van Zweiten, Van Meel JC, Timmermans P. Pharmacology of calcium entry blockers: interaction with vascular alpha-adrenoceptors. Hypertension 1983;5(suppl II):8–17.
297a. Triggle DJ. Pharmacologic and therapeutic differences among calcium channel antagonists: profile of mibefradil, a new calcium antagonist. Am J Cardiol 1996;78 (suppl 9A):7–12.

298. Krebs R. Adverse reactions with calcium antagonists. Hypertension 1983;5(suppl II):125–129.
299. Hansson L. Treatment of hypertension in the elderly. J Cardiovasc Pharmacol 1994; 23(suppl 5):S59–S61.
300. Trenkwalder P, et al. Antihypertensive treatment with felodipine but not with a diuretic reduces episodes of myocardial ischemia in elderly patients with hypertension. Eur Heart J 1994;15:1673–1680.
300a. Pahor M, et al. Long-term survival and use of antihypertensive medications in older persons. J Am Geriatr Soc 1995;43:1191–1197.
300b. Psaty BM, et al. The risk of myocardial infarction associated with antihypertensive drug therapies. JAMA 1995;274:620–625.
301. Malacco E, et al. Systolic hypertension in the elderly: long-term lacidipine treatment. Objective, protocol, and organization. SHELL Study Group. J Cardiovasc Pharmacol 1994;23(suppl 5):S62–S66.
301a. Pahor M, et al. Calcium-channel blockade and incidence of cancer in aged populations. Lancet 1996;348:493–497.
301b. Stason WB, et al. Safety of nifedipine in patients with hypertension. A meta-analysis. Hypertension 1997;30(part 1):7–14.
302. Ben-Ishay D, Leibel B, Stessman J. Calcium channel blockers in the management of hypertension in the elderly. Am J Med 1986;81(suppl 6A):30–34.
303. Erne P, et al. Factors influencing the hypotensive effects of calcium antagonists. Hypertension 1983;5(suppl II):97–102.
304. Rotolo V, Lombardo F, Ciccittini L. Long term effect of oral antihypertensive treatment with verapamil in elderly patients. Clin Ther 1985;15:1–4.
305. Abernathy DR, et al. Verapamil pharacodynamics and disposition in younger and elderly hypertensive patients. Ann Intern Med 1986;105:328–336.
306. Schwartz JB, Abernathy DR. Responses to intravenous and oral diltiazem in elderly and younger patients with systemic hypertension. Am J Cardiol 1987;59:1111–1117.
307. Leonetti, Zamchetti A. Antihypertensive efficacy of nicardipine based treatment in patients of different age and in patients with isolated systolic hypertension. J Hypertens 1988;6(suppl 4):655–657.
308. Krakoff LR. Nicardipine monotherapy in ambulatory elderly patients with hypertension. Am Heart J 1989;117:250–254.
309. Forette F, et al. Nicardipine in elderly patients with hypertension: a review of experience in France. Am Heart J 1989;117:255–261.
310. Littler E. Nicardipine in the elderly hypertensive: a review of experience in the United Kingdom. Am Heart J 1989;117:262–265.
311. Kario K, Shimada K. Differential effects of amlodipine on ambulatory blood pressure in elderly hypertensive patients with different nocturnal reductions in blood pressure. Am J Hypertens 1997;10:261–268.
312. Fagan TC. Blood pressure reduction and tolerability of felodipine ER in older and younger hypertensive patients. J Am Geriatr Soc 1997;45:712–717.
313. Rowe JW. Approach to the treatment of hypertension in older patients. Preliminary results with isradipine. Am J Med 1988;84(suppl 3B):46–50.

314. The British Isradipine Hypertension Group. Evaluation of the safety and efficacy of isradipine in elderly patients with essential hypertension. Am J Med 1989;86(suppl 4A):110–114.
315. Lacourciere Y, et al. Antihypertensive effects of amlodipine and hydrochlorothiazide in elderly patients with ambulatory hypertension. Am J Hypertens 1995;8: 1154–1159.
316. Weinberger MH. Antihypertensive therapy and lipids: evidence, mechanisms and implications. Arch Intern Med 1985;145:1102–1105.
317. Weinberger MH. Antihypertensive therapy and lipids. Paradoxical influences on cardiovascular disease risk. Am J Med 1986;80(suppl 2A):64–70.
318. Weidman P, Gerber A, Mordasini R. Effects of antihypertensive therapy on serum lipoproteins. Hypertension 1986;5(suppl III):120–131.
319. Amery A, Lijnen P. Alterations in lipid metabolism induced by antihypertensive therapy. Drugs 1988;36(suppl 2):1–5.
320. Pollare T, Lithell H, Berne C. A comparison of the effects of hydrochlorothiazide and captopril on glucose and lipid metabolism in patients with hypertension. N Engl J Med 1989;321:868–873.
321. Thakur N, Kochar MS, Thakur RK. Comparison of hypertension control in elderly black and white males. J Clin Pharmacol 1988;28:910A.
322. Sheu WHH, et al. Comparison of the effects of atenolol and nifedipine on glucose, insulin, and lipid metabolism in patients with hypertension. Am J Hypertens 1991;4:199–205.
322a. Giugliano D, et al. Metabolic and cardiovascular effects of carvedilol and atenolol in non-insulin dependent diabetes mellitus and hypertension. Ann Intern Med 1997;126:955–959.
323. Chan P, et al. The effectiveness and safety of low dose pravastatin in elderly hypertensive hypercholesterolemic subjects on antihypertensive therapy. Am J Hypertens 1995;8:1099–1104.
324. Jones E, et al. Prevalence of left ventricular hypertrophy in elderly patients with well controlled hypertension. Clin Exp Pharmacol Physiol 1990;17:207–210.
325. Starr JM, Whalley LJ. Hypertensive old people in Edinburgh (Hope) Study: electrocardiographic changes after captopril and bendrofluazide treatment. Age and Aging 1993;22:343–348.
326. James MA, Fotherby MD, Potter JF. Clinical correlates of left ventricular mass in elderly hypertensives. J Hum Hypertens 1994;8:409–415.
327. Kahn S, et al. Left ventricular hypertrophy on electrocardiogram: prognostic implications from a 10 year cohort study of older subjects: a report from the Bronx longitudinal aging study. J Am Geriatr Soc 1996;44:524–529.
327a. Pearson AC, et al. Echocardiographic evaluation of cardiac structure and function in elderly subjects with isolated systolic hypertension. J Am Coll Cardiol 1991;17: 422–430.
327b. Heesen WF, et al. High prevalence of concentric remodeling in elderly individuals with isolated systolic hypertension from a population survey. Hypertension 1997;29:539–543.
328. Kannel WB. Prevalence and natural history of electrocardiographic left ventricular hypertrophy. Am J Med 1983;75(suppl 3A):4–11.

329. Messerli FH, et al. Hypertension and sudden death increased ventricular ectopy activity in left ventricular hypertrophy. Am J Med 1984;77:18–22.
330. Kannel WB, Levy D, Cupples LA. Left ventricular hypertrophy and risk of cardiac failure. The Framingham Study. Circulation 1986;74(suppl 2):76A.
331. Devereux RB, et al. Cost-effectiveness of echocardiography and electrocardiography for detection of left ventricular hypertrophy in patients with systemic hypertension. Hypertension 1987;9(suppl II):69–76.
332. Messerli F, Losem CJ, Kaesser VR. Left ventricular hypertrophy. Effect of antihypertensive therapy. Drug Ther 1989;7:34–43.
333. Dahlof B, Pennert K, Hansson L. Reversal of left ventricular hypertrophy in hypertensive patients. Am J Hypertens 1992;5:95–110.
333a. Schulman SP, et al. The effects of antihypertensive therapy on left ventricular mass in the elderly. N Engl J Med 1990;322:1350–1356.
334. Applegate WB, Phillips HL, Schnaper H. A randomized controlled trial of the effects of three antihypertensive agents on blood pressure control and quality of life in older women. Arch Intern Med 1995;151:1817–1823.
335. Starr JM, Whalley LJ. Senile hypertension and cognitive impairment: an overview. J Hypertens 1992;10(suppl 2):S31–S42.
336. Applegate WB, et al. Impact of the treatment of isolated systolic hypertension on behavioral variables. Results from the systolic hypertension in the elderly program. Arch Intern Med 1994;154:2154–2160.
337. Croog SH, et al. Effects of antihypertensive medications on quality of life in elderly hypertensive women. Am J Hypertens 1994;7:329–339.
338. Leonetti G, Salvetti A. The effects of cilazapril and nitrendipine on blood pressure, mood, sleep and cognitive function in elderly hypertensives: an Italian multicentre study. Am J Hypertens 1993;6:1132(Abstract 119).
339. Holzgreve H. Managing the elderly hypertensive patient beyond blood pressure reduction. J Hypertens 1995;13(suppl 2):S103–S107.
340. Prince MJ, et al. Is the cognitive function of older patients affected by antihypertensive treatment? Results from 54 months of the medical research council's treatment trial of hypertension in older adults. Br Med J 1996;312:801–805.
340a. Anderson RT, et al. Baseline correlates with quality of life among men and women with medication-controlled hypertension: The trial of nonpharmacologic interventions in the elderly (TONE). J Am Geriatr Soc 1997;45:1080–1085.
341. Starr JM, Whalley LJ, Deary IJ. The effects of antihypertensive treatment on cognitive function: results from the Hope Study. J Am Geriatr Soc 1996;44:411–415.
341a. Okumiya K, et al. J-Curve relation between blood pressure and decline in cognitive function in older people living in a community in Japan. J Am Geriatr Soc 1997;45: 1032–1035.
342. Anderson RJ, Read WG. Current concepts in the treatment of hypertensive urgencies. Am Heart J 1986;111:211–219.
343. Lip GYH, Bewers M, Bewers GD. Complications and survival of 315 patients with malignant phase hypertension. J Hypertens 1995;13:915–924.
343a. Lip GYH, et al. Malignant hypertension in the elderly. Q J Med 1995;88:641–647.
344. Zampaglione B, et al. Hypertensive urgencies and emergencies. Hypertension 1996; 27:144–147.

345. Isles CG, McLay A, Boulton Jones JM. Recovery in malignant hypertension presenting as acute renal failure. Q J Med 1984;53:439–452.
346. Cressman MD, et al. Intravenous labetolol in the management of severe hypertension and hypertensive emergencies. Am Heart J 1984;107:980–985.
347. DeQuattro V. Treating hypertensive crisis: which drug for which patient. J Crit Illness 1987;2:24–35.
348. Ledingham JGG. Management of hypertensive crisis. Hypertension 1983;5(suppl 3):114–1198.
349. Given BD, et al. Nifedipine in severely hypertensive patients with congestive heart failure and preserved ventricular systolic function. Arch Intern Med 1985;145:281–285.
350. Jaker M, et al. Oral nifedipine versus oral clonidine in the treatment of urgent hypertension. Arch Intern Med 1989;149:260–265.
351. Anderson RJ, et al. Oral clonidine loading in hypertensive urgencies. JAMA 1981;246:848–850.
352. Spitalewitz S, Porush JG, Oguagha C. Use of oral clonidine for rapid titration of blood pressure in severe hypertension. Chest 1983;83(suppl):404–407.
353. Haft J, Litterer WE. Chewing nifedipine to rapidly treat hypertension. Arch Intern Med 1984;144:2356–2359.
354. McAllister RG. Kinetics and dynamics of nifedipine after oral and sublingual doses. Am J Med 1986;81(suppl 6A):2–5.
355. Harten JV, et al. Negligible sublingual absorption of nifedipine. Lancet 1987;2:1363–1365.
356. Conen D, Bertel O. Oral calcium antagonist for treatment of hypertensive emergencies. J Cardiovasc Pharmacol 1982;4:S378–S382.
357. Lacche A, Bagagglia P. Hypertensive emergencies: effects of therapy by nifedipine administered sublingually. Curr Ther Res 1973;34:879.
358. Houston MC. Treatment of hypertensive urgencies and emergencies with nifedipine. Am Heart J 1986;111:963–969.
358a. Grossman E, et al. Should a moratorium be placed on sublingual nifedipine capsules given for hypertensive emergencies and pseudoemergencies? JAMA 1996;276:1328–1331.
359. Case DB, et al. Acute and chronic treatment of severe and malignant hypertension with the oral converting enzyme inhibitor captopril. Circulation 1981;64:765–771.
360. Davies AB, et al. Rapid reduction of blood pressure with acute oral labetolol. Br J Clin Pharmacol 1982;3:705–710.
361. Campese WM, Stein D, DeQuattro V. Treatment of severe hypertension with minoxidil: advantages and limitations. J Clin Pharmacol 1979;19:231–241.
362. Danielson M, Dammström BG. The prevalence of secondary and curable hypertension. Acta Med Scand 1981;209:451–455.
363. Melicow MM. One-hundred cases of pheochromocytoma (107) tumors at the Columbia Presbyterian Medical Center 1926–1976. Cancer 1977;40:1987–2004.
364. Modlin IM, et al. Pheochromocytomas in 72 patients: clinical and diagnostic features, treatment and long term results. Br J Surg 1979;66:456–465.
365. Ganguly A, et al. Diagnosis and localization of pheochromocytoma. Am J Med 1979;67:21–26.

366. St John Sutton MG, Sheps SG, Lie JT. Prevalence of clinically unsuspected pheochromocytoma. Mayo Clin Proc 1981;56:354–360.
367. Stenström G, Svärdsudd K. Pheochromocytoma in Sweden 1958–1981. Acta Med Scand 1986;220:225–232.
368. Shub C, et al. Echocardiographic findings in pheochromocytoma. Am J Cardiol 1986;57:971–975.
369. Stenström G, Ernest I, Tisell LE. Long-term results in 64 patients operated upon for pheochromocytoma. Acta Med Scand 1988;223:345–352.
370. Havlik RJ, Cahow EC, Kinder BK. Advances in the diagnosis and treatment of pheochromocytoma. Arch Surg 1988;123:626–630.
371. Cooper ME, et al. Pheochromocytoma in the elderly: a poorly recognized entity? Br Med J 1986;293:1474–1475.
372. Bravo EL, et al. Circulating and urinary catecholamines in pheochromocytoma. N Engl J Med 1979;301:682–686.
373. Bravo E, et al. A reevaluation of the hemodynamics of pheochromocytoma. Hypertension 1990;15(suppl I):128–131.
374. Brunjes S, Johns VJ Jr, Crane MG. Pheochromocytoma. Postoperative shock and blood volume. N Engl J Med 1960;262:393–396.
375. Bravo EL, et al. Blood pressure regulation in pheochromocytoma. Hypertension 1982;4(suppl II):193–199.
376. Pruyo A, et al. Total plasma dopamine and norepinephrine ratio in catecholamine-secreting tumors. Hypertension 1988;11(suppl I):202–206.
377. Tsujimoto G, Manger WM, Hoffman BB. Desensitization of beta adrenergic receptors by pheochromocytoma. Endocrinolgy 1984;114:1272–1278.
378. Lakatta ED. Age-related alterations in the cardiovascular response to adrenergic mediated stress. Fed Proc 1980;39:3172–3177.
379. Bravo EL, Gifford RW Jr. Pheochromocytoma diagnosis, localization and management. N Engl J Med 1984;311:1298–1302.
380. Young JB, et al. Enhanced plasma norepinephrine response to upright posture and oral glucose administration in elderly human subjects. Metabolism 1980;29:532–539.
381. Lenders JWM, et al. Plasma metanephrines in the diagnosis of pheochromocytoma. Ann Intern Med 1995;123:101–109.
382. Ganguly A, et al. Diagnosis and localization of pheochromocytoma. Detection by measurement of urinary norepinephrine excretion during sleep, plasma norepinephrine concentration and computerized axial tomography (CT scan). Am J Med 1979;67:21–26.
383. Levine SN, McDonald JC. The evaluation and management of pheochromocytomas. Adv Surg 1984;17:281–331.
384. Bravo EL. Evolving concepts in the pathophysiology, diagnosis and treatment of pheochromocytoma. Endocrin Rev 1994;15:356–368.
385. McEwan AJ, et al. Radioiodobenzylguanidine for the scintigraphic location and therapy of adrenergic tumors. Sem Nuclear Med 1985;15:132–153.
386. Editorial. Iodobenzylguanidine for location and treatment of pheochromocytoma. Lancet 1984;2:905–907.

387. Hull CJ. Pheochromocytoma. Diagnosis, preoperative preparation and anesthetic management. Br J Anaesth 1986;58:1453–1468.
388. Shapiro B, Fig LM. Management of pheochromocytoma. Endocrinol Metab Clin NA 1989;18:443–447.
389. Proye C, et al. Exclusive use of calcium channel blockers in preoperative and intraoperative control of pheochromocytomas: hemodynamics and free catecholamine assay in ten consecutive patients. Surgery 1989;106:1149–1154.
390. Gröndel S, et al. Adenosine: a new antihypertensive agent during pheochromocytoma. World J Surg 1988;12:581–585.
391. Nadeiros JL, et al. Adrenal pheochromocytoma: a clinicopathologic review of 60 cases. Hum Pathol 1985;16:580–589.
392. Hamada M, et al. Blood pressure response to the Valsalva maneuver in pheochromocytoma and pseudopheochromocytoma. Hypertension 1995;25:266–271.
393. Robertson D, et al. The diagnosis and treatment of baroreflex failure. N Engl J Med 1993;329:1449–1455.
394. Streeten DHP, Tomycz N, Anderson GH Jr. Reliability screening methods for the diagnosis of primary aldosteronism. Am J Med 1979;67:403–413.
395. Bravo EL, et al. Clinical implications of primary aldosteronism with resistant hypertension. Hypertension 1988;11(suppl 1):207–211.
396. Lim RC Jr, et al. Primary aldosteronism: changing concepts in diagnosis and management. Am J Surg 1986;152:116–121.
397. Artaega E, et al. Aldosterone-producing adrenocortical carcinoma. Preoperative recognition and course in three cases. Ann Intern Med 1984;101:316–321.
398. Tarazi RC, et al. Hemodynamic characteristics of primary hyperaldosteromisn. N Engl J Med 1973;289:1330–1335.
399. Carey RM, et al. Idiopathic hyperaldosteronism. A possible role for aldosterone-stimulating factor. N Engl J Med 1984;311:94–100.
400. White EA, et al. Use of computed tomography in diagnosing the cause of primary aldosteronism N Engl J Med 1980;303:1503–1507.
401. Dunnick NR, et al. Localization of functional adrenal tumors by computed tomography and venous sampling. Radiology 1982;142:429–433.
402. Young WR Jr, Klee GG. Primary aldosteronism, diagnostic evaluation. Endocrinol Metab Clin NA 1988;17:367–377.
403. Mantero F, et al. Mineralocorticoid-hypertension due to a nasal spray containing 9 alpha-fluoroprednisolone. Am J Med 1981;71:352–357.
404. Lins PE, Adamson V. Primary aldosteronism. A follow-up study of 28 cases of surgically treated aldosterone-producing adenomas. Acta Clin Scand 1987;221: 275–282.
405. Hofnagels WHL, et al. Spironolactone and amiloride in hypertensive patients with or without aldosterone excess. Clin Pharmacol Ther 1980;27:317–323.
406. Ganguly A, Weinberger MH. Triamterene-thiazide combination;alternative therapy for primary aldosteronism. Clin Pharmacol Ther 1981;30:246–250.
407. Griffing GT, et al. Amiloride in primary aldosteronism. Clin Pharm Ther 1982;31:56–61.
408. Nadler JL, Hsueh W, Horton R. Therapeutic effect of calcium channel blockade in primary aldosteronism. J Clin Endocrinol Metab 1985;60:896–899.

409. Griffing GT, Melby JC. The therapeutic effect of a new angiotensin converting enzyme inhibitor, enalapril maleate, in idiopathic hyperaldosteronism. J Clin Hypertens 1985;1:265–268.
410. Bertagna C, Orth DN. Clinical and laboratory findings and results of therapy in 58 patients with adrenocortical tumors admitted to a single medical center (1951–1978). Am J Med 1981;71:855–875.
411. Donckier J, et al. Successful control of Cushing's disease in the elderly with long-term metyrapone. Postgrad Med J 1986;62:727–730.
412. Aron DC, Tyrell JB. Cushing's syndrome. Endocr Metabol Clin NA 1994;23:451–698.
413. Saruta T, et al. Multiple factors contribute to the pathogenesis of hypertension in Cushing's syndrome. J Clin Endocrinol Metab 1986;62:275–279.
414. Sato A, et al. Glucocorticoid-induced hypertension in the elderly. Am J Hypertens 1995;8:823–828.
415. LaPalio L, et al. Safety and efficacy of metoprolol in the treatment of hypertension in the elderly. J Am Geriatr Soc 1992;40:354–358.
416. Holwerda NJ, et al. Valsartan, a new angiotensin-II antagonist for the treatment of essential hypertension: efficacy and safety compared with placebo and enalapril. J Hypertens 1996;14:1147–1151.

13

Vascular Disease of the Kidney

Both renal arteries and veins can be involved by various disease processes, as summarized in Table 1. The vascular diseases of the degenerative group are the most common cause of renal insufficiency in the elderly.

I. ARTERIAL DISEASE

A. Inflammatory Disease

Inflammatory disease (vasculitis) is discussed in Chapter 7.

B. Degenerative Vascular Diseases

1. Atherosclerosis

a. Incidence and Prevalence. Renal artery stenosis (RAS) secondary to atheromatous disease is common in subjects over the age of 50 years (1,2). In autopsy series, the prevalence of RAS varies between 18% in patients 65 to 74 years and 42–62% for those over the age of 75 (3–5). In studies of older patients undergoing coronary and abdominal angiography, unsuspected RAS (>50% luminal narrowing) is found in 11–23% (6). The incidence is even higher (14–57%) in patients with known aorto-iliac occlusive disease or other forms of peripheral vascular disease (6). RAS may be responsible for end-stage renal disease in 14% of patients over the age of 50 (7), 6.7% for those aged 78–81 years, and 16.5% for those aged 82–85 years (8).

Table 1 Classification of Vascular Disease of the Kidney in the Elderly

Arterial disease
Inflammatory: vasculitis
Degenerative
Atherosclerosis
Embolic disease
Nephrosclerosis (arteriosclerosis)
Venous disease
Renal vein thrombosis

b. Clinical Manifestations and Pathogenesis. Most patients with renal artery disease are asymptomatic. The diagnosis should be considered in any elderly subject with: (a) recent onset of hypertension; (b) worsening of hypertension that was previously controlled; (c) malignant hypertension (particularly in whites); (d) recurrent pulmonary edema in the presence of well-maintained left ventricular systolic function (9); (e) evidence of peripheral vascular disease elsewhere, particularly if the patient is a smoker (10,11); (f) a rapid decrease in renal function despite good blood pressure control, particularly if an ACEI is used (12); (g) diabetes mellitus and hypertension (13). In addition to these criteria, 50% of elderly patients with azotemia and hypertension refractory to two or more drug therapy will have renovascular disease (14,14a). On examination, hypertension is present in 65–70%. Abdominal auscultation may reveal a high-pitched systolic and/or diastolic bruit in the periumbilical area or paravertebrally, with radiation laterally. Bruits over carotid or femoral vessels or an aortic aneurysm are commonly present. In addition, evidence of end-organ damage (retinopathy or left ventricular enlargement) is frequently present (14b).

Urinalysis is generally unremarkable, although proteinuria, even greater than 1 g has been reported (15). Renal insufficiency is present in more than 50% of patients. On kidney-uretero-bladder (KUB) films, renal tomograms, or sonograms, a discrepancy (of >1.5 cm) in kidney size may be found.

Stenosis of the renal arteries may be responsible for two clinical syndromes, renovascular hypertension and ischemic nephropathy, which frequently coexist in the elderly.

i. Renovascular Hypertension. Our understanding of the pathogenesis of renovascular hypertension is based mainly on experimental data (16,16a). During the initiation phase, the elevation in the blood pressure results from an increase in peripheral vascular resistance due to high circulating angiotensin II (AII), originating from the poorly perfused kidney. At a later stage, both an increase in circulating blood volume and peripheral resistance contribute to maintaining the hypertension. The former results from stimulation of aldosterone production by AII as well as other intrarenal mechanisms leading to an increase in renal sodium (Na) reabsorption and volume expansion. An increase in central pressor mechanisms, most likely linked to AII and central sympathetic activation (17), an upregulation of the angiotensin gene expression with increase receptor production (18), downregulation of the vasodilator kallikrein genes (19), and structural changes in systemic blood vessels (remodeling) (20) all contribute to the persistently increased peripheral resistance. Finally, as reviewed elsewhere (16a), there is some evidence that AII may shift the arachidonic acid metabolism from the synthesis of prostaglandins to the synthesis of lipoxygenase products which are vasoconstrictors and could potentially amplify the vasoconstrictive effect of AII.

ii. Ischemic Nephropathy. Ischemic nephropathy is defined as renal insufficiency resulting from a decrease in renal perfusion associated with bilateral RAS or RAS in a solitary kidney (1,2,21–23). On histological examination, glomerular sclerosis, either focal or global, interstitial fibrosis, and tubular atrophy are noted. The mechanism(s) by which RAS alters glomerular filtration rate is not well understood. Computed tomography-derived intrarenal blood flow measurements comparing patients with fibrodysplastic RAS to those with atherosclerotic disease have demonstrated a more marked reduction in whole kidney and renal cortical perfusion in the latter group. Furthermore, no relationship is found between whole or regional kidney perfusion and the severity of the stenosis in the atherosclerotic group, in contrast to the fibrodysplastic group (24). Altered balance among the various locally synthesized vasoactive substances (endothelin, atrial natriuretic peptide, AII, endothelium-derived nitric oxide, etc.), as well as altered intracellular metabolism, probably contribute to nephron death and subsequent renal impairment seen with ischemic nephropathy (25).

c. Diagnosis. The investigation of an elderly patient with suspected renal artery stenosis should start with a determination of kidney function, as assessed by the serum creatinine and/or creatinine clearance, examination of the urine sediment, and 24-hr protein excretion. A renal sonogram will provide an estimate of kidney size and discrepancies in size and also can be used to rule out obstructive uropathy. Time-honored initial screening procedures such as the rapid sequence intravenous pyelogram (IVP), isotope renography, plasma renin activity, and intravenous substraction angiography are now replaced by renography following the oral administration of 50 mg of captopril. Three tracers, ^{99}Tc-DTPA, ^{131}I-hippuran with or without furosemide, and ^{99}Tc-MAG$_3$, are presently in use. The choice of one over the other depends on availability and familiarity with the agent used, since sensitivities of 90–92% and specificities of 92–96% have been reported for all three, particularly in unilateral disease (26,27). A lower sensitivity level (65%) has been reported by others, however (27a). TcMAG$_3$ is best in patients with a serum creatinine greater than 2 mg/dl (27b). Their diagnostic accuracy is limited in the presence of bilateral RAS or RAS to a solitary kidney with or without azotemia.

Renal duplex scanning, by determining the ratio of peak systolic velocities in the renal artery and the aorta, has been found to be the best predicting Doppler parameter for detecting RAS greater than 60%, with a 87% sensitivity and 92% specificity. It has been suggested that a captopril test (determining peripheral plasma renin activity before and 60 min following the oral administration of 50 mg of captopril) in combination with duplex scanning may increase its overall diagnostic accuracy (27c). A small kidney (<8.5 cm) in addition to an absent Doppler signal suggests complete arterial occlusion (26,28). This test, unfortunately, is time consuming and operator dependent. These drawbacks tend to limit its diagnostic usefulness.

Spiral CT angiography offers great promise and is particularly accurate in localizing ostial lesions. However, intravenous contrast is required, and the specificity tends to decrease in the presence of renal insufficiency (29–31). Three-dimension phase-contrast magnetic resonance angiography (MRA) has been found to be quite accurate in depicting disease in the proximal portion of the renal artery. Distal renal artery and its branches are usually poorly visualized. One advantage is that no contrast medium is required (32,32a). This test might eventually become the most useful one for diagnosing renal artery disease in the elderly. Unfortunately, the test is rather expensive and is contraindicated in patients with ferromagnetic implants.

The first question the clinician should answer when facing an elderly patient with a strong suspicion of renal artery disease is whether correction of the lesion (if found) is necessary and feasible. If so, then arteriography should be carried out without preliminary screening tests in order to make a definitive diagnosis (33). Either conventional or intraarterial digital substraction angiography can be used. Because of the increased risk of nephrotoxicity due to contrast agents in the elderly with vascular disease and associated renal insufficiency, it is necessary to take precautions to avoid acute renal failure by preventing dehydration, correcting heart failure if present, and administering furosemide or mannitol (or both) immediately after the injection of the contrast agent (see Chapter 10).

If the index of suspicion for renal artery disease is not very high, one should start with one of the screening tests outlined above. A positive test is an indication for an arteriogram, if therapeutic intervention is anticipated.

d. Natural History and Therapy.

i. Renovascular Hypertension. The presence of a stenotic lesion on the arteriogram does not necessarily indicate that the lesion is causing hypertension (34). In an autopsy study of 114 elderly patients with RAS reported by Holley et al. (35), 66 patients had moderate disease (more than one-third and less than two-thirds involvement of the intimal surface by atheromatous plaques). Five (8%) of the patients with moderate disease were hypertensive, and four of these (80%) had bilateral disease. Fifteen (31%) of the patients with severe disease (greater than two-thirds involvement of the intimal surface) were hypertensive, 13 of whom (87%) had bilateral disease. Physicians have relied on renal vein renin determinations to predict cure or improvement in blood pressure following surgical or angioplastic intervention (36); a ratio of 1.5:1 or greater has been accepted as highly predictive of success. This technique, has a significant false-negative rate and therefore cannot be adopted as the sole criterion in making the decision to intervene (37); however, when combined with a positive captopril renogram, this test is a good predictor of blood pressure response to intervention.

In patients with unilateral RAS and hypertension, four choices of therapy are available: drug therapy, surgery, percutaneous transluminal angioplasty (PCTA), with and without a stent placement. The choice of treatment should be tailored to the individual patient. Since 88% of elderly patients with RAS have generalized atherosclerosis with a high incidence of renal insufficiency or renovascular hypertension superimposed on essential hypertension, a prudent approach is to reserve the invasive interventions for patients whose blood pressure cannot be controlled with an appropriate drug regimen (38). The percentage of patients requiring intervention for blood pressure control alone decreased from 42% during 1975–1980 to 26% during 1981–1984 (39). Patients who fail to respond to medical therapy and those who have complete occlusion of the renal artery with postocclusion retrograde filling may benefit from either surgery or PCTA with or without stent placement. Surgery consists of either endarterectomy or revascularization (aortorenal, splenorenal, or hepatorenal bypass). In some patients, simultaneous aortic surgery (aneurysm repair) may be necessary. Those with a small kidney (<8 cm in length), with little or no function assessed by differential nuclear scanning, should probably have a nephrectomy (21,40). Surgery in the elderly does not appear to be associated with a higher risk compared to younger patients, if patients are carefully selected. Therefore, criteria such as co-morbid conditions and surgical expertise rather than age per se should be taken into consideration when making a decision about surgery (1,2,11,21,40).

PCTA consists of a controlled disruption of the arterial wall, performed with a fluoroscopically placed balloon. The latter is inflated to a diameter approximately 1 or 2 mm greater than the internal diameter of the healthy portion of the renal artery. Dilatation occurs by splitting the atheroma and making radial and longitudinal tears between the intima and media of the artery, with the adventitia (the portion of the vessel wall most resistant to dilatation) stretched and ballooned outward (41,42). This technique has been used successfully in elderly patients with renovascular hypertension by several groups (43–47). The overall technical success rate is 40–82%, and improvement in blood pressure is noted in approximately 60%, but cure is achieved in only 8–14% (46–49), similar to the results reported with surgical intervention (50–51). The lowest success rate was found in patients with ostial lesions, which are present in 80–85% of the elderly with renal artery disease. We share Vidt's recommendation that PCTA should be restricted to patients with focal, nonostial lesions (52). Complications include acute renal failure (which is not always reversible), hematomas (either retroperitoneal or at the puncture site), and microembolization of the kidneys, bowel, and lower extremities by atheromatous fragments. Renal artery occlusion and rupture have been reported; thus, the surgical team should be prepared to intervene on an emergency basis whenever PCTA is attempted (53,54). Recurrent stenosis does occur, the incidence varying from 0 to 23% (47,55).

Endovascular stent insertion with or without PTCA should be given strong consideration in elderly with an ostial lesion in whom surgery is not feasible or when PCTA has failed. Technical success rates in stent placement as high as 95% have been reported (56,56a). Restenosis occurs during the first 6–11 months in 20–30% of patients and often can be managed by PTCA. The percentage of patients with cure or improvement in blood pressure following the procedure varies between 16% and 64%, somewhat lower than surgery or angioplasty, probably because of bias in deciding which patients require the procedure (56–60a). Following stenting, patients should be maintained on ticlopidine, 250 mg twice daily, or clopidogrel 75 mg once daily, and aspirin, 100 mg twice daily, rather than coumadin (61). When ticlopidine is used, the white blood cell count should be monitored every other week, since neutropenia, not always reversible, tends to occur 3–4 weeks after initiating therapy. The drug is usually discontinued after 4 weeks.

Patients with unilateral RAS and renovascular hypertension should be followed closely, since 14–17% will develop de-novo stenosis in the contralateral kidney within 28 months, and 27% will develop it within 56 months (51,62).

ii. Ischemic Nephropathy. Ischemic nephropathy is present in 50–80% of elderly subjects with atheromatous disease of the renal arteries (1,2,21–23, 39,63,63a). Although no large prospective study has compared the long-term outcome with the therapeutic options discussed above, a variety of retrospective series suggest that patients managed medically have poorer long-term renal function and survival than those treated with either surgery or angioplasty (64–66). In one study, the 2-year patient survival was 74% for medically treated patients with bilateral stenosis and 47% for those with unilateral occlusion plus contralateral stenosis. In these two groups, 68% and 55%, respectively required dialysis within a 2-year period (63a). The poor prognosis in these patients is probably explained by the progressive nature of atherosclerotic disease, but may also be worsened by cholesterol embolization (23,67). In a group of 85 medically treated patients with RAS followed by Schreiber and associates (68), serial arteriograms indicated progression of the stenosis in 44%. In patients with less than 50% stenosis, progression was noted in 31% (5% developed complete occlusion). In lesions with greater than 75% stenosis, approximately 40% progressed to complete occlusion. Similar findings have been reported by Zucchelli et al. (5), Tollefson and Ernst (62), and Zierler et al. (69). Progression tends to occur relatively early, usually within 2 years following the initial arteriography, and is usually manifested clinically by a reduction in kidney size and a decrease in renal function in those with bilateral disease (70). The cumulative incidence of progression to occlusion in arteries with greater than 60% stenosis was found to be 4–5% at 1 year, 4–11% at 2 years, and 7% at 3 years (69,69a).

At the present time, the best approach in terms of timing and type of intervention in the elderly with ischemic nephropathy remains to be determined. Part of the difficulty lies in the fact that there is no reliable way to predict which patients will benefit from intervention (69b,69c). In general, better outcome may be expected in those who have a positive captopril renal scan and lateralization of renal veins renin (47), those who have collateral circulation (which may be visualized by angiography) that is adequate to maintain organ survival but insufficient to maintain adequate excretory function, and those who had a rapid worsening in kidney function, at times severe enough to require dialytic therapy (71–76b). In contrast, patients with a serum creatinine greater than 4 mg/dl (22,77–80), small kidneys (<7 cm), and those with macroalbuminuria (albumin excretion greater than 200 μg/min) do not fare as well (81).

The choice among surgery, PCTA, or stenting should be individualized. Consideration should be given to the presence of a significant contraindication to surgery (advanced coronary disease, poor general condition), the local expertise and technical success rate for each approach, and the location of the lesion(s) (ostial lesions for the most part should not be treated by PCTA). The degree of success (defined either as improvement or stabilization of kidney function) for the three therapeutic modalities has varied among different investigators. Most of the reports are retrospective, making it difficult to compare the modalities (51,56,57, 77–79,82–83a). Fifty-five percent of the patients managed surgically improve, 31% stabilize, and 14% deteriorate (83b). Following PCTA, 43% of the patients improve; the remaining 57% either stabilize or deteriorate (83c). In the elderly, revascularization is associated with a 40% major morbidity (respiratory failure, cardiovascular complications) and a mortality rate of 6%, somewhat higher than for younger patients undergoing the same procedure, and increases with the severity of the renal disease (63,83d,83e). In general, patients who improve do so early following intervention; however, long-term follow-up is sorely needed in these patients. Kidney function generally continues to deteriorate in those patients who did not improve following surgery (83a).

In a recent study evaluating the long-term anatomical results of PCTA with serial duplex ultrasonographic examination, the cumulative incidence of restenosis was found to depend on the initial anatomic result. In patients with a successful (100%) dilatation, the cumulative incidence of restenosis to greater than 60% was 13% at 1 year and 55% at 2 years. In those patients where only partial dilatation (to less than 60% stenosis) was achieved, the cumulative incidence of restenosis to greater than 60% was 44% at 1 year and 55% at 2 years. Better initial results were found with PCTA associated with stent placement, but the long-term results were a lot worse in the stented vessels (83f). The restenosis rate was 44% in the stented arteries and 18% in the nonstented vessels. Better results of stenting have been reported by Blum et al. (60a), who noted that restenosis to more than 50% occurred in only 11% of their patients followed for an average of 27 months.

The patients who undergo surgery, PCTA, or stenting should be followed on a regular basis with periodic determination of serum creatinine or creatinine clearance, nephrotomographic studies to follow kidney size, and either Doppler or MRA studies. Deterioration in kidney function or a reduction in kidney mass is an indication for repeat angiography to determine the need for further intervention.

2. *Embolic Disease*

a. Renal Artery Embolism of Cardiac Origin. Renal artery embolism has been found in 1.4% of 4411 autopsies reported by Hoxie and Coggin (84). The elderly account for approximately 36% of reported patients (85,86). Seventy percent of the patients have atrial fibrillation at the time of diagnosis. In the remaining 30%, renal artery embolization was associated with a recent acute myocardial infarction, cardiomyopathy with associated congestive heart failure, or bacterial endocarditis. The disease usually presents with a sudden onset of flank pain associated with nausea and vomiting. On physical examination, low-grade fever, costovertebral angle tenderness, moderate abdominal guarding, and hypoactive bowel sounds are usually present. Hypertension is also quite frequent. Patients with bilateral embolization or embolization to a solitary kidney (50% of patients) may be oliguric or anuric. Mild to moderate leukocytosis and an elevated serum lactic dehydrogenase (LDH) are found in most patients. The rise in LDH occurs within 24 hr of renal infarction and persists for up to 14 days. Renal insufficiency is found in 90%. The urinalysis usually reveals proteinuria (1–4+) and hematuria. On renal scan, there is absence of blood flow to an entire kidney or segment of a kidney.

The differential diagnosis of renal artery embolization includes acute pyelonephritis (which most often presents with pyuria and bacteriuria) and acute nephrolithiasis, with or without obstruction, which should always be ruled out by a KUB and sonographic studies. The definitive diagnosis is made angiographically (87–90), with the demonstration of an occlusion or a filling defect in the renal artery. Once the diagnosis has been made, therapy should be initiated with intraarterial streptokinase at a dose of 9000 U/hr for the first hour, followed by a maintenance dose of 5000 U/hr until the clot lyses or 36 hr (whichever comes first) (91). Higher doses have been used by others—200,000 U intravenously given over 20–30 min, followed by 100,000 U/hr given by a constant-infusion pump for 8 hr (92). Once the desired therapeutic effect has been achieved, intravenous heparin at the usual dose, followed by oral Warfarin is indicated (93). The kidney salvage rate, which does not necessarily correlate with the duration of occlusion, with this approach is approximately 75%, and compares favorably with the 83% salvage rate reported with embolectomy (93a,93b). Transluminal angioplasty or surgery should be reserved for patients who fail to improve with lysis therapy (94). Long-term anticoagulation should be continued in every patient.

b. Cholesterol Embolization. Cholesterol embolism is part of the entity referred to as atheromatous renal disease by Meyrier and colleagues (23), in which the renal disease is due either to atheromatous stenosis of the renal artery alone (69% of cases), or cholesterol emboli alone (6% of cases), or a combination of both (25% of cases). In another study of 24 patients with biopsy-proven renal cholesterol emboli, renal artery stenosis (either unilateral or bilateral) was found in 19 (79%) (67). The true incidence of cholesterol embolism-induced renal failure in the elderly is not known, but the elderly account for 63% of the reported cases, with males outnumbering females by a ratio of 8.6:1.4 (67,95–100). Renal cholesterol embolization usually develops in patients with extensive atherosclerosis of the aorta as well as clinical and laboratory evidence of vascular disease elsewhere (101). It may occur following spontaneous detachment of atheromatous plaques from the aorta (102) or following aortic surgery (103,104), aortography (105–107), percutaneous transluminal angioplasty of coronary (108) or renal vessels (109), and after thrombolytic therapy for an acute myocardial infarction (110). Renal cholesterol emboli were found at autopsy in 30% of patients who die within 6 months following aortography (111). Embolization occurs in 25% of patients undergoing repair for an aortic aneurysm and in 1.4–30% of patients following angioplasty (109). Spontaneous cholesterol embolization occurs in 0.8–4.2% of the general population (111,112).

The diagnosis of cholesterol embolism should be suspected whenever renal failure develops in an elderly patient subjected to any of the procedures described above, particularly if other systemic manifestations are present, such as skin discoloration (purple toes, livedo reticularis), retinal embolism, or multiple visceral involvement, including the small and large bowel and the pancreas. The central nervous system and the spinal cord may also be involved as part of the so-called multiple cholesterol embolization syndrome (113).

Renal dysfunction may become manifest anytime from hours to 2–6 weeks following the initial event. The kidney disease tends to be progressive to end-stage kidney disease requiring dialysis; in some patients, however, the disease follows a more indolent course, and there is subsequent improvement in function, occasionally even after maintenance dialysis has been initiated (95,98). In the majority of elderly hypertensive patients with cholesterol emboli, acute worsening of hypertension is seen, which is often difficult to control, probably related to activation of the renin-angiotensin system (114). The erythrocyte sedimentation rate and the white blood cell count are usually elevated. Eosinophilia has been reported (115), as well as hypocomplementia (97). It is postulated that atheromatous emboli activate complement either directly by surface contact or indirectly through enzymes of the coagulation system. In fact, the eosinophilia may be related to activation of the complement system, since C5a is chemotactic for eosinophils (116). The urinary sediment is nonspecific. Proteinuria, when present, is minimal, although values greater than 3 g per 24 hr have been reported (101,117). In some of these patients, a variant of focal segmental glomerulosclerosis (epithelial cell proliferation and capillary loop collapse) may be present on histological examination of the kidneys (117a).

Definitive diagnosis of renal cholesterol embolization depends on the demonstration in the kidney biopsy of the biconcave, needle-shaped clefts (which remain after dissolution of the cholesterol crystals during routine histological preparation) in the arcuate or interlobular arteries or glomerular tufts, associated with corresponding ischemic changes in the renal parenchyma (118). In patients with livedo reticularis and renal failure, a punch biopsy of the affected skin may reveal similar intravascular clefts (98), obviating the need for kidney biopsy.

In patients who present with hypertension, multiple organ involvement, eosinophilia, and proteinuria, cholesterol embolization may mimic polyarteritis nodosa or other vasculitides involving the kidneys. An active urinary sediment (hematuria, RBC casts) and/or a positive antineutrophilic cytoplasmic autoantibody (ANCA) favors the diagnosis of vasculitis; otherwise, angiographic or histological confirmation is necessary. Contrast medium-induced acute renal failure must be ruled out in patients who have undergone angiography. Dye-induced renal failure, in contrast to cholesterol embolism, is not accompanied by systemic manifestations and follows a shorter and more benign course, with recovery generally taking place in 7–14 days (see Chapter 10). Left atrial myxoma and bacterial endocarditis may occasionally present a clinical picture similar to that of cholesterol embolization. These conditions usually can be diagnosed by physical examination, echocardiography, and blood culture.

The management of renal failure in patients with cholesterol embolization is similar to that of other forms of renal disease. Anticoagulation is of no benefit and may even be harmful, since inhibition of thrombus formation on ulcerated or traumatized atheromatous plaques may render them more brittle and prone to release even more cholesterol crystals (95). Patients who develop acute symptoms and signs of cholesterol embolization following an invasive procedure do very poorly, and the majority of them die with multiple-organ infarction. Those in whom the embolization is spontaneous or have a subacute or chronic course do better and, as noted earlier, may in time recover enough kidney function to discontinue maintenance dialysis, if started (95,99).

3. Nephrosclerosis

Hypertensive nephrosclerosis is a histological diagnosis made when occlusive changes, consisting of myointimal hypertrophy of the interlobular arteries and hyaline thickening of the walls of the afferent arterioles, are found in the kidney of a hypertensive patient with renal insufficiency (119), since these findings could also be a part of aging per se. Clinically, the diagnosis is entertained in a patient with long-standing hypertension who presents with renal insufficiency and proteinuria of less than 1–1.5 g per 24 hr, after other causes of renal disease such as ischemic nephropathy, obstructive uropathy, congenital disease (polycystic kidney disease), and various tubulointerstitial nephritides have been ruled out. Primary glomerulopathies are usually recognized by the presence of relatively large amounts of protein in the urine (more than 2 g per 24 hr). Occasionally, patients with biopsy-proven nephrosclerosis may have this degree of proteinuria (120,121).

The pathogenesis of hypertensive nephrosclerosis is not clear. The rate of decline in renal blood flow seen with age is accelerated in the presence of hypertension (122). Lindeman et al. (123) have shown that a significant correlation exists between the mean arterial blood pressure and the rate of decline in creatinine clearance with time in subjects aged 22–97 years who have been followed serially. Also, the prevalence of serum creatinine concentrations equal to or greater than 1.5 mg/dl increases with age in the hypertensive population (124). This suggests strongly that the histological changes seen in nephrosclerosis result from the hypertension leading to glomerular sclerosis. Glomerular overproduction of transforming growth factor $beta_1$ ($TGF\beta_1$) may contribute to the tubulointerstitial injury by stimulating the synthesis of various extracellular matrix proteins (124a). Other factors, such as genetic susceptibility, metabolic abnormalities, and local immune factors, might also be at work (124b). Even though nephrosclerosis appears to be a leading cause of chronic renal insufficiency in the elderly [72% of patients with hypertensive nephrosclerosis at time of renal biopsy are over the age of 50 years (120)], there is still some controversy about whether clinically significant renal insufficiency occurs in patients with essential hypertension in the absence of malignant or accelerated hypertension (125,126). The problem exists because most patients with the diagnosis of nephrosclerosis do not undergo a kidney biopsy, and often renovascular disease is not adequately excluded (23,127). Furthermore, even when a biopsy has been performed, arteriolarnephrosclerosis may be seen in conjunction with other forms of advanced renal disease, which are no longer diagnosable because of severe glomerulosclerosis, tubular atrophy, and interstitial fibrosis (end-stage kidney). Despite these drawbacks in assessing the incidence of nephrosclerosis and renal failure, there is little doubt that hypertension represents a strong independent risk factor for end-stage renal disease, particularly in blacks (128). Nephrosclerosis was found to be overdiagnosed in 60% of elderly whites with end-stage renal disease in one study (129), but not in elderly blacks (130).

The management of elderly with renal insufficiency secondary to nephrosclerosis requires aggressive blood pressure control. In fact, it has been suggested, but not proven, that the blood pressure be lowered to 135/85 or less (particularly in blacks). Other approaches geared toward slowing the progression of renal failure, as discussed in Chapter 11, should also be introduced in these patients. In our experience and that of others (131), the disease tends either to stabilize or follow a very slow course once BP has been controlled, even when advanced renal insufficiency is present. In some patients, primarily elderly black males, rapid deterioration in renal function occurs despite what has been considered good blood pressure control (132,133). The mechanism responsible for a higher incidence of this phenomenon in blacks is not clear, but appears to be related to several factors including insulin resistance, greater salt sensitivity, a higher vascular sensitivity to various adrenergic stimuli (134), and, perhaps, inadequate lowering of the blood pressure for these patients.

II. VENOUS DISEASE

A. Renal Vein Thrombosis

Renal vein thrombosis may be associated with severe volume contraction, extension of thrombotic disease of the vena cava, involvement of the renal vascular pedicle by cancer or other retroperitoneal disease, and various glomerular diseases associated with the nephrotic syndrome (135). The association of renal vein thrombosis with the nephrotic syndrome is important because it may acutely alter the natural history of the various glomerulopathies and may add significantly to morbidity, as discussed in Chapter 6.

REFERENCES

1. Delin K, et al. Surgical treatment of renovascular hypertension in the elderly patient. Acta Med Scand 1982;211:169–174.
2. Olin JW, et al. Renovascular disease in the elderly: an analysis of 50 patients. J Am Coll Cardiol 1985;5:1232–1238.
3. Vetrovec GW, et al. Frequency of renal artery stenosis in hypertensive patients undergoing coronary angiography. Clin Res 1986;34:205A.
4. Schwarts CJ, White TA. Stenosis of renal artery: an unselected necropsy study. Br Med J 1964;2:1415–1421.
5. Zucchelli P, Zuccala A. Ischemic nephropathy in the elderly. In: Sessa A, Meroni M, Battini G, eds. Glomerulonephritis in the Elderly. Basel, Karger: Contrib Nephrol 1993;105:13–24.
6. Grego BA, Breyer JA. The natural history of renal artery stenosis: who should be evaluated for suspected ischemic nephropathy? Sem Nephrol 1996;16:2–11.
7. Scoble JE, et al. Atherosclerotic renovascular disease causing renal impairment—a case for treatment. Clin Nephrol 1989;31:119–122.
8. Mailloux LU, et al. Predictors of survival in patients undergoing dialysis. Am J Med 1988;84:855–862.
9. Pickering TG, et al. Recurrent pulmonary edema in hypertension due to bilateral renal artery stenosis. Treatment by angioplasty or surgical revascularization. Lancet 1988;2:551–552.

10. Nicholson JP, et al. Cigarette smoking and renovascular hypertension. Lancet 1983; 2:765–766.
11. Van Bockel JH, et al. Surgical treatment of renovascular hypertension caused by arteriosclerosis. II. Influence of preoperative risk factors and postoperative blood pressure response on late patient survival. Surgery 1987;101:468–477.
12. Textor SC, et al. Critical perfusion pressure for renal function in patients with bilateral atherosclerotic renal vascular disease. Ann Intern Med 1985;102:308–314.
13. Sawicki PT, et al. Prevalence of renal artery stenosis in diabetes mellitus—an autopsy study. J Intern Med 1991;229:489–492.
14. Ying CY, et al. Renal revascularization in the azotemic hypertensive patient resistant to therapy. N Engl J Med 1984;311:1070–1075.
14a. Van Jaarsveld BC, et al. Hypertension resistant to two-drug treatment is a useful criterion to select patients for angiography: the Dutch Renal Artery Stenosis Intervention Cooperative (DRASTIC) study. In: Zoccali C, ed. Clinical Hypertension in Nephrology. Basel, Karger: Contrib Nephrol 1996;119:54–58.
14b. Losito A, et al. Comparison of target organ damage in renovascular and essential hypertension. Am J Hypertens 1996;9:1062–1067.
15. Eiser AR, Katz SM, Swartz C. Reversible nephrotic range proteinuria with renal artery stenosis: a clinical example of renin-associated proteinuria. Nephron 1982;30: 374–377.
16. Martinez-Maldonado M. Pathophysiology of renovascular hypertension. Hypertension 1991;17:707–719.
16a. Romero JC, et al. New insights into the pathophysiology of renovascular hypertension. Mayo Clin Proc 1997;72:251–260.
17. Sawamura T, Nakada T. Role of dopamine in the striatum, renin-angiotensin system and renal sympathetic nerve on the development of two-kidney, one-clip Goldblatt hypertension. J Urol 1996;155:1108–1111.
18. Modrull JG, et al. Upregulation of angiotensin II type 1 receptor gene expression in chronic renovascular hypertension. J Surg Res 1995;59:135–140.
19. el-Dahr SS, et al. Renin, angiotensinogen and kallikrein gene expression in two-kidney Goldblatt hypertensive rats. Am J Hypertens 1993;6:914–919.
20. Lee RM, et al. Pathophysiology of smooth muscle in hypertension. Can J Physiol Pharmacol 1995;73:574–584.
21. Geyske CGM, et al. Renovascular hypertension: The small kidney updated. Q J Med 1988;251:203–217.
22. Bedoya L, et al. Baseline renal function and surgical revascularization in atherosclerotic renal artery disease in the elderly. Clev Clin J Med 1989;56:415–421.
23. Meyrier A, et al. Atheromatous renal disease. Am J Med 1988;85:139–146.
24. Lerman LO, et al. Computed tomography-derived intrarenal blood flow in renovascular and essential hypertension. Kidney Int 1996;49:846–854.
25. Kellerman PS. Cellular and metabolic consequences of chronic ischemia on kidney function. Sem Nephrol 1996;16:33–42.
26. Mann JFE. Detection of renovascular hypertension. State of the art 1995. Nephrol Dial Transplant 1995;10:1285–1286.
27. Dondi M. Captopril renal scintigraphy with ^{99}m-TC-Mercapto acetyl triglycine (^{99}mTc-MAG_3) for detecting renal artery stenosis. Am J Hypertens 1991;4:7275–7405.

27a. Van Jaarsveld BC, et al. The place of renal scintigraphy in the diagnosis of renal artery stenosis. Arch Intern Med 1997;157:1226–1234.

27b. Erbsloh-Moller B, et al. Furosemide I-hippuran renography after angiotensin-converting enzyme inhibition for the diagnosis of renovascular hypertension. Am J Med 1991;90:23–29.

27c. Miralles M, et al. Captopril test and renal duplex scanning for the primary screening of renovascular disease. Am J Hypertens 1997;10:1290–1296.

28. Miralles M, et al. Value of Doppler parameters in the diagnosis of renal artery stenosis. J Vasc Surg 1996;23:428–435.

29. Elkohen M, et al. Evaluation of spiral computed tomography of the renal arteries alone or combined with Doppler ultrasonography in the detection of renal artery stenosis. Prospective study of 114 renal arteries. Arch Mal Coeur Vaiss 1995;88: 1159–1164.

30. Olbricht CJ, et al. Minimally invasive diagnosis of renal artery stenosis by spiral computed tomography angiography. Kidney Int 1995;48:1332–1337.

31. Kaatee R, et al. Atherosclerotic renal artery stenosis: ostial or truncal? Radiology 1996;199:637–640.

32a. Postma CT, et al. Magnetic resonance angiography has a high reliability in the detection of renal artery stenosis. Am J Hypertens 1997;10:957–963.

32. deHaan MW, et al. Renovascular disease in patients with hypertension detection with systolic and diastolic gating in three-dimensional, phase-contrast MR angiography. Radiology 1996;198:449–456.

33. Carmichael DJS, et al. Detection and investigation of renal artery stenosis. Lancet 1986;1:667–670.

34. Eyler WR, et al. Angiography of the renal areas including a comparative study of renal artery stenosis in patients with and without hypertension. Radiology 1962;78: 879–891.

35. Holley KE, et al. Renal artery stenosis: a clinical-pathologic study in normotensive and hypertensive patients. Am J Med 1964;37:14–22.

36. Vaughan JED. Renovascular hypertension. Kidney Int 1985;27:811–827.

37. Pickering TG, et al. Differing patterns of renal veins renin secretion in patients with renovascular hypertension and their role in predicting the response to angioplasty. Nephron 1986;44(suppl 1):8–11.

38. Lawrie GM, et al. Renovascular reconstruction. Factors affecting long term prognosis in 919 patients follow-up to 31 years. Am J Cardiol 1989;63:1085–1092.

39. Novick AC. Trends in surgical revascularization for renal artery disease. Ten years experience. JAMA 1987;257:498–501.

40. Anderson GS, et al. Treatment of renovascular hypertension by unilateral nephrectomy: a follow-up study in patients above 60 years of age. Scand J Urol Nephrol 1986;20:51–56.

41. Sos TA, et al. Technical aspects of percutaneous transluminal angioplasty in renovascular disease. Nephron 1986;44(suppl):45–50.

42. Kinney TB, et al. Transluminal angioplasty: a mechanical-pathophysiological correlation of its physical mechanisms. Radiology 1984;153:85–89.

43. Canzanello VJ, et al. Percutaneous transluminal renal angioplasty in management of atherosclerotic renovascular hypertension: results in 100 patients. Hypertension 1982;13:163–172.

44. Grim CE, et al. Percutaneous transluminal dilatation in the treatment of renal vascular hypertension. Ann Intern Med 1981;95:439–442.
45. Kuhlman U, et al. Renovascular hypertension: treatment by percutaneous transluminal dilatation. Ann Intern Med 1980;92:1–6.
46. Sos TA, et al. Percutaneous transluminal renal angioplasty in renovascular hypertension due to atheroma or fibromuscular dysplasia. N Engl J Med 1983;309:274–279.
47. Jensen G, et al. Treatment of renovascular hypertension: one year results of renal angioplasty. Kidney Int 1995;48:1936–1945.
48. Brown LA, Ramsay LE. Is improvement real with percutaneous transluminal angioplasty in the management of renovascular hypertension? Lancet 1987;2:1313–1316.
49. Ramsey LE, Waller OPC. Blood pressure response to percutaneous transluminal angioplasty for renovascular hypertension: an overview of published series. Br Med J 1990;300:569–572.
50. Dean RH, et al. Evolution of renal insufficiency in ischemic nephropathy. Ann Surg 1991;213:446–456.
51. Weibull H, et al. Percutaneous transluminal renal angioplasty versus surgical reconstruction of atherosclerotic renal artery stenosis: a prospective randomized study. J Vasc Surg 1993;18:841–852.
52. Vidt DG. Geriatric hypertension of renovascular origin: diagnosis and management. Geriatrics 1987;42:59–70.
53. Tegtmeyer CJ, Kellum CD, Ayers C. Percutaneous transluminal angioplasty of the renal artery. Results and long term follow-up. Radiology 1984;153:77–84.
54. Mahler F, et al. Complication in percutaneous transluminal dilatation of renal arteries. Nephron 1986;44(suppl):60–63.
55. Wise KL, et al. Renovascular hypertension. J Urol 1988;140:911–924.
56. Rees CR, et al. Palmaz stent in atherosclerotic stenosis involving the ostia of the renal arteries. Preliminary report of a multicenter study. Radiology 1991;181:507–514.
56a. Rundback JH, Jacobs JM. Percutaneous renal artery stent placement for hypertension and azotemia: pilot study. Am J Kidney Dis 1996;28:214–219.
57. Kuhn FP, et al. Renal artery stenosis: preliminary results of treatment with Strecker stent. Radiology 1991;180:367–372.
58. MacLeod M, et al. Renal artery stenosis managed by Palmaz stent insertion: technical and clinical outcome. J Hypertens 1995;13:1791–1795.
59. Dorros G, et al. Follow-up of primary Palmaz-Schatz stent placement for atherosclerotic renal artery stenosis. Am J Cardiol 1995;75:1051–1055.
60. Van de Ven PJG, et al. Transluminal vascular stent for ostial atherosclerotic renal artery stenosis. Lancet 1995;346:672–674.
60a. Blum U, et al. Treatment of ostial renal-artery stenosis with vascular endoprosthesis after unsuccessful balloon angioplasty. N Engl J Med 1997;336:459–465.
61. Schömig A, et al. A randomized comparison of antiplatelet and anticoagulant therapy after the placement of coronary artery stents. N Engl J Med 1996;334:1084–1089.
62. Tollefson DFJ, Ernst CB. Natural history of atherosclerotic renal artery stenosis associated with aortic disease. J Vasc Surg 1991;14:327–331.
63. Hansen KJ, et al. Management of renovascular hypertension in the elderly population. J Vasc Surg 1989;10:266–273.

63a. Connolly JO, et al. Presentation, clinical features and outcome in different patterns of atherosclerotic renovascular disease. Q J Med 1994;87:413–421.
64. Hunt JC, et al. Renal and renovascular hypertension: a reasoned approach to diagnosis and management. Arch Intern Med 1974;133:988–999.
65. Dean RH, et al. Renovascular hypertension: anatomic and renal function changes during drug therapy. Arch Surg 1981;116:1408–1415.
66. Chiarni C, et al. The time problem in renovascular hypertension (RVH): renal ischemia. Kidney Int 1985;28:247A.
67. Vidt DG, et al. Atheroembolic renal disease: association with renal artery stenosis. Clev Clin J Med 1989;56:407–413.
68. Schreiber MJ, Pohl MA, Novick AC. The natural history of atherosclerotic and fibrous renal artery disease. Urol Clin NA 1984;11:383–392.
69. Zierler RE, et al. Natural history of atherosclerotic renal artery stenosis: a prospective study with duplex ultrasonography. J Vasc Surg 1994;19:250–258.
69a. Zierler RE, et al. A prospective study of disease progression in patients with atherosclerotic renal artery stenosis. Am J Hypertens 1996;9:1055–1061.
69b. Pohl MA, et al. Does renal revascularization preserve renal function in patients with atherosclerotic renal artery stenosis? An ongoing prospective study. J Am Soc Nephrol 1991;2:242.
69c. Webster J, et al. Prospective randomized trial of interventional angioplasty versus medical therapy in hypertensive patients with atheromatous renal artery stenosis. Am J Hypertens 1995;8:38A.
70. Scarpelli PT, et al. Chronic total renal artery occlusion: a diagnostic challenge. Eur Urol 1984;10:178–182.
71. Zinman L, Libertino JA. Revascularization of the chronic totally occluded renal artery with restoration of renal function. J Urol 1977;118:517–521.
72. Schefft P, et al. Renal revascularization in patients with total occlusion of the renal artery. J Urol 1980;124:184–186.
73. Elmore JR, et al. Renal failure and advanced atherosclerotic lesions. Salvage by vascular reconstruction. Arch Surg 1988;123:610–613.
74. Jamieson GG, et al. Reconstructive renal vascular surgery for chronic renal failure. Br J Surg 1984;71:338–340.
75. Bilfinger TW, Gore DC, Wolma FJ. Renal revascularization in anuric patients. Determinants of outcome. South Med J 1989;82:558–562.
76. Kaylor WM, et al. Reversal of end stage renal failure with surgical revascularization in patients with atherosclerotic renal artery occlusion. J Urol 1989;141:486–488.
76a. Pattison JM, et al. Percutaneous-transluminal renal angioplasty in patients with renal failure. Q J Med 1992;85:883–888.
76b. Hansen KJ, et al. Surgical management of dialysis-dependent ischemic nephropathy. J Vasc Surg 1995;21:197–209.
77. Hansen KJ, et al. Contemporary surgical management of renovascular disease. J Vasc Surg 1992;16:319–331.
78. Hallett JW, et al. Renovascular operations in patients with chronic renal insufficiency. Do the benefits justify the risks? J Vasc Surg 1987;5:622–627.
79. Bredenberg CE, et al. Changing patterns of surgery for chronic renal artery occlusive diseases. J Vasc Surg 1992;15:1018–1024.

80. Socard G, et al. Improved renal function after renal artery revascularization. J Cardiovasc Surg 1985;26:157–161.
81. Halimi JM, et al. Albuminuria predicts renal functional outcome after intervention in atheromatous renovascular disease. J Hypertens 1992;13:1335–1342.
82. Libertino JA, et al. Renal revascularization to preserve and restore renal function. J Urol 1992;147:1485–1487.
83. O'Donovan RM, et al. Preservation of renal function by percutaneous renal angioplasty in high-risks elderly patients: short-term outcome. Nephron 1992;60:187–192.
83a. Cambria RP, et al. Renal artery reconstruction for the preservation of renal function. J Vasc Surg 1996;24:371–382.
83b. Rimmer JM, Gennari J. Atherosclerotic renovascular disease and progressive renal failure. Ann Intern Med 1993;118:712–719.
83c. Meyrier A, et al. Vascular nephropathies and nephrosclerosis: epidemiology and pathophysiology. Adv Nephrol 1996;26:207–245.
83d. Reilly JM, et al. Revascularization of the solitary kidney: a challenging problem in a high risk population. Surgery 1996;120:732–737.
83e. Donohoe P, et al. A four-year audit of interventional treatment for atheromatous renal artery stenosis. In: Zoccali C, ed. Clinical Hypertension in Nephrology. Basel, Karger: Contrib Nephrol 1996;119:78–82.
83f. Tullis MJ, et al. Results of percutaneous transluminal angioplasty for atherosclerotic renal artery stenosis: a follow-up study with duplex ultrasonography. J Vasc Surg 1997;25:46–54.
84. Hoxie HJ, Coggin CB. Renal infarction. Statistical study of two hundred and five cases and a detailed report of an unusual case. Arch Intern Med 1940;65:587–594.
85. Moyer JD, et al. Conservative management of renal artery embolus. J Urol 1973; 109:138–143.
86. Lessman RK, et al. Renal artery embolism. Clinical features and long-term follow-up of 17 cases. Ann Intern Med 1978;89:477–482.
87. Selli C, Turini D, Berni G. Embolism in a single functioning kidney: report of two cases. Br J Urol 1976;48:419–425.
88. Buckspur MB, Goldberg MR. Renal artery embolism: diagnosis and treatment. Can J Surg 1978;21:362–366.
89. Barry JM, Hodges CV. Revascularization of totally occluded renal arteries. J Urol 1978;119:412–415.
90. Fletcher S, et al. Acute embolic bilateral renal artery occlusions in an elderly patient. Case report: importance of early diagnosis. Gerontology 1984;30:178–181.
91. Rudy DC, et al. Segmental renal artery emboli treated with low dose intra-arterial streptokinase. Urology 1982;19:410–413.
92. Zucchelli P, et al. Acute renal failure due to renal artery occlusion. In: Eliahou E, ed. Clinical Acute Renal Failure. London: John Libbey, 1982:152–255.
93. Wu KK. New pharmacologic approaches to thromboembolic disorders. Hosp Pract 1985;20:101–120.
93a. Gasparini M, Hofmann R, Stoller M. Renal artery embolism: clinical features and therapeutic options. J Urol 1992;147:567–572.
93b. Salam TA, Lumsden AB, Martin LG. Local infusion of fibrinolytic agents for acute renal artery thromboembolism: report of ten cases. Ann Vasc Surg 1993;7:21–26.

94. Nicholas CG, DeMuth WE. Treatment of renal artery embolism. Arch Surg 1984; 119:278–281.
95. Smith MC, Ghose MK, Henry AR. The clinical spectrum of renal cholesterol embolization. Am J Med 1981;71:174–180.
96. Drost H, et al. Cholesterol embolism as a complication of left heart catheterization. Br Heart J 1984;52:339–342.
97. Cosio FG, Zager RA, Sharma HML. Atheroembolic renal disease causes hypocomplementemia. Lancet 1985;2:118–121.
98. McGowan JA, Greenberg A. Cholesterol atheroembolic renal disease. Am J Nephrol 1986;6:135–139.
99. Siemons L, et al. Peritoneal dialysis in acute renal failure due to cholesterol embolization: two cases of recovery of renal function and extended survival. Clin Nephrol 1987;28:205–208.
100. Hendell RC, et al. Multiple cholesterol emboli syndrome. Arch Intern Med 1989; 149:2371–2374.
101. Thadhani RI, et al. Atheroembolic renal failure after invasive procedures. Natural history based on 52 histologically proven cases. Medicine 1995;74:350–358.
102. Gore J, Collins DP. Spontaneous atheromatous embolization. Review of the literature and a report of 16 additional cases. Am J Clin Pathol 1960;33:416–426.
103. Thurbeck WM, Castleman B. Atheromatous emboli to kidneys after aortic surgery. N Engl J Med 1957;257:442–447.
104. McCombs PR. Acute renal failure following resection of abdominal aortic aneurysm. Surg Gynecol Obstet 1977;148:175–179.
105. Harrington JT, Somers SG, Kassirer JP. Atheromatous emboli with progressive renal failure. Ann Intern Med 1968;68:152–159.
106. Gaines PA, et al. Cholesterol embolization: a lethal complication of vascular catheterization. Lancet 1988;1:168–170.
107. Colt HG, et al. Cholesterol emboli after cardiac catheterization. Medicine 1988; 67:389–400.
108. Tilley WS, et al. Renal failure due to cholesterol emboli following PCTA. Am Heart J 1985;110:1301–1302.
109. Weitz Z, et al. Cholesterol emboli in atherosclerotic patients: report of five cases occurring spontaneously or complicating angioplasty. and renal bypass. J Am Geriatr Soc 1987;35:357–359.
110. Rosman HS, et al. Cholesterol embolization: clinical findings and implications. J Am Coll Cardiol 1990;15:1296–1299.
111. Ramirez G, et al. Cholesterol embolization, a complication of angiography. Arch Intern Med 1978;138:1430–1432.
112. Kealy WF. Atheroembolism. J Clin Pathol 1978;31:984–989.
113. Rosansky SJ, Deschamps EG. Multiple cholesterol emboli syndrome after angiography. Am J Med Sci 1984;288:45–48.
114. Delakos TG, et al. Malignant hypertension resulting from atheromatous embolization predominantly of one kidney. Am J Med 1974;57:135–138.
115. Kasinath BS, et al. Eosinophilia in the diagnosis of atheroembolic renal disease. Am J Nephrol 1987;7:173–177.

116. Kay AB, Shin HS, Austen KF. Selective attraction of eosinophils and synergism between-eosinophil chemotactic factor of anaphylaxis (ECF-A) and a fragment cleaved from the fifth component of complement (C_5). Immunology 1973;24:969–976.
117. Haggie SS, Urizar RE, Singh J. Nephrotic-range proteinuria in renal atheroembolic disease: report of four cases. Am J Kidney Dis 1996;28:493–501.
117a. Greenberg A, et al. Focal segmental glomerulosclerosis associated with nephrotic syndrome in cholesterol atheroembolism: clinical correlations. Am J Kidney Dis 1997;29:334–344.
118. Jones DB, Iannaccone PM. Atheromatous emboli in renal biopsies. Am J Pathol 1975;78:261–276.
119. Tracy RE, et al. The evolution of benign arterionephrosclerosis from ages 6 to 70 years. Am J Pathol 1990;136:429–439.
120. Mujais SK, et al. Marked proteinuria in hypertensive nephrosclerosis. Am J Nephrol 1985;5:190–195.
121. Innes A, et al. Clinical features of benign hypertensive nephrosclerosis at time of renal biopsy. Q J Med 1993;86:271–275.
122. Schmieder RE, Schachinger H, Messerli FH. Accelerated decline in renal perfusion with aging in essential hypertension. Hypertension 1994;23:351–357.
123. Lindeman RD, Tobin JD, Shock NW. Association between blood pressure and the rate of decline in renal function with age. Kidney Int 1984;26:861–868.
124. Shulman NB, et al. Prognostic value of serum creatinine and effect of treatment of hypertension on renal function. Hypertension 1989;13(suppl 1):180–193.
124a. Razzaque MS, Harada T, Taguchi T. Significance of increased accumulation of type VI collagen and transforming growth factor beta 1 in tubulo interstitial damage in hypertensive nephrosclerosis: an immunohistochemical study. J Intern Med Res 1996;24:199–208.
124b. Zucchelli P, Zuccala A. The diagnostic dilemma of hypertensive nephrosclerosis, the nephrologist's view. Am J Kidney Dis 1993;21(suppl 2):87–91.
125. Freidman BI, Iskandar SS, Appel RG. The link between hypertension and nephrosclerosis. Am J Kidney Dis 1995;25:207–221.
126. Baldwin DS, Neugarten J. Treatment of hypertension in renal disease. Am J Kidney Dis 1985;5:A57–A70.
127. Kasiske BL. Relationship between vascular disease and age-associated changes in the human kidney. Kidney Int 1987;31:1153–1159.
128. Rostand SG, et al. Renal insufficiency in treated essential hypertension. N Engl J Med 1989;320:684–688.
129. Zuccheli P, Zuccala A. Primary hypertension: How does it cause renal failure? Nephrol Dial Transplant 1994;9:223–225.
130. Fogo A, et al. Accuracy of the diagnosis of hypertensive nephrosclerosis in African Americans: a report from the African American Study of kidney disease (AASK) trial. Kidney Int 1997;51:244–252.
131. Toto RD, et al. "Strict" blood pressure control and progression of renal disease in hypertensive nephrosclerosis. Kidney Int 1995;48:851–859.
132. De Leeuw PW. Renal function in the elderly: results from the European working party on high blood pressure in the elderly trial. Am J Med 1991;90(suppl 3A):45S–49S.

133. Kirk KA, Rutsky EA, Pate BA. Racial differences in the incidence of treatment for end-stage renal disease. N Engl J Med 1982;306:1276–1279.
134. Tracy RE. Renovasculopathies of hypertension and the rise of blood pressure with age in blacks and whites. Sem Nephrol 1996;16:126–133.
135. Keating MA, Althansen AF. The clinical spectrum of renal vein thrombosis. J Urol 1985;133:938–945.

Index

About the Authors

Pierre F. Faubert is an Attending Physician, Division of Nephrology and Hypertension, Brookdale University Hospital and Medical Center, Brooklyn, New York, and an Associate Professor of Clinical Medicine, State University of New York Health Science Center at Brooklyn. The author or coauthor of numerous key professional publications, he is a Fellow of the American College of Physicians and a member of the American and International Societies of Nephrology, among others. Dr. Faubert received the M.D. degree (1973) from the University of Sherbrooke, Quebec, Canada.

Jerome G. Porush is the Director, Division of Nephrology and Hypertension, Brookdale University Hospital and Medical Center, Brooklyn, New York, and a Professor of Medicine, State University of New York Health Science Center at Brooklyn. The author or coauthor of over 100 original publications, reviews, and book chapters, he is a Fellow of the American College of Physicians and the American College of Clinical Pharmacology. Dr. Porush received the M.D. degree (1955) from the State University of New York Health Science Center at Brooklyn.